When the Body Become

Note on Author

Phillip B. Zarrilli is well known for his teaching of kalarippayattu, yoga, and t'ai ch'uan, especially for performers. He conducts training at his own kalari/studio in West Wales, throughout the U.K., and with such organizations as the Centre for Performance Research (Wales), Passe Partout (Netherlands), Gardzienice Theatre (Poland). He is currently Professor in the Department of Drama at the University of Exeter, U.K. where he teaches these disciplines as part of the B.A. and M.A. (Theatre Practice) degrees. His numerous other books include *Kathakali Dance-Drama: Where Gods and Demons Come to Play* (Routledge Press, 2000); editor of *Acting (Re)considered: Theories and Practices* (Routledge Press, 1995); editor of Richmond and Darius Swann of *Indian Theatre: Traditions of Performance* (University of Hawaii Press, 1990), among others. He is also a noted theatre director, and his recent productions of the plays of Samuel Beckett in Austria with Theatre Asou, and in Los Angeles with Patricia Boyette have won critical acclaim.

When the Body Becomes All Eyes

Paradigms, Discourses and Practices of Power in Kalarippayattu, a South Indian Martial Art

Phillip B. Zarrilli

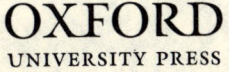

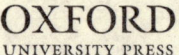

YMCA Library Building, Jai Singh Road, New Delhi 110 001

Oxford University Press is a department of the University of Oxford. It furthers the
University's objective of excellence in research, scholarship, and education
by publishing worldwide in

Oxford   New York

Athens   Auckland   Bangkok   Bogota   Buenos Aires   Cape Town
Chennai   Dar es Salaam   Delhi   Florence   Hong Kong   Istanbul   Karachi
Kolkata   Kuala Lumpur   Madrid   Melbourne   Mexico City   Mumbai
Nairobi   Paris   São Paulo   Shanghai   Singapore   Taipei   Tokyo   Toronto   Warsaw

with associated companies in Berlin Ibadan

Oxford is a registered trade mark of Oxford University Press
in the UK and in certain other countries

Published in India
By Oxford University Press, New Delhi

© Oxford University Press 1998

The moral rights of the author have been asserted

Database right Oxford University Press (maker)

Oxford India paperbacks 2000
Second impression 2001

All rights reserved. No part of this publication may be reproduced,
stored in a retrieval system, or transmitted, in any form or by any means,
without the prior permission in writing of Oxford University Press,
or as expressly permitted by law, or under terms agreed with the appropriate
reprographics rights organization. Enquiries concerning reproduction
outside the scope of the above should be sent to the Rights Department,
Oxford University Press, at the address above

You must not circulate this book in any other binding or cover
and you must impose this same condition on any acquirer

ISBN 019 565538 9

Typeset by Eleven Arts, Keshav Puram, Delhi 110 035
Printed in India by Saurabh Print-O-Pack, Noida, U. P.
Published by Manzar Khan, Oxford University Press
YMCA Library Building, Jai Singh Road, New Delhi 110 001

To Gurukkal Govindankutty Nayar
C.V.N. Kalari, Thiruvananthapuram

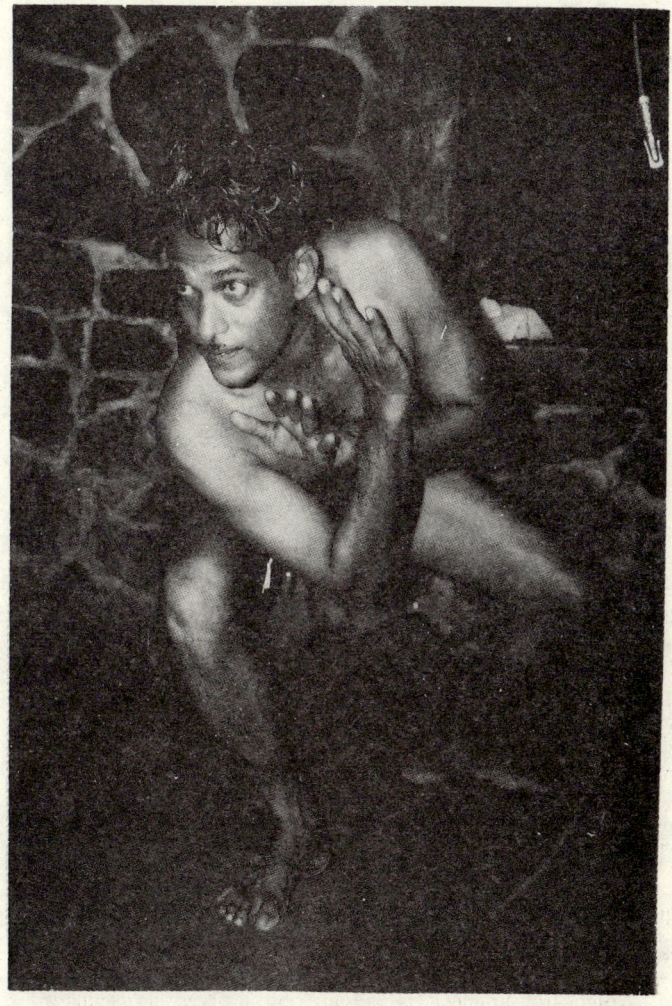

Figure 0.1

Preface

In the well-known *Bhagavad Gita* section of India's *Mahabharata* epic, Krishna elaborates a view of duty and action intended to convince Arjuna that, as a member of the warrior caste (*ksatriya*), he must overcome all his doubts and take up arms, even against his relatives. As anyone familiar with either the *Mahabharata* or India's other great epic, the *Ramayana*, knows, martial arts have existed on the South Asian subcontinent since antiquity. Both epics are filled with scenes describing how the princely heroes obtain and use their humanly or divinely acquired skills and powers to defeat their enemies—by training in martial techniques under the tutelage of great gurus like the brahman master, Drona; by developing super human strength like Bhima; by practising austerities and meditation techniques which give a martial master access to subtle powers to be used in combat; and/or by receiving a gift or a boon of divine, magical powers from a god.

Although there has been a great deal of scholarly and popular interest in South Asian philosophy and religion, culture, medicine (Ayurveda), and performance, little is known about the traditional South Asian martial arts, many of which are still practised.[1] This monograph is an ethnographic study of one South Indian martial art, *kalarippayattu* (literally 'place of exercise') practised in Kerala (Figure 0.2), as a set of practices through which experience and meaning are created.[2] Some attention is also given to the closely related Tamil martial art, *varma ati* (literally, 'hitting the vital spots'). Other martial arts not discussed in this monograph include Tamil Nadu's form of staff fighting (*silambam*) (Raj 1971, 1975, 1977), north Indian stick fighting (*dandi*), *malkhambh* (wrestler's post exercise, Staal 1983–4, 1993) and *kusthi* (wrestling, Alter 1992).

From at least the twelfth century, kalarippayattu was practised throughout Kerala and contiguous parts of Coorg (Kodagu) district, Karnataka, in south-western coastal India. The practice of kalarippayattu was especially associated with subgroups of Hindu Nayars whose duty it was to serve as soldiers and

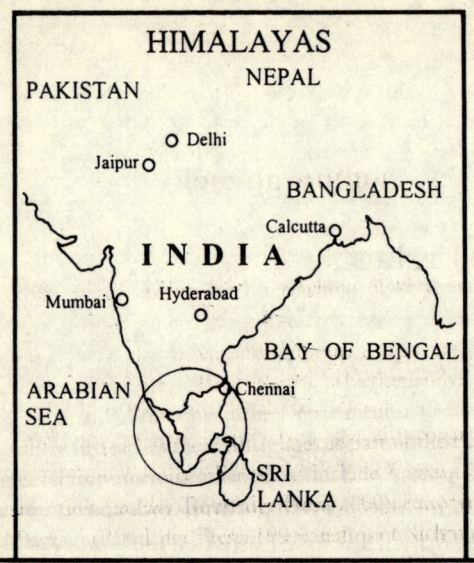
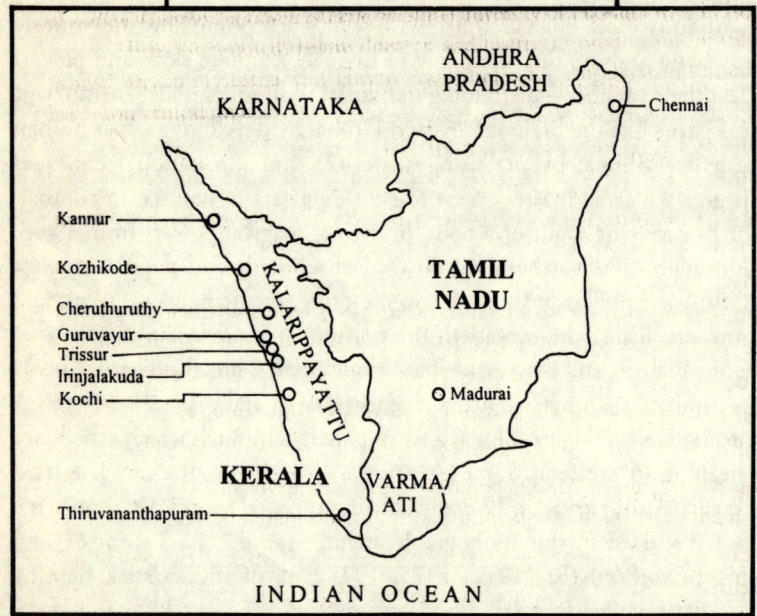

Figure 0.2: Location of Kerala and Tamil Nadu in South Asia. Within Kerala the northern (Malabar region of Kozhikode and Kannur), central (Kochi) and southern (Travancore/Thiruvananthapuram) regions each had its own distinctive styles of kalarippayattu practice.

healers at the behest of the village head, district ruler or local *raja*, having vowed to serve him to death as part of his retinue. Along with Nayars, some Cattar (or Yatra) Brahmans, one subgroup of the Ilava caste given the special title of *chekor*, as well as some Christians and Muslims learned, taught and practised the martial art.

Kalarippayattu declined after the introduction of firearms but survived under the tutelage of a few masters in scattered regions of Kerala. During the modern era kalarippayattu was first brought to general public attention during the 1920s in a wave of rediscovery of indigenous arts. Despite increasing public awareness within the north Malabar region, however, kalarippayattu continued to be little known as a practical martial and healing art to the general public in Kerala and in India as late as 1976 when I began field research and my own training.[3]

This ethnographic monograph provides the first comprehensive account of kalarippayattu as an integral part of Kerala culture and an evolving Malayali identity. It is based on extensive interviews, fieldwork and personal engagement in long-term training and practice conducted in Kerala in between 1976 and the present: 1976–7 (ten months), 1980 (three months), 1983 (seven months), 1985 (two months), 1988–9 (eight months), and 1993 (7 months). A complete list of *kalari* visited and interviews conducted is found in Appendix II. Regarding citation, when appropriate I name the master quoted. Given the secrecy and sensitivity surrounding certain aspects of martial practice, some masters requested either (1) that I *not* include 'secrets' in this book, or (2) that their names not be mentioned directly when sensitive information or interpretations were shared. No information is provided here which any master requested remain secret. When specific names are not cited, either the information is common to at least three masters, or it was inappropriate to name the specific master. During interviews, some masters consulted, read from, and/or allowed me to copy sections of their personal manuscripts. The nature of these manuscripts is discussed in Appendix I, and a list of manuscripts is found at the conclusion of the Bibliography.

Readers interested in kalarippayattu as a practical martial discipline may wish to skim or skip the more theoretical aspects of Chapter 1.

Acknowledgements

I am indebted to numerous individuals and institutions for their assistance, guidance, and support. Thanks first to the kalarippayattu practitioners who have generously assisted me in research and training since 1976. My first and greatest thanks to Gurukkal Govindankutty Nayar of the C.V.N. Kalari, Thiruvananthapuram who introduced me to kalarippayattu, and has so graciously continued to teach me. Among those students who practised with me and therefore taught me, I thank Aravindakshan Nayar, Rajashekaran Nayar, Sathyan Narayanan, Peter, Hari and Gopi among others.

To C. Mohammed Sherif of the Kerala Kalarippayattu Academy, Kannur, I owe not only friendship, but much of my understanding of the intricacies and power of kalarippayattu's practical applications, of differences in styles, of the unique nature of the central Kerala style, and of the esoteric nature of Sufi practice. Thanks to Chandran Gurukkal, Azhicode and Sreejayan Gurukkal of Chembad, who shared with me their teaching of yoga and/or massage. Without the friendship and brotherhood of Sensei Moses Thilak (Marma Adi Research Martial Arts Academy, Madras), his wife Usha, as well as Balachandran Master (Indian School of Martial Arts, Thiruvananthapuram) I would never have been exposed to the intricacies of varma ati and many of its masters in Thiruvananthapuram district and Tamil Nadu. Thanks to Raju Asan of Y.N.K. Kalari, Vizhinjam, who introduced me practically to his version of 'southern style' kalarippayattu. Special thanks also to all those masters who shared their practice, hospitality, and homes with me over the years: P.P. Narayanan Gurukkal, K. Achutan Gurukkal, N.V. Narayanan Nayar, Kallada Balakrishnan, Gurukkal C.M.M. Vaidyar, M.K. Bhaskaran Gurukkal, K.K. Krishnan Gurukkal, K.T. Achuthan Gurukkal, E.P. Kunnu, P. Dasan Gurukkal, Karunan Gurukkal, K.V. Choyikutty Gurukkal, K.V. Chandu, Thomas Muttam, V.K. Madhavan Panikkar (deceased), P.M. Neelakandhan Namboodiripad, B. Kunhi

Moideen Gurukkal, K. Narayanan Nayar Gurukkal, Haji N.M. Kutty, C. Sankaranarayanan Menon Gurukkal, P.K. Balan Gurukkal, Sakhav P.V. Mohamedunni Gurukkal, C.T. Balamenon Gurukkal, P.S. Higgins Master, E.P. Vasu Gurukkal, S. Krishnankutty Nayar, S. Alisan Kunju Asan, A. Kumaran Asan, Masters David and Richard Strarthern, Kottakkal Kunnasan Asan, Kunnan Asan K., K.K. Muthu Asan, Ustaz Haji Hamzh Haji Abu, Kalathil Krishnan Vaidyar Gurukkal, K. Kunhikannan Gurukkal, Moolachal Narayanan Asan, Sadasivan Asan, Chelayan Asan, and Dr Gnanidass.

Several individuals have served as indefatigable companions, research assistants, and translators over the years, including Shaju Joseph, Kunju Vasudevan Namboodiripad, James Devi Raj (assistance with Tamil source materials), and Jose George. Deborah Neff provided assistance with research on medical aspects of the system.

Parts of this manuscript were previously published. Chapter 6 was originally published as 'To Heal and/or To Harm: The Vital Spots (*Marmmam/Varmmam*) in Two South Indian Martial Traditions', Parts I and II in *Journal of Asian Martial Arts*, 1, 1 (36–67) and 1, 2 (1–16), 1992. Sections of Chapter 4 and 5 were first published as 'Three Bodies of Practice in a Traditional South Indian Martial Art', in *Social Science and Medicine*, 28, 12 (1289–1309), 1989. Sections of the Introduction and other chapters were published as follows: 'Repositioning the Body: Practice, Power, and Self in an Indian Martial Art', in *Consuming Modernity: Public Culture in a South Asian World*, edited by Carol A. Breckenridge (Minneapolis: University of Minnesota Press, 1995); 'Doing the Exercise: The In-Body Transmission of Performance Knowledge in a Traditional Martial Art', *Asian Theatre Journal*, 1, 2 (191–206); and 'Between Text and Embodied Practice: Writing and Reading in a South Indian Martial Tradition', in *Shastric Tradition in Indian Arts*, ed. A.L. Dallapiccola (Stuttgart: Franz Steiner, 1989: 415–24).

I acknowledge with thanks the following research grants which made this book possible: a Fulbright Dissertation Fellowship (1976–7), American Institute of Indian Studies short-term and long-term fellowships (1980, 1983), University of Wisconsin-Madison Graduate School grants (1980, 1983, 1988–9), the Richard Carley Hunt Memorial Post-Doctoral Fellowship of the Wenner-Gren Foundation for Anthropological Research (1985), a fellowship from the Social Science Research Council (1985), a National Endowment for the Humanities Senior Research Fellowship through the American Institute of Indian Studies (1988–9), and Fulbright and Guggenheim Fellowships (1993) which allowed time to think about and reflect upon the 'emotions' (Chapter 7) and states of being.

Thanks to my students who have always been eager to know more about kalarippayattu, and to my colleagues in the Department of South Asian Studies at the University of Wisconsin-Madison for their interest in my work, especially David Knipe, Kirin Narayan and V. Narayana Rao. Thanks especially to Peter Claus, Francis Zimmermann, and Joan Erdman who have read and critiqued my research on kalarippayattu over the years, and to Dilip Menon for his thorough reading of a draft of this manuscript and his suggestions for final revisions. To Sharon Grady, much appreciation for her support during a number of the years it took to complete this manuscript.

NOTE ON TRANSLITERATION

The comprehensive glossary provides concise definitions of all Malayalam, Tamil, and Sanskrit terms. At the request of the publisher diacritical marks have not been included. Commonplace usage is adopted for names of familiar deities, epics, etc.

Contents

Preface		vii
Acknowledgements and Note on Transliteration		x
List of Illustrations		xiv
Chapter 1.	Introduction: Repositioning the Body, Practice, Power and Self	1
Chapter 2.	History, Kingship and the Heroic: Kalarippayattu and the Invention of a Past	24
Chapter 3.	The Ritual Life of the Kalari and its Deities: Protecting and Empowering the Body-in-Practice	61
Chapter 4.	'First the Outer Forms': The Physical Body and the First Fruits of Practice	84
Chapter 5.	'Then the Inner Secrets': The Subtle Body (*Suksma Sarira*), The Vital Energy (*Prana-Vayu*) and Actualizing Power (*Sakti*)	123
Chapter 6.	To Heal and/or To Harm: The Vital Spots of the Body and Practice	154
Chapter 7.	When the 'Body is all Eyes': Attaining a State of Transformative 'Fury', 'Doubtlessness' and 'Mental Power'	201
Chapter 8.	Repositioning the Body, Practice, Power and Self in the Ethnographic Present	215
Appendix I:	Texts in the Kalarippayattu Tradition	243
Appendix II:	Interviews, Personal Correspondence—Kalarippayattu and Varma Ati Masters	246
Endnotes		254
Bibliography		273
Glossary		299
Index		308

List of Illustrations

0.1 Gurukkal Govindankutty Nayar of the C.V.N. Kalari, Thiruvananthapuram, in the 'lion' pose. Ideally, the 'body is all eyes'.

0.2 Location of Kerala and Tamil Nadu in South Asia. Within Kerala the northern (Malabar region of Kozhikode and Kannur), central (Kochi) and southern (Travancore/Thiruvananthapuram) regions each had its own distinctive styles of kalarippayattu practice.

1.1 *New Thrill's* 'Deadly Art of Locks and Throws' with the author in a karate-style uniform demonstrating traditional kalarippayattu techniques. Hamzah is pictured in the centre and several of his students lower right.

1.2 Japanese advertisement featuring Sathyan Narayanan competing with a Japanese actor as they perform a 'high kick' to tout a product which 'replenish[es] Vitamin B–1 when your body is all worn out'.

1.3 A traditional dug-out 'pit' *kalari* with a thatched roof. Sreejayan Gurukkal's kalari in the village of Chembad.

1.4 Gurukkal Govindankutty Nayar's C.V.N. Kalari, Thiruvananthapuram with its modern design. It houses a pit kalari, separate massage area, clinic, and upstairs apartment and rooms.

1.5 The first of eight leg exercises, 'straight leg' kick (*nerkal*), in which the leg powerfully and fluidly touches the shoulder (Sathyan Narayanan). The body 'becomes as flexible as a band'.

1.6 Sword and shield practice: Gurukkal Govindankutty Nayar and Rajashekaran Nayar of the C.V.N. Kalari, Thiruvananthapuram.

2.1 An early woodblock print showing Nayar soldiers wielding the sword and shield, and use of bow and arrow. Both wear the *kacca* wrapped

List of Illustrations • xv

tightly around the hips to provide firm support to the abdominal region.

2.2 *Kuttysasthan*—one of many 'hero' *teyyam* in which deified ancestors/ heroes are propitiated in the north Malabar region of Kerala. Most infamous among these is Tacoli Otenan.

2.3 Kottakkal Karnaran Gurukkal (1850–1935) (seated, right) with his student C.V. Narayanan Nayar (1905–44) (seated, left), and students at their kalari—probably during the early 1930s.

2.4 Tacholi Otenan's story in comic-book form.

3.1 Measurements for construction of a kalari.

3.2 Interior of the S.N.G.S. Vallabhata Kalari Chavakkad: On the left is the 'permanent' seven-tiered stone *puttara* where the guardian deity is lodged—here Chandika Devi, a form of the goddess. Along the western wall to the right of the *puttara* is a lamp representing Ganapadi, wooden *pitham* representing past teachers, low wooden platform for Siva, low wooden platform for Sakti or Parvati, and the red cloth on the wall behind the sickle sword of Bhovaneswari or mother earth (Bhumi Devi). Krishnadass, son of C. Sankaranarayana Menon Gurukkal, faces the goddess in the south west corner as he executes part of the *puttara tol*—worshipping the goddess with his bodymind and, as explained in Chapter 5, activating the internal energy joining Siva and Sakti.

3.3 The location of the deities of the C.V.N. Kalari, Thiruvananthapuram.

3.4 The *pitham* (seat, pedestal or tripod) represents past gurus at the C.V.N. Kalari, Thiruvananthapuram. Located on the western side of the kalari facing the auspicious east, arrayed on either side of the *pitham* are weapons used in training.

3.5 Deities of the Sree Narayanan Guru Kalari, Chavakkad.

3.6–3.7 Some of the special rituals conducted at the C.V.N. Kalari, Thiruvananthapuram to celebrate Navaratri Mahotsavam, the annual celebration of new beginnings. Facing the temporarily installed Saraswati, Durga and Mahalakshmi, a local brahman pujari performs weapons puja (3.6). In front of the goddesses are the master's traditional texts—sources of knowledge. Behind and to the sides of the goddesses are the weapons—the tools of the trade. Each new student presents the teacher with *daksina*, and receives his blessings (3.7).

4.1 Gurukkal Govindankutty Nayar gives the first main stroke in foot massage (*kal uliccil*) across the small of the back while holding on to ropes suspended from the ceiling.

4.2 Sreejayan Gurukkal administers deep strokes to a student's thighs while keeping his legs open with his feet.

4.3 It takes days to prepare oils through cooking and decoction. Decoction results in a highly concentrated oil applied externally. Cooking oils in the kitchen at the C.V.N. Kalari, Thiruvananthapuram.

4.4 Gurukkal Govindankutty Nayar corrects a young student learning the 'lion pose' as part of the first body exercise sequence by attempting to get the student to lengthen and straighten his spine—part of a process that leads to correct spinal alignment, 'centering', and activation of the internal energy.

4.5 A young female student performs the 'sitting leg' (*iruttikal*) at the C.V.N. Kalari, Thiruvananthapuram.

4.6 The eight basic leg exercises of the C.V.N. Kalari, Thiruvananthapuram.

4.7–4.8 Students of Sreejayan Gurukkal of Chembad performing the first section of a body exercise sequence which combines poses, steps, kicks and jumps in complex combinations performed back and forth across the kalari floor.

4.9 The eight basic poses in two styles.

4.10–4.13 Poses (*vadivu*) are comparable to yoga *asana*, but they are dynamic—the practitioner moves to and from them. Some of the poses as practised by Gurukkal P.K. Balan of Kecheri:

    4.10 An advanced student demonstrates the horse pose in which the practitioner 'concentrates all (his) powers centrally' while jumping forward and thrusting with the elbow in an attack.

    4.11 The peacock pose in which the practitioner, like the peacock, 'spreads its feathers and raises its neck, and dances by steadying itself on one leg'.

    4.12 The serpent pose where the practitioner, like the serpent, always keeps its tail 'on the ground without movement' so that 'he can turn in any direction' to attack or defend.

4.13   Gurukkal P.K. Balan demonstrates the cock pose—a position from which he lifts 'one leg and shakes his feathers and neck, fixing his gaze on the enemy and attacking'.

4.14   One of kalarippayattu's many jumps and body turns: As demonstrated by Sathyan Narayanan, in the 'turning jump' when fully executed the body is extended in a straight line, horizontal to the floor. This same turning cut is later applied as a slashing sword cut. (Photograph courtesy of Sathyanarayanan Nayar.)

4.15–4.16   Sreejayan Gurukkal uses kalarippayattu's basic steps learned 'innocently' as part of the first body exercise to block an attack, enter his opponent and throw him to the ground.

4.17   The seventh of eighteen empty-hand attacks practised by C. Mohammed Sherif, Kerala Kalarippayattu Academy, Kannur: literally 'right (palm or butt of the hand) to chin'.

4.18   The fifteenth empty-hand attack—a 'right inside chop'.

4.19   *Kalam* are rice powder drawings created each morning outside homes or temples. They range from simple white diagrams which are decorative and/or symbolic, to complex large three dimensional motifs used in ritual performances and into which a deity's presence is invoked. C. Mohammed Sherif draws and discusses a simple kalam used in central and southern style kalarippayattu practice—a series of straight lines joining loops at the four corners, with a circle in the middle. These simple kalam are used for training in basic steps. (Photo courtesy of Kerala Kalarippayattu Academy.)

4.20–4.22   Part of the second, 'peacock' form of *cumatadi* as practised by P.K. Balan Gurukkal. In this part of the sequence, the students have moved into the peacock stance (4.20) from which they move quickly back into an extended leg position (4.21) from which a very strong, vigorous forward doubled-fisted thrust is made (4.22).

4.23   *Vandana cuvattu*—Sadasivan Asan's son performs the salutation in four directions with his left foot stationary. Here he begins a right arm slashing cut from left to right.

4.24–4.26   *Otta cuvatu*—single foot steps. Some masters, like Raju Asan, draw a kalam of five circles on the floor within which the basic steps are taken. One foot, usually the left, remains stationary while the other moves in all four directions to defend and/or counter attack from the four basic directions. Raju Asan performing part of the second of twelve otta cuvatu sequences—a left cut (4.24), followed by an attack ninety degrees to his right with the right fist and toe (4.25–4.26). Figure 4.26 shows the application to an opponent.

4.27 C. Sankaranarayana Menon consults one of his original family *grandam*.

4.28 Training with long staff (*kettukari*). Achuthan Gurukkal trains a young boy to defend his ribs with the long staff.

4.29 Basic techniques with short stick (*ceruvadi*) usually include twelve basic sequences taught as codified forms. Rajashekharan Nayar and Aravindakshan Nayar practising attack to and defence of a blow to the ankle.

4.30–4.31 In otta practice the practitioner must keep spinal alignment while staying deep in position. The author (right) prepares to defend against an attack from Rajashekharan Nayar. The author (left) defends an attack from Rajashekharan Nayar (right). Otta requires the practitioner to keep spinal alignment while staying very deep in the position. (Photographs by Ed Heston.)

4.32 Practice with dagger: Sathyanarayanan Nayar (left) defends against a thrust from Hari at the C.V.N. Kalari, Thiruvananthapuram.

4.33 One of the few specialists in spear techniques, Velayudan Asan (left) attacks his student, Jayakumar (right).

4.34 Jayakumar (right) delivers a double-hand cut upward toward his opponent's groin with the traditional double-edged sword (*curika*).

4.35 Govindankutty Nayar thrusts with his spear as Aravindakshan Nayar defends with his shield.

4.36 The flexible sword (*urmui*) is swung with a slashing circling action around the head, warding off opponents from any direction or attacking an opponent also wielding an urumi. Here Gurukkal Madhavan Panikkar attacks Mohammedunni Gurukkal.

5.1 The mediating action of vital energy (*prana* or *prana-vayu*).

5.2 The 'correct' way to perform the 'lion pose' (*simhavadivu*):

(a) With the hands/arms crossed over the chest and 'ready', the movement originates in the 'centre' at the navel—the leg is kicked up, the prana-vayu flowing up from the navel out through the knee and through the foot as it extends upward . . .

(b) to the forehead level with the big toe extended.

(c) The leg descends down the stationary leg along the line of the body, the energy flow returning to the navel region as the leg descends.

(d) The natural extension of the descent of the leg is a forward step in which the foot is firmly planted on the earth.

(e) The firmly planted foot provides the base for a jump, executed as the weight is taken on the forward foot, as the hands extend behind the body, and supported by the navel/hip region.

(f) Landing from the jump the energy is recycled and drawn into the navel region as . . .

(g) the final position is assumed with the hands in front of the chest, in the 'lion' pose.

5.3 The flow of energy and movement in the lion pose: a summary of Figures 5.2 (a–g).

5.4 The oppositional flow of energy in the final position of the lion pose. The arrows indicate the direction in which the energy is flowing. This opposition creates the triangle which is the lion pose's solid base and source of strength. Note also that the central axis of the spine follows the long line of the triangle. The spinal column and the interior 'subtle channel' of the body is thought to be the central axis through which the prana is channelled.

5.5 Sreejayan Gurukkal applies a firm slap with the palm to the top of the head where *sahasrara cakra* is located to 'awaken the senses'.

5.6 Vasu Gurukkal performs *brahyamanaka pranayama* in which he moves the breath through various parts of the body while repeating the root *mantram* 'aum' and performing *vira* (the heroic) *mudra* with his hands.

5.7 Especially in central-style empty-hand practice, basic floor patterns are not only a pattern for steps, but are also understood as mystical *yantra* (diagrams). By meditating on yantra the secrets of the application of steps, locks, etc. are revealed. In the first kalam the two basic constituents of the design are the straight line (a) and curved loop (b). For Hindus the straight line is interpreted as Siva (the lingam), and the loop as Sakti (the yoni) which, when combined give the practitioner access to power. For Muslims the straight line is interpreted as *alif*, the first letter of the Arabic alphabet, and the loop as *lam*. In (c) four of these patterns are joined representing a combination of basic footwork patterns.

In (d) is depicted a pattern of five basic squares, which constitutes a seldom taught and secretive internal style of central practice. In this yantra, there are four gates to the four cardinal directions, each of which when discovered and accomplished reveals a set of offences or defences to the practitioner.

5.8 Sufi Master Abdul Kadar leads a late-night *ratheeb* which, through group chanting, leads to atonement with Allah and the concentration and focus of greater spiritual powers for the martial practitioner. (Photo courtesy of Kerala Kalarippayattu Academy.)

6.1 A master demonstrates the principle of attacking the vital spots by pressing one of the vital spots of a rooster, rendering the rooster limp in his hands. He then revives the rooster with a counter-application.

6.2 Location of the *marmans* of *Susruta Samhita* as interpreted by Fedorova (1989).

6.3 Assisted by his son, C. Sankaranarayanan Gurukkal places a new cast on a broken arm. Once a broken bone is set in a temporary plaster, the patient returns every three days to have the limb massaged with medical oils, and a new cast applied. The cotton bandages have been soaked in medicinal oils and are being wrapped around splints.

6.4 One important massage therapy in the repertory of many practitioners is application of cloth bags (*kili*) of specially prepared medicine herbs for injuries, such as this 'catch' in the student's chest. Here Gurukkal K. Narayanan Nayar gives a treatment to one of his students.

6.5 Comparative chart of vital spot distribution in the body.

6.6 The locations of the vital spots on the body according to one kalarippayattu text, the *Marmmanidanam*.

6.7 Chandran Gurukkal demonstrates how he precisely locates *nabhimarmmam* (at the navel) by measuring the correct distance from *hrttamarmmam*.

6.8 Using a stiff piece of straw, Balachandran Master demonstrates one method of teaching students the locations of the vital spots—in this case, *tilartakalam*, one of the twelve death spots in the *varma ati* system.

6.9 Comparative locations of kalarippayattu's 'practical vital spots' (*kulabhyasamarmmam*).

6.10–6.11 Gurukkal Madhavan Panikkar of Pallikkar in Malappuram district demonstrates how he defends an attack to his forehead with his left hand and returns an attack to his opponent's *sankapuspam marmmam* located between the breasts with an elbow thrust.

6.12 An alternative counterattack is made to *mukkatappan marmmam* located between the eyes at the bridge of the nose. After blocking with the left hand, Madhavan Panikkar attacks with the right hand, hitting downward with the outer edge of the bone.

6.13–6.14 After defending an overhead blow with crossed fists, Madhavan Panikkar counterattacks with a left forward step behind the attacker's right leg and an elbow thrust to *tarippan marmmam* ('jellyfish vital spot') located in the middle of the thigh.

6.15 Higgins Master of the P.B. Kalari, Trissur, who specializes in empty-hand techniques and applications, illustrates how he defends against a knife attack, and counterattacks by grabbing the attacker's hair with the left hand to expose *manya marmmam* on the neck for attack with his right elbow.

6.16–6.17 Two styles of *cottoccan*: small sticks designed to be easily concealed in the hand. The first style is rounded at both ends, occasionally tipped with brass, and held in the palm of the hand for either forward or backward thrusts to the vital spots. The second is more like a small billy club held at the gripping end. The vital spots are attacked either with thrusts or with a quick flick of the wrist.

6.18 Having defended against an attack with the right fist, Sadasivan Asan demonstrates a counterattack to the vital spot located at the bridge of his opponent's nose (*paalmarmmam* or *mukkuvarmam*).

6.19–6.20　Balachandran Master demonstrates a threefold counterattack beginning with a right elbow attack to *nermarmmam* located between the breasts (6.19), followed by a blow to *tilartakalam* between the eyes with the right knuckle, and concluding with a fist attack to the two *vittiumarmmam* located on the scrotum (6.20).

6.21　Raju Asan, student of Chelayan Asan, demonstrates how he stimulates *kavalikalam* by applying pressure with his thumb.

6.22　When spasms occur and/or the face begins to contort, Raju Asan demonstrates how Chelayan Asan simultaneously stimulates *amakalam* in the calf and *koncanimarmmam* in the ankle.

6.23–6.27　This set of photographs illustrates one of Chelayan Asan's complex sets of counter-applications for penetration of *nermarmmam* located between the breasts. Pressure is first applied with the knee against *vayukalam* in the small of the back (6.23) while the patient is supported on the opposite side at *nermarmmam*. The master rubs down along the patient's sides (6.24). Lifting up the head under the chin (6.25), he slaps the top of the head on *unnimarmmam* (6.26), and concludes by reaching under the patient's shoulders from behind, gripping, lifting sharply (6.27), and shaking.

6.28　The thirty-two yoga *marmmam*.

7.1　Noted Kathakali actor, Gopi Asan, playing the role of Rugmamgada in *pacca* make-up, enters a state of transformative 'fury' with loosened hair.

8.1　Ustaz Hamzah (left) demonstrates a left-hand block of a punch delivered by one of his black belt students in Kuala Lumpur, Malaysia.

8.2　Ustaz Hamzah's 'yellow belt' syllabus.

8.3　An action-packed photograph typical of those used to advertise kalarippayattu as an effective street-wise self-defence martial art.

8.4　The increasing theatricalization of kalarippayattu is evident at demonstrations such as this one in 1983 at Palakkad, where one student performed this leaping right side-kick over three classmates to break three clay tiles.

Chapter

1

Introduction: Repositioning the Body, Practice, Power and Self

In mid-January 1984, I came to the end of seven months of field research and training in Kerala, India, on the region's martial/medical art, *kalarippayattu*. After a brief two-week stopover on my way home, in Kuala Lumpur to visit Ustaz Haji Hamzah Haji Abu's 'International Kalari-Payat Dynamic Self-Defence Institute',[4] I returned to Madison, Wisconsin, to receive a copy of the 11 January 1984 issue of *New Thrill* which had been forwarded to me by my Malaysian host. *New Thrill* is a bi-weekly English language tabloid published in Kuala Lumpur which, according to its subtitle, 'prob[es] the unknown, the mysterious and the exciting', for its presumably young, and primarily male Malaysian readership. Framed by moral platitudes and distanced by the veneer of an investigative report, the cover story 'Mai-Pen-Rai' provocatively described the lives of several young Thai prostitutes with detail sufficient to titillate male Malaysian readers who might either travel to Thailand for sex, or at least fantasize doing so.[5]

I leafed through the tabloid skimming other stories which probed 'the unknown, mysterious, and exciting' including 'The (Hollywood) Stars Who Live in Fear', i.e. Olivia Newton John, Kate Jackson, Robert Redford and Barbara Streisand; an article about how Jackie Bisset, Raquel Welch and Joan Crawford were 'Waitresses while waiting for stardom'; two stories in the 'Probe the Unknown' section on 'Orgone energy' and 'The Druid who Learned to Fly'; and finally an article with the bold headline: 'Kalari-Payat: Deadly Art of Locks and Throws'. Among the photographs illustrating the article (Figure 1.1) were a complex set of images–four photographs of myself costumed in a karate-style uniform and (honorary) black belt given to me by my Malaysian host Hamzah, demonstrating four of kalarippayattu's traditional poses; a head-shot of Ustaz Haji Hamzah himself, the Mahaguru and founder of this new street-wise self-defence version of kalarippayattu in Malaysia; and a photograph of two of Hamzah's Malay-Indian students demonstrating an action-packed kalarippayattu style side-kick. When performed in a karate-style uniform with the action stopped at the moment of full extension and impact, this final image has the glamour of the more familiar karate or kung-fu style kicks worthy of a Bruce Lee.

Between my first trip to Kerala in 1976 and my last in 1995, kalarippayattu practitioners and/or various producers of culture have either presented or represented the martial art in numerous new contexts for a variety of new publics. In addition to the Malaysian tabloid's sensational representation of

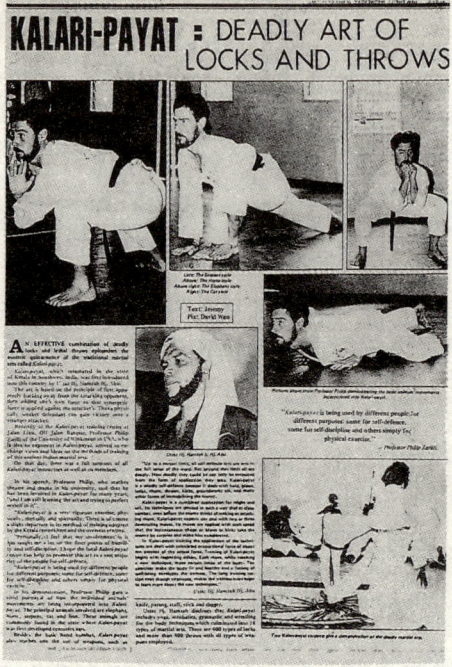

Figure 1.1: New Thrill's *'Deadly Art of Locks and Throws'* with the author in a karate-style uniform demonstrating traditional kalarippayattu techniques. Hamzah is pictured in the centre and several of his students lower right.

kalarippayattu as a 'deadly art of self-defence', the many other ways kalarippayattu has been represented to diverse audiences include: for a Japanese television/print media audience as a humorously exotic vehicle through which to sell a vitamin which is touted as 'replenish[ing] Vitamin B-1 when your body is all worn out' (Figure 1.2); for the American television viewing public watching 'PM Magazine' as an ancient, orientalized, tradition-bound art through which a holistic unity and 'at-onement' might be achieved; and for Malayali newspaper readers as an encapsulation of Kerala's cultural, mytho-historical heritage whose story of single-minded devotion and dedication to practice is paralleled by the dedication of today's South India Bank.

Although such print and visual media representations of kalarippayattu

Introduction • 3

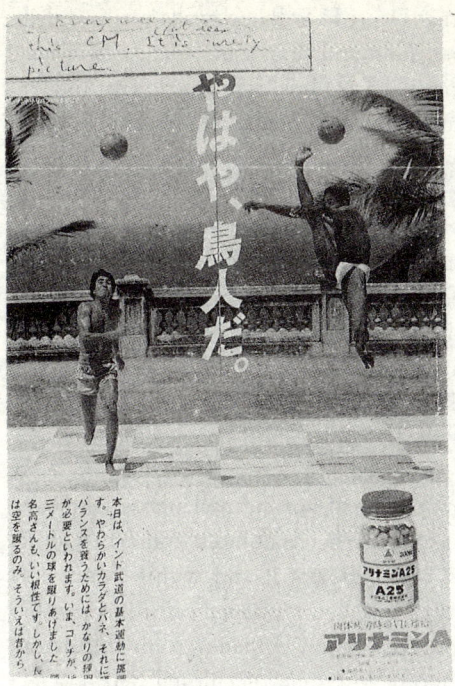

Figure 1.2: Japanese advertisement featuring Sathyan Narayanan competing with a Japanese actor as they perform a 'high kick' to tout a product which 'replenish[es] Vitamin B-1 when your body is all worn out'.

are recent developments, this martial art has a long history of being adapted for practice and/or presentation in a variety of contexts other than for interstate warfare and duels. This includes the training of Kerala's Kathakali dance-drama performers, the inclusion of martial techniques in the propitiation of ancestral heroes in Hindu *teyyam* ritual performances in northern Kerala, its use in training the first Indian (Malayali) circus performers in the late nineteenth century, staged performances as part of government-sponsored Festivals of India throughout the world, the dance choreography of the now internationally known Madras-based choreographer Chandralekha (Bharucha 1995) and my own use of kalarippayattu (along with tai chi ch'uan) in training American performers (1993).

The current history and practice of kalarippayattu cannot be considered without taking into account the emergence of Asian martial/self-defence arts as a global form of cosmopolitanism, a phenomenon attributable to the spread of popular martial-arts films and other forms of popular literature on the martial arts. V. Pandian summarized the situation in India:

> Ever since the mid-70s, when Bruce Lee took the movie-going public by storm with his exploits in *Enter the Dragon*, there has been a virtual renaissance of the martial arts (1983a).
>
> In recent times, moviegoers—particularly in India—have been enthralled by the amazing feats performed by exponents of the martial arts. In fact, people like Bruce Lee and Liu Chia Hui have become household names in India (1983b).

Although it was as early as 1933 that Dr M.H.S. Barodawalla was awarded his black belt after studying karate, judo and jujitsu in Japan, it was not until the 1970s and the influx of martial-arts films from abroad that Indian students travelled east in large numbers to train themselves, returning home to open karate or karate-style schools throughout the subcontinent. By the early 1980s karate-style fight scenes had become ubiquitous in popular Indian films; karate stories, complete with action-packed photographs of brick-breaking and gang fights had become regular fare in newspapers and popular magazines; karate schools could be found not only in major cities but also in small towns and villages throughout India; and state-wide police forces were receiving regular training in karate (Fernandes 1982; Katiyar 1983). Within Kerala, practitioners of kalarippayattu compete with teachers of karate, kung-fu, and modern composite forms of self-defence for students as well as the public.

These examples illustrate how one mode of cultural praxis takes on new and highly divergent meanings in the heteronomous contexts within which kalarippayattu is practised and performed, and within which its images are produced. Kalarippayattu is being shaped within a set of arenas that South Asian anthropologist Arjun Appadurai and historian Carol Breckenridge call 'public culture'—'a zone of cultural debate . . . characterized as an arena where other types, forms, and domains of culture are encountering, interrogating and contesting each other in new and unexpected ways' (1988: 6). The public culture terrain which kalarippayattu inhabits in the late twentieth century is contested by an increasingly diverse group of 'producers of culture and their audiences', many of whom make use of the mass media in shaping their version of martial practice (ibid.: 6–7).

What interests me most about this phenomenon is the dynamic and shifting relationship between the body, bodily practice[s], knowledge, power, agency and the practitioner's 'self' or identity, *as well as* the discourses and images of the body and practice created to represent this shifting relationship. In each context of its practice, presentation or representation the kalarippayattu practitioner's body, practice, power and self are constantly being repositioned for the practitioner himself, the teacher, and/or cultural consumers, thereby making available quite different images, discourses of power and agency, experiences, knowledge and meanings for them all.

THEORETICAL FRAMEWORK: AN ETHNOGRAPHY OF THE BODY IN PRACTICE

This monograph is a performance ethnography of kalarippayattu as one mode of cultural praxis through which bodies, knowledges, powers, agency and selves/identities have been and are repositioned through practice.[6] Practices are those modes of embodied doing through which everyday as well as extra-daily experiences, realities and meanings are shaped and negotiated.[7] As discussed by Mauss (1973), de Certeau (1984) and Bourdieu (1977) everyday practices include such habitualized and routined activities as walking, driving, hygienic practices, etc.[8] Extra-daily practices are those practices such as rituals, dances, theatre performances, the recitation of oral narratives, meditation and/or religious practices, martial arts, etc., which require the practitioner to undergo specialized body training in order to become accomplished in attaining a certain specialized state of consciousness, body, agency, power, and so on. Extraordinary energy, time and resources are often invested by a society to create cultural specialists whose embodied practices are the means by which personal, social, ritual and/or cosmological realities are created and enacted.

Because practices are not things, but an active, embodied doing, they are intersections where personal, social and cosmological experiences and realities are negotiated.[9] To examine a practice is to examine these multiple sets of relationships and experiences. A practice is not a history, but practices always exist within and simultaneously create histories. Likewise, a practice is not a discourse, but implicit in any practice are one or more discourses and perhaps paradigms through which the experience of practice might be reflected upon and possibly explained.

Martial arts, like other overt techniques of disciplining the body including aerobics, weight training, contact improvisation, etc. are 'incorporating practices' through which the body, and therefore experience and meaning are 'culturally shaped in its actual practices and behaviours' (Connerton 1989: 104).[10] These are 'technologies' [of the body] in Foucault's sense, i.e. practices through which 'humans develop knowledge about themselves' (1988: 18). Psychophysiological techniques are practised in order for the practitioner to be transformed to attain a certain normative and idealized relationship between the 'self', 'agency', 'power', and behaviour. Ideally, the practitioner's 'self' is reconstituted through long-term practice to achieve agency, power and a type of behaviour which can be deployed personally, socially, even cosmologically. Such a transformation can only be actualized through the body-in-practice.

As cultural theorist Richard Johnson asserts, 'subjectivities are produced, not given, and are therefore the objects of inquiry, not the premises or starting points' (1986: 44). Following both Johnson and anthropologist Dorrine Kondo's thoughtful ethnographic study of the self,[11] I bracket 'self', 'agency', 'power', 'body' and 'behaviour' with quotation marks to suggest the problems with Western essentialization and reification, and in order to emphasize that all five should always be considered provisionally, i.e. they are dynamically 'crafted' in the constantly unfolding temporal creation of the self in particular contexts of experience.[12] As Kondo asserts regarding self/identity, I would assert that self as well as agency, power, body and behaviour are 'nodal points repositioned in different contexts. Selves [agency, power, bodies, and behaviour], in this view, can be seen as rhetorical figures and performative assertions enacted in specific situations within fields of power, history, and culture' (1990: 304). The martial arts are techniques of bodily practice which allow an individual to gain agency and power, and to act *within certain specific contexts, in very certain ways.*

Given this processual view of the ongoing temporal constitution of the self, and, therefore, of experience and meaning, the 'body' too must be viewed as provisional. John Blacking noted long ago that 'there is no such thing as "*the body*", there are many kinds of body, which are fashioned by the different environments and expectations that societies have of their members' bodies (1985: 66). As environments and expectations change, so do the kinds of bodies which societies produce. Although both body and self are always in the process of being crafted and are therefore provisional, I agree with medical anthropologists Lock and Scheper-Hughes that it is

> reasonable to assume that all humans are endowed with a self-consciousness of mind and body, with an internal body image, and with what neurologists have identified as the proprioceptive or sixth sense, our sense of body self-awareness, of mind-body integration, and of being-in-the-world as separate and apart from other human beings (1990: 57).[13]

In this proprioceptive sense, the martial practitioner assumes *a* body in his practice, but 'the body' he assumes is a palimpsest of many different sets of assumptions about the body, practice, power, etc.

Anthropologist Michael Jackson has also argued persuasively and passionately for bringing the body and lived experience back into anthropological discourse so that culture will no longer be viewed as disembodied (1989). This is similar to the view expressed by Margaret Drewal (1991) in that both insist upon a more processual, phenomenological, performative view of the constitution of meaning and experience than previous anthropologies of the body; the latter tended to 'interpret embodied experience in terms of cognitive and linguistic models of meaning' (Jackson 1989: 122). An alternative is to develop a phenomenology of the lived body, a recognition that for the cultural actor

> the body as an experienced phenomenon is primordially presented not as a representable object but in the immediacy of its lived concreteness. The experienced body is not an object for the abstractive gaze; it is the body *as lived, as lodged in the world* as a base of operations from which attitudes are assumed and projects deployed. The body as object, which has its limited natural justification in the anatomical and physiological sciences, is the body excepted from its living involvements and quoted out of context (Schrag 1969: 186).

I assume with Bryan S. Turner a constant dialectic between the lived experience of the body (Leib) and 'the body as representation' (Korper) (Turner 1992: 57); therefore I assume that practitioners speak from their experience of the body-in-practice (Leib), that these explanations are discursive representations of the body (Korper), and that there is a constant process of negotiation between experience, the set of discursive formations available and how an individual thinks and talks about the experience of practice at any given moment.

It is through the experience-generating body-self in practice that one's self, agency and power are 'disciplined' or transformed. As Johnson points out, the 'who I am' shaped in practice cannot be divorced from the 'who we are', i.e. individual experience and collective identity form a dialectic which is the arena through which the 'self' is forged *in practice* (1986: 44; see also Synnott 1993). Therefore, this monograph also discusses some of the institutional and social contexts which shape the experience of the body and self in practice, and the ever-changing set of paradigms of the body *per se* and the body-in-practice which influence martial practice today.

Through their body-based techniques, practitioners of disciplines like the martial arts attain three context-specific types of socially circumscribed abilities—in Foucault's words, they learn 'to produce, transform, or manipulate things', i.e. they obtain agency; to 'determine the conduct of individuals and submit them to certain ends or domination', i.e., they obtain power[s]; and 'to transform themselves in order to attain a certain state', i.e. they create a self (1988: 18). Simultaneously, through their practice, the body becomes a semiotic system producing certain context-specific 'signs, meanings, symbols, or signification' (ibid.).

Power is manifest when it is exercised on a particular body in a particular context, i.e. 'power' comes into being as it is practised—most vividly in the terrifying aspects of torture (Scarry 1985). It is locatable as it happens. But power also exists as a set of context-specific discursive fields of possibilities. A manifestation of a particular type of power in a particular context is read as 'power-full' through an implicit discourse of power which allows interpretation of the event. Between each discourse of power and the (potential) exercise of that power there exists what might be called a 'field of possibilities'—the possibility that particular discursive constructions of power will actually be exercised on a body in space and time. It is this 'field of the possible' which accounts for the 'agency' inherent in discourses of power. The elocutionary force of such discourses is lodged in the *possibility* (and probability) of the exercise of that power in a specific context by a specific practitioner. To the extent that the possibility of the exercise of a particular power is assumed to be present in a discourse of power, that discourse may itself constrain or influence behaviour, actions, etc., *in a specific context where that power might be exercised.*

Modes of extra-daily cultural practice like kalarippayattu are not practices reducible to their obvious set of virtuosic body-techniques; rather, modes of cultural practice exist as a set of potentialities of self, power and agency inherent in the complex *set* of practices, discourses and representations through which a practitioner's experience of practice is historically and contextually negotiated. Through entrainment and embodiment, complex, extra-daily cultural practices and performances 'structure the structure' of experience and meaning (Kapferer 1986: 202)—a structure which can never be static, but is always *in a process of negotiation*, or in Bourdieu's sense, a form of 'tactical improvisation' (Jenkins 1992: 51). The view of improvisation and process adopted here is multi-faceted—tactical improvisation occurs both 'within' a specific process of practice like kalarippayattu, as well as between practice as received and the horizon of its possibilities which stretches toward an 'undetermined' future.[14] It is within this potentially 'undetermined' future field of the possible that the individual practitioner constantly [re]constitutes his own practice, thereby subtly or overtly shifting and recreating the paradigms (of body, self, agency, power, behaviour) assumed and potentially manifest in his practice.

Each specific context within which a version of kalarippayattu is practised, performed and represented assumes one or more paradigms of the body and of practice which contest other available paradigms as they seek both the attention of practitioners and their audiences.[15] No mode of martial practice is necessarily restricted to a single paradigmatic set of assumptions about the body or the exercises/techniques which constitute the practice. Similarly, a paradigm of the body-in-practice is not completely circumscribed by its context, i.e. practising 'traditional' kalarippayattu exercises in a 'traditional' *kalari* (Chapters 3–7) does not mean that the paradigm[s] of the body assumed in practice are restricted to 'traditional' assumptions. Rather, the body-in-practice today is shaped by all the competing (traditional and non-traditional) paradigms available to the practitioner.

Consequently, kalarippayattu is best considered a complex nexus of four interactive arenas:

(1) *the literal arenas* of practice including the kalari itself where training goes on daily and the contest is for accomplishment and the attention of the master, annual competitions between and among kalari where the contest is for recognition among peers, and the arena of the public stage where the contest is for public recognition of a particular style of practice;

(2) *social arenas* including the Sangham (governing body), which oversees the running of the kalari (where the contest is over who controls the setting of rules), the kalari identified as part of a common lineage or style of practice (where the contest is for recognition among peer institutions and teachers), and the formal associations of kalari (where factions jockey for power within an organizational framework);

(3) *the arenas of cultural production* which generate either live or mediated presentations and representations of the martial art such as brochures, newspaper reports, popular films, traditional cultural performances including calendrical or seasonal festivals, etc.; here the contest is to arrest attention and create symbolic impressions or meanings; and

(4) *the arena of experience and self-formation*—the crucible of the individual's experience where embodied practice helps shape a self, as well as his own style and interpretation of the body-in-practice.

None of these particular arenas operates in isolation from the others—the student practising at the Navajivan Kalari in Malappuram district may also compete in the annual state-wide competitions of the Kerala Kalarippayatt Association, may attend a performance of the rival Kerala Kayikabhyasa Kalari Sangham in Palakkad, see demonstration versions of the martial art on local television performed by the C.V.N. Kalari of Thiruvananthapuram and see Ustaz Hamzah demonstrate his version of kalarippayattu as a form of street-wise self-defence when Hamzah comes from Malaysia to

Malappuram for further training; the student may read the advertisement for the South Indian Bank in his local newspaper, may see kalarippayattu performed by a rival group at the district Onam celebrations, attend a Bruce Lee or Jackie Chan movie and, finally, just might create his own unique mode of embodied martial practice.

Operative within the literal, social, cultural production and personal arenas are five major paradigms which shape practice, its experience, or its public presentations and representations: kalarippayattu as an ancient martial art encapsulating Kerala's unique cultural, mytho-historical heritage (Chapter 2); as a traditional psychophysiological discipline, practice of which cultivates mental, physical and spiritual benefits (Chapters 3–7); as an effective, practical fighting art whose realization depends on the development of subtle, internal skills through correct practice of the basic forms (Chapters 3–8); as a 'scientific' system of physical-culture training beneficial to the modern sportsman and physical culturalist; and kalarippayattu as a street-wise cosmopolitan form of bare-hand self-defence comparable in effectiveness to any of the better known East Asian fighting arts (Chapter 8). If the 'lived body' in its concreteness is the site of experience and source of knowledge for the practitioner, contemporary discourses and representations of the body and martial practice play a crucial role in shaping the fundamental assumptions a kalarippayattu practitioner has about his body and the experience of practice.

To summarize my argument, depending upon how a particular individual is positioned within a system of practice within a particular socio-historical location, the martial arts are one technology of the body through which self, agency, power, the body and behaviour are, in Kondo's terms, 'crafted' and which 'offer culturally, historically specific pathways to self-realization as well as to domination' (1990: 305).[16] This monograph examines the multiple paradigms, representations and practices through which the bodies, agency, power, selves and behaviours of kalarippayattu martial arts practitioners have been and are being repositioned in the past, as well as today. Therefore, following Tyler, my purpose is 'not to reveal the other in univocal descriptions which allegorically identify the other's difference as our interest', but rather to provide 'a fantasy of identities, a plurivocal evocation of difference . . .' (Tyler 1987:102) which are worked out by each individual martial practitioner in the context of his own practice.

OUTLINE OF THE BOOK

In the remainder of this chapter I introduce the reader to my own initial experience of kalarippayattu practice in Kerala, and to the fieldwork on which it is based. The first of kalarippayattu's many identities is explored in Chapter 2—how its significance for Malayalis arises out of history, kingship and concepts of the heroic in the construction of a Kerala history. Chapters 3 through 7 constitute an account of what one master described as 'the deeper understanding about the body and mind [in] practice of kalarippayattu, the spirit of which is vastly different from its visible surface', i.e., the 'lived body' in its concreteness, and the multiple 'traditional' paradigms that inform the lived experience of practice. Following Bruner, my primary concern here is with the 'relationship between experience and its expressions' where 'experience structures expressions . . . [and] expression also structures experience' (1986: 5). In some ways this part of my account cannot be other than an 'ideal-typical picture of the core . . . activities' (Marglin 1985), expressions, and assumptions which characterize the body, practice, and the experience of practice in many, but not all kalari today. It is 'ideal-typical' in that it is not the account of a single Malayali practitioner, but rather is constructed from fieldwork, observations, practice and interviews with numerous practitioners throughout Kerala solicited under my prompting as an 'outside-insider'. As such it is not an account which can be found to exist in its entirety in any *one* kalari.

The palimpsest of the 'traditional' notions of body, practice, power and self presented in these chapters would be incomplete without Chapter 8—the counterpoint against which the ideal-typical account of Chapters 3 to 7 must be read. I explore in detail how practice today negotiates between the more traditional paradigmatic assumptions and alternative paradigms and assumptions which masters and students alike encounter today.[17]

FIELDWORK AND RESEARCH TECHNIQUES

Entering the Field: First Blood

This monograph is based on ethnographic fieldwork conducted primarily in Kerala. In August 1976, I arrived in Kerala, in south-western coastal India for the first time to conduct research on the history and process of training in Kathakali, an elaborate and highly conventionalized dance-drama which enacts stories from the epics and *puranas* in all-night performances (Zarrilli 1984b, 2000). As a performance scholar and ethnographer, theatre director and actor-trainer, I was interested in how Malayali actor-dancers understood their training process, and how that process enabled them to embody Kathakali's aesthetic principles.

During the cool monsoon season beginning in the first week of June each year, Kathakali students undergo vigorous training in 'body control exercises' (*meyyarappatavu*) and full body massage (*uliccil*) meant to provide the performer with a psycho-physiological foundation for developing his art. Kathakali performers and connoisseurs alike insisted that the source of this preliminary training was the region's martial art, kalarippayattu; however, they also lamented the fact that kalarippayattu was no longer taught.

At a New Delhi Fulbright conference two months later, I was surprised to learn from Richard Schechner, Professor of Performance Studies at New York University, and founder of The Performance Group (one of the most important 1960s avant-garde experimental theatre companies), that he was coming to Kerala to observe a variety of traditional arts, including kalarippayattu. On 11 November 1976, during the north-east monsoon in Kerala, an eclectic entourage set out by bus from the village of Cheruthuruthy—home of the Kerala Kalamandalam (the state arts academy) where I was living and Schechner was visiting. Our group included Schechner, Wayne Ashley (an American research scholar studying *teyyam* ritual performance), M.P. Sankaran Namboodiri (my Kathakali teacher at the Kalamandalam) and Vasudevan Namboodiripad (then Superintendent of the Kalamandalam and advisor for my research project). In spite of the fact that Sankaran and Vasudevan were both extraordinarily knowledgeable about Kerala cultural traditions, they had never seen kalarippayattu before; therefore, they journeyed with us to Badagara near Tellicherry in northern Kerala. Along the way we were joined by folklorist, historian and host, Professor K.K.N. Kurup of the University of Calicut who had arranged the kalarippayattu and other demonstrations for Schechner.

When we arrived in the village near Badagara for the martial arts demonstration, we were greeted by various village and kalari officials, and taken to the local kalari. It was a traditional pit (*kuli*) style kalari (Figure 1.3) dug out of the ground, about five feet deep with a pounded earth floor and woven palm-leaf roof. From the entrance on the east of the kalari, we descended the earthen steps carved out of the ground into the pit. As our guests guided us toward folding chairs set up along the southern wall of the rectangular space, the rain began to pour outside, its patter muffled by the plaited palm leaves overhead. To my left, in the south-west corner, was the *puttara*, a seven-tiered platform carved out of the clay-earth where the

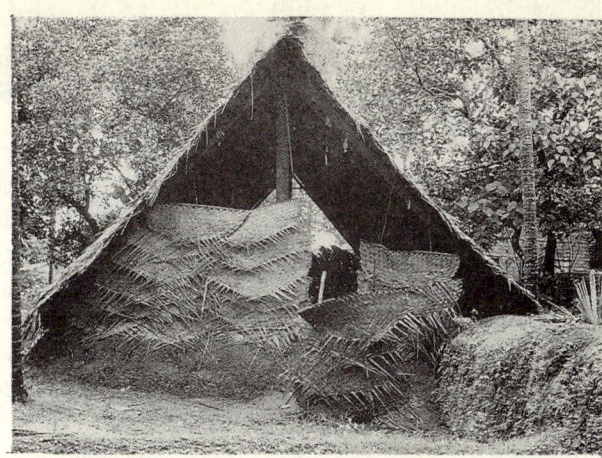

Figure 1.3: A traditional dug-out 'pit' kalari, with a thatched roof. Sreejayan Gurukkal's kalari in the village of Chembad.

guardian deity of the kalari resides (either a form of the goddess Bhagavati or Bhadrakali or a combination of Siva-Sakti). Simple puja (worship) had been done with lighted lamps, incense and flowers.

After being introduced to the master of the kalari and officially welcomed, students demonstrated items in the traditional repertoire including body exercise sequences intended to render the body flexible, balanced and controlled, performing to the cadences of a master's commands (*vayttari*); the use of *otta*, a curved wooden elephant-tusk-shaped weapon meant to attack the body's vital spots, three-span stick, long staff, dagger, sword and shield, and finally, the use of the flexible double-edged sword (*urumi*) were demonstrated. Having spent my first several months observing the virtuosity of many of the trained performers of the Kalamandalam, and given my own cosmopolitan preference for clear focus, concentration and skill in performance, I was disappointed by what I saw—many of the students were out of shape as they gasped for breath while performing the exercises. What followed made me even more uncomfortable. When the students began to demonstrate with weapons, they were not fully focused—the blows often missed and lacked any degree of power or force.

The last item demonstrated was the urumi, a vicious and dangerous flexible double-edged sword approximately five feet in length, which is uncurled from the waist. Two practitioners faced each other and unleashed a string of slashing cuts whipping the urumi round their heads and bodies in figure-eight patterns with the sound of a whirlwind as the blades sliced through the humid, monsoon air, striking the opponent's metal shield. Sitting inches from the slashing blades, and with the audience packed into the small rectangular space, I sank further back into my chair. No sooner had I recoiled than the quick exchange was over. There was commotion among the participants—one of the young men had been hurt, his toe bleeding from a cut opened by one of the blades, either his own or that of his opponent. The teacher of the kalari applied an unguent from his repertoire of traditional treatments to stop the bleeding. Even though the injury was not serious, I left the demonstration shaken, as we moved to a local public school room for the reception planned to honour our visit.

Second Glimpse

One week before my departure for Badagara, I read in the 3 November 1976 *Indian Express* (Kochi edition) that '"Kalari payattu", Kerala's dying art of unarmed combat, is being revived with the inauguration (in Thiruvananthapuram) of a model kalari training centre.' I wrote to the master, Gurukkal Govindankutty Nayar, and received permission to visit his school and observe the training in December. Arriving by autorickshaw at the Thiruvananthapuram kalari located near the busy city bus stand and a block from the famous Sri Padmanabhaswamy Temple, I found a brand new two-storey concrete and brick building of modern design (Figure 1.4). On the first floor were a waiting room and consultation office where the master received potential students, patients seeking treatment requiring his hands-on therapy, members of the press or outsiders like me. A distinguished man of forty-five, Govindankutty Nayar sat across from me at his desk. Behind him was a large old photograph of a young man clad in a leopard-skin-style garment seated on a table, surrounded by an array of weapons

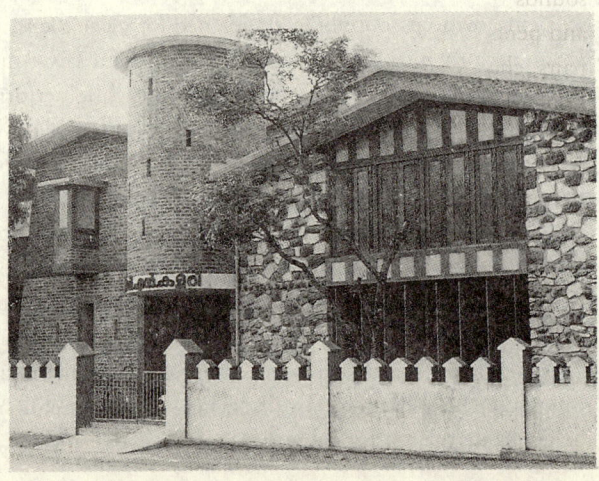

Figure 1.4: Gurukkal Govindankutty Nayar's C.V.N. Kalari, Thiru-vananthapuram with its modern design. It houses a pit kalari, separate massage area, clinic, and upstairs apartment and rooms.

and trophies—Govindankutty Nayar's father. 'You may see the training tomorrow morning at 6:00 a.m.', he told me, his eyes bright, penetrating.

I walked the block from my hotel near the temple to the kalari early next morning. At 6:00 a.m. I was led down a short flight of steps to the pit-style kalari. I entered an area set off behind a structure resembling a retaining wall on the north side of the rectangular room which divided the space for training from this small, narrow area where massage is given, where students change clothes and apply oil to their body, and where occasional spectators like me sit to observe the training.

In the unhurried atmosphere of a day of regular training, I noticed that the air was rich with many scents—wicks lit and burning in gingili oil cupped in brass oil lamps, freshly burning incense, oils applied to the body and sweat. Some students were already exercising in the training space. After descending the steps, each student stepped into the earth-floored training space with his right foot first, touched the floor, his forehead and chest with his right hand, and then crossed to the far south-west corner where a raised, seven-tiered stone platform was located. Touching the base of the platform, some of the students stood silent for a brief moment with hands folded, and then touched a number of other icons or carved stones located around the perimeter of the training space. Others were more perfunctory when paying their respects to the kalari deities.

Sunken below ground level and protected by its high inner walls made of rough-cut stone and set in the midst of the audible early morning hubbub of Thiruvananthapuram city with its careening, noisy buses, cars, trucks and autorickshaws, the kalari seemed quiescent, even though the irrepressible sounds of the increasing stream of morning traffic hung above the space, and penetrated it at times. Students continued to arrive individually and in pairs, changing from street clothes into a *lengotti* (loin-cloth), touching the floor when entering the training space, applying gingili oil or the specially prepared kalari *mukutt* ('slippery') oil to their entire body and beginning their exercises until their bodies began to bead with sweat and glisten under the dim, muted early morning light.

At about 6:30 Gurukkal Govindankutty Nayar arrived. Descending the steps he entered the kalari like his students, stepping with his right foot and touching the floor, and then crossing to the far corner. The students temporarily interrupted their exercises, and came to him to touch his feet. He, in turn blessed each, touching their heads.

All the students gathered at the eastern or students' end of the pit. Commanding their respect and attention, the master began to lead them through the more strenuous exercise sequences (*meippayattu*). His verbal commands led small groups of students through increasingly complex combinations of kicks, steps and jumps, performed as they moved back and forth across the floor. The commands were firm and energetic, and most of the students moved in unison in response to the calls.

When beginners performed, their efforts were laboured and appeared to require great exertion like the students at Badagara. But when advanced students or the master himself performed an exercise, the movements appeared effortless. For advanced students executing one leg kick, the leg seemed to rise effortlessly to the shoulder, extending straight above the head and touching the upraised hand with a quick flick and slap (Figure 1.5). Executing the gymnastic combination of kicks, steps, turns and jumps which comprise the sequences, these students moved with a grace and ease which belied the obvious difficulty with which beginners performed the same exercises. At least this master and his advanced students, moved through these exercises with a concentrated, effortless flow of energy. In that seemingly effortless flow I sensed the potential to unleash deadly force and power. The practical fighting efficacy of these techniques lurked behind the beauty of the forms.

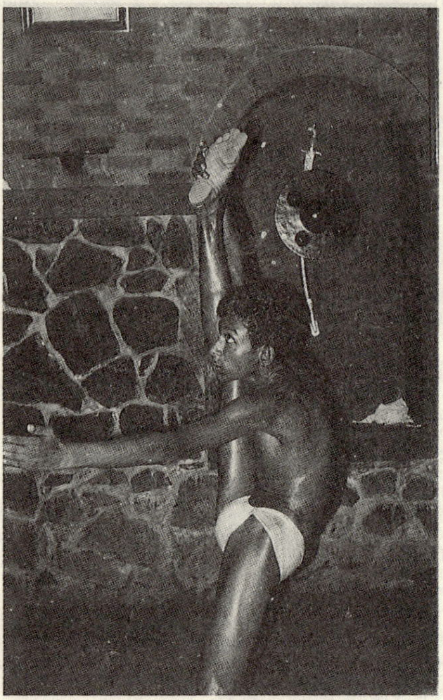

As the class went on, relatively inexperienced students took up practice of a long staff, slowly and haltingly executing blows and defences in response to the instructions of either the master or a senior student. When two advanced students took up short sticks, I was unprepared for their lightning-fast, fluid exchange of blows, clearly filled with potentially deadly force. The two short-sticks attacked or defended in rapid succession

Figure 1.5: The first of eight leg exercises, 'straight leg' kick (nerkal), *in which the leg powerfully and fluidly touches the shoulder (Sathyan Narayanan). The body 'becomes as flexible as a band'.*

temples, ribs, hands, heads, stomachs, ankles—the two sticks striking out in loud acclaim the solid power of each hit.

At some point during the week Gurukkal Govindankutty Nayar began to practise sword and shield, one of the most deadly weapons in the repertory, with one of his most advanced students—an incredibly flexible and well-trained student of about eighteen years. After 'saluting' each other by performing a series of prostrations with the entire body, they began an exchange of jumps, turns and slashing cuts both in set forms and free style, moving back and forth across the kalari floor (Figure 1.6). The master's eyes opened wide (Figure 0.1), sparks literally flew from the student's shield from the tremendous force of the torrent of blows to the head, ribs and ankles he delivered as he backed the student into a corner of the kalari.

The exchange momentarily took my breath away. At the time I could not explain why. I did not have an appropriate language with which to express what I had witnessed. In retrospect, my breath was taken away, not out of a sense of danger for either myself or the student practising, but for the fluidity and virtuosity of the exchange, the single-point focus, as well as the manifest power and 'danger' in the master's attack. But it was a 'danger' different from what I had experienced at Badagara where I had been afraid *for* students, not *of* the manifest (but controlled) power that was being unleashed, and that could and would do harm if unleashed. In the context of these routine daily classes, these practitioners embodied an extraordinary intuitive sense of control, and the master a sense of actualized power that was palpable.

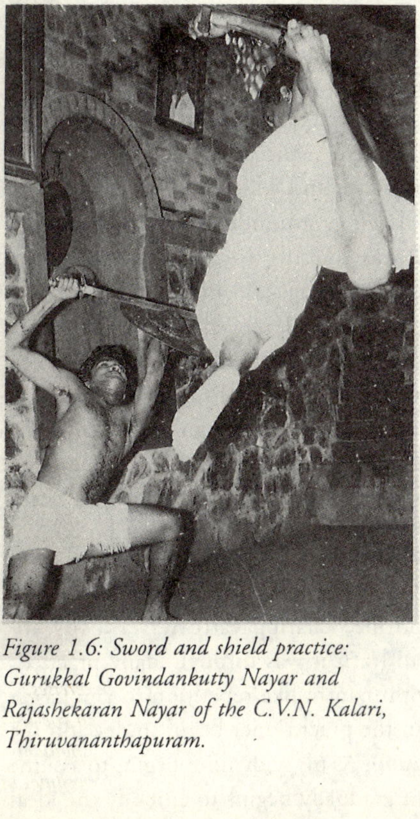

Figure 1.6: Sword and shield practice: Gurukkal Govindankutty Nayar and Rajashekaran Nayar of the C.V.N. Kalari, Thiruvananthapuram.

Immersion

I wondered how they, and the master in particular, had gained such virtuosic accomplishment, whether this manifest control was limited to their practice of kalarippayattu or was understood to have changed their lives in some way outside the kalari, and if so, how this change was understood to have taken place. I sensed in the control, focus, flow of energy and release of potentially deadly power all the requisite traits of the consummate preposessed presence of a master performer. Therefore, my wonder was prompted not simply by my research, but equally by my desire to learn these exercises and use them in training performers. Kalarippayattu became the object of my double desire to experience as well as understand this art. After a week of observations and discussions in Thiruvananthapuram, I knew that it would be impossible to satisfy either desire without immersing myself in the practice of kalarippayattu.

Given my interest in virtuosity and control, I was naturally more attracted to Govindankutty Nayar's practice than that demonstrated at the Badagara kalari. As Edwin Bruner has observed, 'we choose those informants whose narratives are most compatible with our own—just as, I am sure, informants select their favorite anthropologists based on the same criterion of compatibility (1986: 151). The narrative of the 'bodymind'[18] written in practice at the Thiruvananthapuram kalari, and which I interpreted in my own Western terms as 'virtuosic, flowing, grounded and centred', was certainly compatible with what I was looking for. I asked Gurukkal Govindankutty Nayar if I could begin training, and he accepted me as a student. Six weeks later, after my family and I moved our household to Thiruvananthapuram, I began my own intensive training—training which has continued each time I have returned to Kerala. Immersing myself in daily kalarippayattu training meant much more to me than simply engaging in 'participant observation'—it gradually repositioned my own experience and understanding of my body, mind, their relationship, and what it means to 'know' through the body (mind) rather than the 'mind' (less body).

Beginning with the 'Body'

As my teacher and many others told me, kalarippayattu was a 'body art' (*meyyabhyasam*), and the only way to learn it was through 'daily practice'. 'Daily practice' is *the* phrase used with mantra-like repetition to emphasize the fact that only with repetition can the practitioner begin to develop the proper 'body expression' (*deham bhavam*). As his bodymind begins to assume this appropriate expression, a student gradually begins to embody the ideal state of accomplishment assumed in practice—a state where, according to the popular folk expression, like Lord Brahma, the thousand-eyed, 'the body becomes all eyes' (*meyyu kannakuka*). This is an optimal state of awareness and readiness, often compared to the intuitive, instinctual state of an animal in its natural environment where it is ready to respond to any stimuli in that environment. I shall return to this later.

These expressions clearly establish the bodymind as the site of experience and source of knowledge for Malayali practitioners, and certainly from the point of view of practice they would agree with phenomenologist Calvin Schrag's assertion, quoted earlier, that 'The body as an experienced phenomenon is primordially presented not as a representable object but in the immediacy of its lived concreteness' (1969: 186). The occasional bruised knuckle, pulled muscle, or bloodied toe requiring treatment by the master, the experiences of flow or exhilaration during deep exercise, the potential tedium in the constant process of repetitive correction as well as the manifestation of the master's body 'becoming all eyes' convinced me that the practitioner's body was the lived body which should not and could not be 'quoted out of context'. The body and the experience of the body were a place from which to begin an account of this subcultural system, and the kalari was the practical arena within which assumptions about the body, mind and practice became both apparent and palpable to me.

Gurukkal Govindankutty Nayar and his advanced students 'flowed like a river' when they performed their serpentine, graceful, yet powerfully grounded movements. It seemed an unapproachable state of embodiment. When I began my own training in 1976, my body did anything *but* flow. At twenty-nine, I was physically 'tight', wiry and awkward. Unlike the young boys who could throw themselves easily into the training, and like a few of the other 'older' students closer to my age, I was unable to perform any of the exercises with comfort or ease. I was only beginning to learn Malayalam, and was confused by the verbal commands. I felt myself an incongruous, inept presence in the kalari, as well as in my body. To my knowledge I was only the second Westerner to undergo kalarippayattu training, and I was certainly an anomaly and curiosity to many, if not most of the students and visitors to the kalari. Govindankutty Nayar found my ineptitude humorous, as also my appearance. Dressed in the traditional kacca in the kalari, my white skin had become a multi-coloured rainbow, with my neck and shoulders bright pink from the Kerala sun, my arms tanned and browned, my usually unexposed stomach and thighs white, and my calves and feet browned from sun and dirt.

Although a figure providing comic relief during my first months of training, my bodymind began the long process of assimilating two foreign languages—those of the body and of the word. Malayalam provides guidance in the form of verbal commands (*vayttari*), and correction in the form of reprimands, but it is the student's bodymind that must speak through its actions. Reflection and questions have no place in the training space, though for me as a reflexive Westerner this was a lesson long in the learning.

My overt physical ineptitude was matched by my equal naïveté about how to learn through my body, and how that body was related to my mind. I physically 'attacked' the kalarippayattu exercises. I tried to force the exercises into my body; my body into the forms. I was determined to learn each exercise, no matter how difficult. There in the Indian kalari was my Akron, Ohio Buchtel Griffin's high school football coach yelling at me:

> Zarrilli, hit him harder. Get up and let's see you move! And I mean really move this time! Get up and do it again–right, this time![19]

Given this approach, my body was filled with tensions, and my mind was filled with unnecessary intentions and distractions prompted by my aggressive attempt to control and assert my will on what my body was trying to do. I half-facetiously wondered whether my body would ever be the same again. Little did I know that neither my 'body' nor my 'mind' would be the same.

Through the initial months of aching muscles and ineptitude, I eventually made progress; however, by the time of my departure in 1977 I was far from being able to embody 'correct practice'. It was clear that to embody kalarippayattu more correctly would require years of practice. Consequently, I have returned to Kerala to continue both research and training as often as possible. After years of practice, the landscape of my own bodymind in practice, as well as my understanding of that relationship began to alter. I emphasize 'beginning' because every day of practice in Kerala I could watch a master like Govindankutty Nayar actualize this optimal state of 'the body becoming all eyes'. When he performed a kalarippayattu pose like the lion, in that moment of stillness when he fully assumed and held the position, behind its stasis was a palpable inner 'fulness' reflected in his concentrated gaze and in his readiness to respond to the immediate environment.

When demonstrating the martial art or when acting, I eventually found myself able to enter a state of readiness and awareness more consistently—

I no longer 'attacked' the activity or the moment. My body and mind were being positively 'disciplined', or, more appropriately, 'cultivated' toward engagement in the present moment, not toward an end or goal. My initial physical tensions and mental inattentions gradually gave way to sensing myself simultaneously as 'flowing' yet 'power-full', 'centred' yet 'free', 'released' yet 'controlled'.

Simultaneously, through the long process of repetition of basic forms of practice, I also began to sense a shift in the quality of my relationship to my bodymind in exercise or on stage—I was discovering what I later identified from accounts of Malayali practitioners as an 'internal energy', which I was gradually able to control and modulate physically and vocally, whether in performance or when extending my breath or 'energy' through a weapon, when delivering a blow or a massage stroke. I was moving from a concern with external form to awareness of a new understanding of the 'internal', dynamic dimension of my psycho-physiological relationship to my bodymind *in practice*. I was beginning to learn how to enter a state of heightened awareness of, and sensitivity to, both my bodymind and breath in action, as well as the immediate environment. My exposure to Malayali assumptions about the body, mind, their relationship, exercise, physiology and medicine began to make sense to me not only outside, but inside the kalari.[20]

How Malayalis thought and talked about practice gave me a second language with which to interpret what I was both seeing and doing. Gradually, my research began to inform my practice as much as my practice informed my research. They were becoming integrally linked in a series of interwoven hermeneutic *and* experiential circles—my teacher's embodiment of the ideal mode of practice, my own attempts to embody it, observations of other students' attempts to embody it, observations of other teachers' and their students' practice, and the many interpretations offered about what I both observed and experienced.

Watching and Being Watched

Recognizing that kalarippayattu cannot be contained or represented by one arena of practice, or by one particular version of experience, in 1983 I expanded my field of research beyond the Thiruvananthapuram C.V.N. Kalari. Travels to Palakkad, Kunnamkulam, Kachery, Chavaggad and numerous other village and town kalari exposed me to both similar as well as different styles, nuances of interpretation, paradigms and assumptions about practice.[21] As I travelled the length and breadth of Kerala to document training and interview teachers in numerous kalari, I received numerous invitations to attend demonstrations, and to inaugurate functions by giving short speeches on kalarippayattu and its value. Practitioners seeking public validation and new forms of patronage for an art they felt was being neglected by the government, recognized my value as a legitimizing outsider, and called attention to my presence. The higher my public profile, the more I began to attract the attention of Kerala's voracious journalists—I was being watched as carefully as I was watching. For an article focusing on my research ('Kathakali influenced by "kalari payattu"') the 5 September 1980 *Indian Express* (Kochi edition) featured a photograph of me practising long staff with Rajashekaran Nayar in the C.V.N. Kalari, with the caption, 'Not a scene from a film on "Thacholi Othenan" (a well-known popular folk hero trained in the martial art)—It is Dr. Zavrilli (*sic*) practising payattu (exercises)'. Others, like Suresh Awasthi, placed a high value on my application of kalarippayattu to performer training in the United States (see Zarrilli 1993). In his article appearing in *Namaskaar* (a traditional mode of greeting in which one folds the hands across the chest; here the title of the in-flight magazine of Air-India) Awasthi calls attention to the 'regrettable' fact that

> Kalari remains confined to Kerala and is not taught at any of the important sports and military training centres in the country . . . It is also unfortunate that Kalari has not received the attention of actors, dancers and performers since it could be profitably included in training programmes . . . It is only the young drama teacher and director, Phillip B. Zarrilli . . . who after receiving training in kalari at the Trivandrum Centre uses its exercises for training in acting (1982–83: 14).[22]

Inevitably my presence became one factor contributing to a resurgence of interest in kalarippayattu among Malayalis, Indians in general, as well as foreigners. A growing number of academic and popular accounts of kalarippayattu, both my own and those of others, have attracted both non-Malayalis and foreigners to the study of kalarippayattu. Since 1980 many of my students have travelled to Kerala to study. In 1983 an Irishman living in Brazil read my 1978 article on kalarippayattu, and travelled to Kerala to begin training. At a 1983 conference, a Bombay little-theatre director learned about kalarippayattu from me and set out the next year for Chavakkad to train at the Sri Narayana Guru Kalari in order to apply her study of the martial art to her contemporary theatre work. Indeed, by 1980 the foreign tourists visiting the C.V.N. Kalari in Trivandrum as part of their tour of South India were as likely to see one or more westerners training as they did Malayalis—a fact not always appreciated when taking photographs or videotapes of 'natives' practising a 'traditional' art.

It is to the ways in which Malayalis interpret kalarippayattu as part of Kerala history, kingship and the heroic, that I now turn our attention in Chapter 2.

Chapter 2

History, Kingship and the Heroic: Kalarippayattu and the Invention of a Past

Although a complete account of the history and development of south Indian martial arts must be left to historians, in this chapter I begin with a brief overview of the two major source traditions which shaped the emergence of kalarippayattu—Tamil (Dravidian) traditions dating from early Sangam culture, and the Sanskrit Dhanur Veda traditions; the central role that kalarippayattu played in medieval Kerala culture through the nineteenth century; and the contemporary history of kalarippayattu and *varma ati* as practised today within a new socio-political and economic order, especially in the post-independence period. I then examine how kalarippayattu, as a highly visible mode of cultural performance practice, has been creatively negotiated in several closely related narratives in which Malayalis recount their martial art—its role in their collective past, and the role of that past in the present—and has thereby become one of the key contemporary symbols of Malayali collective and commemorative identity (Connerton 1989, passim). I focus on how kalarippayattu has been used to create an idealized image of Malayali manhood as part of the 'Kerala heritage', how this historical discourse has been central to the formation of modern Kerala state as a political entity, and to Malayali identity as a distinct socio-political formation. Moreover, I examine how the particular version of kalarippayattu associated with the 'Kerala heritage' is that of a 'traditional' and 'ancient' art descended from the sage who founded Kerala, Parasurama, and is therefore an apt symbol of Malayali identity.

WHAT'S IN A NAME?

Implicit in the act of naming is a narrative (Turner and Bruner 1986; Kaviraj 1993). My immediate concern is to tell the story behind the use of the compound, kalari-payattu, to represent the regional system of martial practice peculiar to Kerala. It is a story that encompasses the role of kalarippayattu in Kerala history as told by modern historians, as well as the story of how certain parts of this now standard history are being used to legitimize and popularize the art itself or the art as it symbolized a 'traditional' socio-cultural past that no longer exists.

In Malayalam kalari means 'place, open space, threshing floor, battlefield' (Burrow and Emeneau 1961: 98). It derives from the Tamil *kalam* meaning 'arena, area for dramatic, gladiatorial, or gymnastic exhibitions, assembly, place of work or business' (ibid.).[23] In Malayalam kalari also idiomatically refers to the special place where martial exercises are taught. The root of the Malayalam payattu is Tamil *payil*, 'to become trained, accustomed, practise', while its nominative form means 'practice, habit, word' (Burrow and Emeneau 1961: 265). In Malayalam payil becomes *payiluka*, 'to learn, speak'; *payttuka*, 'to exercise in arms, practice', and finally payattu having the idiomatic meaning, 'fencing exercise, a trick' (ibid.).

Although the Tamil roots of both kalari and payattu are antique and can be traced to the first century (Burrow and Emeneau 1961; Burrow 1947), their specific idiomatic Malayalam meanings may be no older than the eleventh or twelfth centuries when, it is probable, that the systems of martial practice assumed a structure and style akin to those extant today. Belying the assumption that the compound itself might have an equally antique use as the singular kalari and payattu, the Malayalam Lexicon notes that the earliest use of the compound, kalarippayattu is in Ulloor Parameswaram's early twentieth-century drama, *Amba* (Nambudiripad 1976: 502–3). Kalarippayattu does not appear as a compound word in the northern ballads,[24] in the early European descriptions of the martial art and its practitioners, or in twentieth-century scholarly accounts of Kerala customs, including such early works as K.P. Padmanabha Menon's 1924 *History of Kerala*, or M.D. Raghavan's 1929 and 1947 descriptions of the tradition and its practice.

The compound only began to appear with regularity in the twentieth century as it became necessary to represent the martial art for public consumption either in stage demonstrations and/or popular literary and journalistic accounts in order to represent the art, popularize it or draw audiences for public programmes. The compound appeared parenthetically in a translation of C.V. Narayanan Nair's 1933 article published in the *Kerala Society Papers*. In keeping with the closest British colonial analogue available at the time, it was translated as 'the art of fencing (*kalarippayattu*), i.e. the scientific handling of a sword, dagger, spear or stick in attack or self-defence...' (1933: 347). It also appeared in several newspaper accounts of the 1940s and 1950s, and by the 1960s was commonplace in the popular media and among practitioners. For example, the 13 May 1945 English language *Bombay Chronicle Weekly* published an article by K.A. Cherian, '"Kalari Payat"—the Fighting Art of Kerala'. During this post-World War II period, as the term 'martial arts' gained currency as a descriptor for East Asian fighting techniques, the same term began to be used for kalarippayattu as in the 19 January 1956 *Illustrated Weekly of India* article entitled, 'Kalari Payattu: Kerala's Ancient Martial Art'. Before the journalistic need for mass representation, it was unnecessary to name or classify a system of practice which was known to all as an integral part of village life and through the deeds of local heroes.

Whether scholarly or popular, all the above sources use 'kalari', 'payattu' or 'kalarippayattu' to refer to the system of martial practice belonging primarily to Kerala, and contiguous parts of Tulu-speaking Coorg district, South Kanara (see map).[25] Among practitioners of a variety of styles (*arappukai*, *pillatanni* and *vatten tirippu*) and lineages of practice, the common elements in this martial system include preliminary techniques of exercise (*meippayattu*) which, when combined with seasonal full-body massage and application of oils, prepare the practitioner's bodymind for advanced practice and fighting; combat with a variety of wooden practice or combat weapons; techniques of empty-hand fighting used primarily for disarming an opponent; special breathing and meditation exercises (not universal today); knowledge of the body's vital spots (*marmmam*) which one must learn to attack and defend; a specific class of medical treatments (kalari or *marmma cikitsa*) for injuries received in training or combat (bruises, muscle pulls, broken bones, penetration of the vital spots) or diseases affecting the wind humour; and rituals circumscribing practice and combat (not universal today). All these were practised in a 'kalari'—the idiomatic term for the roofed pits where a variety of types of exercises or techniques were practised and known by their specific technical names—meippayattu, 'body exercise', *kuntam* payattu, 'spear exercise/fight', *val* payattu, 'sword exercise/ fight', etc.[26]

The kalari was a centre for training and healing in villages or with royal households, and also served as a temple where the guardian deity was either a form of the goddess or Siva/Sakti in combination. By oral and written tradition, sage Parasurama is believed to be the founder of the art and the first kalari. The system of treatment and massage, and the assumptions about practice are closely associated with Ayurveda, the 'science' by knowledge of which 'life' (*ayuh*) can be prolonged. Masters in this system are usually known as *gurukkal* (but only occasionally as *asan*), and were often given honorific titles, especially Panikkar. Many masters possess palm leaf manuscripts on which was recorded a variety of technical information, most important the colloquial verbal commands recited when students practise basic forms of body exercises and weapons, vital spots and their treatment.

Practising the martial art, especially at advanced levels when learning combat weapons, was an exclusive right and privilege for those designated to serve a ruler. From the eleventh or twelfth century this particular right and duty was most associated with specific subgroups of Nayars; however, at least one subcaste of brahmans, as well as some Christians and Muslims were given this right and duty. In addition, one specific subgroup of Illavas (also known as Tiyyas) were given the right and duty of training in arms to fight in duels to the death.

As Sreedharan Nayar (1963: 9) asserts, other regional styles of kalarippayattu were also historically practised in central and southern Kerala, where masters were more often called asan and the title given was likely to be Kurup.[27] During the nineteenth and twentieth centuries, the continuity of practice was not as strong in central and southern Kerala as in the north, and by the 1960s the distinctive styles of these regions, such as *dronamballi sampradayam*, were no longer practised by Nayars (ibid.: 11–12).

The kalarippayattu styles practised in the old Travancore region of southern Kerala and adjacent Kanyakumari district of present-day Tamil Nadu became a virtually lost legacy among Nayars; however, some sets of techniques which may at one time have been part of southern kalarippayattu continued to be practised by non-Nayar castes including Nadars, as well as some Sambavar. Known generically as *ati murai* (the 'law of hitting'), these preliminary empty-hand techniques are also known as *ati tata* (hit/defend). Application to the vital spots with these techniques is known as *varma ati* (hitting the vital spots), and sometimes as *chinna ati* (Chinese hitting). Some general features of these techniques clearly distinguish them from the kalarippayattu of the more distant 'northern' styles. These southern arts are decidedly Tamil, and at least for several hundred years have been practised primarily by Nadars who claim an ancient heritage as warriors.[28] They do not practise in special roofed pits but rather in the open, or in an unroofed enclosure of palms. Masters are known as asans. The founder and patron saint is believed to be the sage Agastya rather than Parasurama. Much less ritual circumscribes practice and treatment. Practice and fighting techniques emphasize empty-hand techniques from the first lesson, and initial steps are immediately combined with attacks and defences aimed at the body's vital spots. Some practitioners include fighting with sticks, especially long staff. At some point these practitioners also began to take up weapons whose use at one time may have been the exclusive privilege of Nayars. A similar set of treatment is practised by masters of this system, but it is identified as Dravidian Siddha medicine and not with Ayurveda. Still extant are numerous palm leaf texts in old Tamil which focus on the *varma* and medical treatment.

The linguistic, social, religious, historical, technical and geographical differences briefly recounted suggest that ati murai techniques were either sets of empty-hand and stick techniques which were separate from the kalarippayattu practised by Nayars in old Travancore, *or* techniques practised by both Nayars as well as Nadars and some Sambavar. It is certainly a very closely related if not distinct system of martial practice, and clearly is a Tamil, Dravidian-based system of martial practice. Kalarippayattu in all respects has, like the entire socio-cultural milieu of north and central Kerala in particular, received the distinctive imprint of Aryan brahmanical culture, and was an exclusive privilege and right of certain groups of practitioners. Historically, it is likely that the degree of relationship between these arts depended on geographical proximity, with the kalarippayattu styles and traditions of Malabar more distinct from those of the Nadars, while those in Travancore in the south were not only similar, but may have been common or mixed styles of practice.

During the past thirty years the mixing of styles and arts has increased in direct proportion to mobility. The styles of kalarippayattu traditionally practised in the north in 'pit' kalari can be found in southern Kerala; likewise, a few masters trained in Tamil arts live, practise and teach their arts in north and central Kerala. A number of masters intentionally practise and freely mix both. Somewhat anachronistically, my own training took place in Thiruvananthapuram, the capital city of Kerala located in the far south, but the style is strictly 'northern' kalarippayattu taught by a master whose family home is in Tellicherry, north Malabar. Consequently, the system of practice I have described as kalarippayattu is identified by many practitioners and journalists alike today as 'northern' kalarippayattu, while the martial arts of Travancore and Kanyakumari district, which I have identified as ati tada or ati murai, are called 'southern' kalarippayattu. For reasons to be detailed later, this type of genre blurring is sociologically important;

nevertheless, in this monograph I shall follow Sreedharan Nayar and keep these related sets of techniques distinct (1963: 18).[29] I will use kalarippayattu to refer to the specific system of martial art associated with Kerala, and most recently with the continuity of practice found in old Malabar. I will use the colloquial Tamil ati tata or varma ati to refer to the one or more sets of techniques practised today by the Nadar and some Sambavar of south Travancore and Kanyakumari district, and which may at one time have been practised by Nayars in the region.

THE EARLY TAMIL MARTIAL TRADITIONS

From the early Tamil sangam 'heroic' (*puram*) poetry we learn that from 4 BC to AD 600 a warlike, martial spirit predominated across southern India. According to historian M.G.S. Narayanan, during this era, three major monarchical kingdoms, the Cera, Cola and Pandya were involved in 'a continuous struggle for supremacy and domination' (1977: 7). Ponmudiar wrote concerning the young warriors of the period:

> it is my prime duty to bear and bring him up, it is his father's duty to make him a virtuous man . . . it is the duty of the blacksmith to provide him with a lance; it is the duty of the king to teach him how to conduct himself (in war). It is the son's duty to destroy the elephants and win the battle of the shining swords and return (victorious) (Subramanian 1966: 127).

Each practitioner received 'regular military training' (Subramanian 1966: 143–4) in target practice and horse riding, and specialized in use of one or more of the important weapons of the period including lance or spear (*vel*), sword (val) and shield (*kedaham*), bow (*vil*) and arrow. The importance of the martial hero in the Sangam age is evident in the deification of fallen heroes through the planting of hero-stones (*virakkal*; or *natukal*, 'planted stones') which were inscribed with the name of the hero and his valorous deeds (Kailasapathy 1968: 235) and worshipped by the common people of the locality (Subramanian 1966: 130).[30]

The heroes of the period were 'the noble ones' whose principal pursuit was fighting, and whose greatest honour was to die a battlefield death (Kailasapathy 1968; Hart 1975, 1979). The heroic warriors of the period were animated by the assumption that power (*ananku*) was not transcendent, but immanent, capricious and potentially malevolent (Hart 1975: 26, 81). War was considered a sacrifice of honour, and memorial stones were erected to fallen heroic kings and/or warriors whose manifest power could be permanently worshipped by one's community and ancestors (Hart 1975: 137; Kailasapathy 1968: 235).

Shifting Circumstances and Influences

Although Sangam age combat techniques were the earliest precursors of kalarippayattu and varma ati, what eventually crystallized as kalarippayattu combined indigenous Dravidian techniques with the martial practices and ethos brought by brahman migrations from Saurastra and Konkan down the west Indian coast into Karnataka and eventually Kerala (Kesavan 1976: 25). By the seventh century, with the founding of the first Kerala brahman settlements, a 'new cultural heritage' (Narayanan 1972, passim) had been introduced into the south-west coastal region which subtly transformed the socio-religious heritage of the area. The Kerala brahmans shared with other coastal settlers the belief that their land had been given to them by Parasurama (Figure 2.1), the axe-wielding brahman *avatar* of Vishnu. The Kerala legend records how

> Parasurama threw his axe (*parasu*) from Gokarnam to Kanyakumari (or from Kanyakumari to Gokarnam according to another version) and water receded up to the spot where it fell. The tract of land so thrown up is said to have constituted the Kerala of history, otherwise called *Bhargavakshetram* or *Parasuramakshetram* (Menon 1979: 9).

The establishment of brahman settlements gradually brought in the emergence of brahman ritual and socio-economic dominance through the establishment of a complex system of hierarchically ranked service and marital relationships based on relative ritual purity among castes, especially in the northern and central regions of Kerala (A.K.B. Pillai 1987: 1–119). Important among early brahman institutions for this discussion were the *salai* or *ghatika*, i.e.

> institutions mostly attached to temples where the *cattar* or *cathirar*, proficient in *Vedas* and *sastras* and also military activities, lived under the patronage of kings who considered their establishment and maintenance a great privilege (Narayanan 1973: 33).[31]

Drawing on inscriptional evidence, M.G.S. Narayanan has established that students at these schools were *cattar*, who functioned under the direction of the local village brahman assembly (sabha), recited the Vedas, observed restrictions on diet and behaviour (*brahmacarya*) and served as a 'voluntary force' to defend the temple and school if and when necessary (ibid.: 25–6). Narayanan has also established the continuity between the Kerala cattar of the salai and the cattar mentioned in the eighth-century Jain Prakrit work, *Kuvalaymala* by Udyotanasuri from Jalur in Rajasthan (ibid.: 29). This work records a clear picture of the nature of these educational institutions where students learned not only painting, musical instruments, staging of plays and dancing, but also 'archery, fighting with sword and shield, with daggers, sticks, lances, and with fists, and in duels' (Shah 1968: 250–2).

Along with other brahman institutions, these salai and the cattar trained in them must have played some role in the gradual formation of the distinctive linguistic, social and cultural heritage of the south-west coastal region, although the degree of influence was certainly in direct proportion to the density of brahmanical settlement and influence. M.G.S. Narayanan dates this period of change between the founding of a second or new Cera capital at Makotai under Rama Rajesekhara (*c.* 800–44) and its break up after the rule of Rama Kulasekhara (AD 1089–1122). Before the founding of the Makotai capital, Kerala was 'a region of Tamilakam with the same society and language'. However, in the post-Makotai period Kerala became distinctive in many ways from the rest of Tamilakam (1976b: 28).

This watershed period of Kerala history culminated in the disintegration of the second Cera kingdom at Makotai after a protracted hundred-year war of attrition with the Cola empire. At the end of the war, Rama Kulasekhara (the Perumal) abdicated, and the hitherto centrally controlled Cera kingdom was dismembered and split into numerous smaller kingdoms and principalities.

It is to this extended period of warfare in the eleventh century, when military training was 'compulsory . . . to resist . . . the continuous attacks of the Cola army . . .' that Elamkulam Kunjan Pillai attributes the birth of the martial tradition now known as kalarippayattu (1970: 241).[32] During the war, some brahmans were trained in arms themselves, taught others and actively participated in fighting the Colas (ibid.: 155, 243–4).

Although the salai declined with the end of the Cera kingdom and the division of Kerala into principalities, brahman engagement in the practice of arms continued among at least one subcaste. Known as cattar or yatra brahmans, who were considered degraded or 'half' brahmans because of their vocation in arms, for several centuries they continued to train in, teach, fight with, and rule through the martial arts.[33] Written from a brahmanical point of view to legitimize dominance, the legendary Kerala brahman chronicle, *Keralopathi*, confirms brahmanical subcaste involvement in teaching and bearing arms. It tells how Parasurama gave the land to the brahmans to be enjoyed as '*brahmakshatra*', i.e. a land where brahmans take the role of ksatriyas also. The chronicle adds that

> 3600 brahmans belonging to different settlements or *gramas* accepted the right to bear arms from Parasurama. They are described as *ardhabrahmana* or half-brahmans and *valnampis* or armed brahmans, and their functions are mentioned as *padu kidakka* (restrain offenders), *pada kuduka* (military service) and *akampadi nadakukkuka* (guard service). They are said to be divided into four *kalakams* [a colloquial form of *ghatika*, or the organizations of brahman *cattar* to defend the land] called Perincallur, Payyanur, Parappur and Chengannur respectively. These *kalakams* nominated four preceptors or rakshapurushas for the duration of three years with the right to collect . . . revenue (1973: 37–8).

Some kalarippayattu masters have manuscripts which record the *Keralopathi* account of history, pay homage to brahman masters of the past and thereby accept brahman hegemony. One master's manuscript tells how

> Long ages ago, the sage Parasurama brought 166 *katam* [one *katam* equals five miles] from the sea and consecrated 108 idols. Then in order to defeat his enemies he established forty-two kalari, and then brought some *adhyanmar* [high caste brahmans] in order to conduct worship (puja) at the kalari. Then he taught twenty-one masters of the kalari how to destroy their enemies.

The text also mentions that among the deities to be meditated upon in the kalari are 'the famous past kalari gurus of the Nambootiri houses known as Ugram Velli, Dronam Velli, Ghoram Velli, and Ullutturuttiyattu'.

Although the cattar continue to be mentioned in Kerala's heavily Sanskritized Manipravalam literature, between the thirteenth and fifteenth centuries these formerly well-respected brahman scholars and practitioners in arms are depicted as living a decadent life. References find them 'wearing weapons with fresh blood on them', engaging in combat, demonstrating feats with their swords, describing the martial prowess of Namboodiri chieftains (such as Tirumalaseri Namboodiri of Govardhanapuram) and touting the prowess of cattars in combat (E.K. Pillai 1970: 275). A few of these brahmans continued their practice of arms into the Portuguese period of Kerala history, the Edapalli Nambiadiri (a special designation for a Namboodiri leader) serving as commander of the Zamorin of Calicut's army and navy in the early wars with the Portuguese.

THE DHANUR VEDIC TRADITION

It is likely that at least some of the distinctive traits of Kerala's kalarippayattu crystallized during the intensive period of warfare between the Colas and Ceras, and that such developments were at least in part attributable to the mingling of indigenous Dravidian martial techniques dating from the Sangam age with techniques and an ethos influenced by brahmans and practised in their salai. Some masters trace their lineages of practice to 'Dhanur Veda', and claim that the texts in which their martial techniques are recorded derive from Dhanur Vedic texts.

Although the Dhanur Veda to which present-day kalarippayattu masters refer literally means the 'science of archery,' it encompassed all fighting arts. Among them bow and arrow was considered supreme and empty-hand fighting least desirable (Gangadharan 1985: 645). The *Visnu Purana* describes Dhanur Veda as one of the traditional eighteen branches of knowledge. Both of India's epics, the *Mahabharata* and *Ramayana*, make it clear that Dhanur Veda was the means of education in warfare for all those called upon to fight. Drona, the brahman guru of the martial arts, was the teacher of all the princely brothers in the *Mahabharata*.[34] Although the earliest extant Dhanur Veda text is a collection of chapters (249–52) in the encyclopaedic *Agni Purana*, dating no earlier than the eighth century, historian G.N. Pant also argues that an original Dhanur Veda text dates from the period prior to or at least contemporary with the epics (*c.* 1200–600 BC) (1978: 3–5).[35]

Although late, these Dhanur Vedic texts are an important record of this earlier system of martial practice which influenced the development of kalarippayattu. The four Dhanur Veda chapters in *Agni Purana* appear to be an edited version of one or more earlier manuals briefly covering a wide range of techniques and instructions for the king who must prepare for war by training his soldiers in arms.[36] Like the *purana* as a whole, the Dhanur Veda chapters provide both 'sacred knowledge' (*paravidya*) and 'profane knowledge' (*aparavidya*) of the subject. The text catalogues five training divisions for war (chariots, elephants, horseback, infantry and wrestling) and five types of weapons to be learned—projected by machine such as arrows or missiles, thrown by the hands (spears), cast by hands yet retained (noose), permanently held in the hands (sword) and the hands themselves (249: 1–5). Either a brahman or a ksatriya 'should be engaged to teach and drill soldiers in the art and tactics of the Dhanurveda' because it is their birthright. A sudra can be called upon to take up arms when necessary if he has 'acquired a general proficiency in the art of warfare by regular training and practice', and 'people of mixed castes' might also be called upon if needed by the king (249: 6–8) (M.N. Dutt Shastri 1967: 894–5).

Beginning with the noblest of weapons (bow and arrow), the text describes practical techniques. There are ten lower-body poses to be assumed when using bow and arrow, and a specific posture to assume when the disciple pays obeisance to his preceptor (249: 9–19). Instructions are given on how to string, draw, raise, aim and release the bow and arrow (249: 20–9).

The second chapter records how a brahman should ritually purify weapons before they are used, as well as more advanced and difficult bow and arrow techniques (250). Implicit in this chapter is the manual's leitmotif—how the martial artist achieves a state of interior mental accomplishment. The archer is described as 'girding up his loins' and tying in place his quiver after he has 'collected himself'. He places the arrow on the string after 'his mind [is] divested of all cares and anxieties' (M.N. Dutt Shastri 1967: 897). Finally, when the archer has become so well practised that he 'knows the procedure', he is instructed to 'fix his mind on the target' before releasing the arrow (J.L. Shastri 1984: 648). The consummate martial master progresses from training in basic body postures, through technical mastery of techniques, to single-point focus, to even more subtle aspects of mental accomplishment:

> Having learned all these ways, one who knows the system of karma-yoga [associated with this practice] should perform this way of doing things with his mind, eyes, and inner vision since one who knows [this] yoga will conquer even the god of death (Yama).
>
> Having acquired control of the hands, mind, and vision, and become accomplished in target practice, then [through this] you will achieve disciplined accomplishment (*siddhi*) (Dasgupta 1993a).

Having achieved such single-point focus and concentration, the martial artist must apply this knowledge in increasingly difficult circumstances—hitting targets above and below the line of vision, vertically above the head, while riding a horse and shooting at targets further and further away, and hitting whirling, moving or fixed targets one after the other (250:13–19; 251).

The remainder of the text briefly describes postures and techniques for using a variety of other weapons: noose, sword, armour, iron dart, club, battle axe, discus, trident and wrestling. A short passage near the end of the text returns to the larger concerns of warfare and explains the use of war elephants and men. The text concludes with a description of how to send the well-trained fighter off to war:

> The man who goes to war after worshipping his weapons and the Trailokyamohan Sastra [one which pleases the three worlds] with his own *mantra* [given to him by his preceptor], will conquer his enemy and protect the world (Dasgupta 1993a).

The Dhanur Vedic tradition was a highly developed system of training through which the martial practitioner was able to achieve accomplishment in combat skills to be used as duty demanded. Practice and training were circumscribed by ritual, and the martial practitioner was expected to achieve a state of ideal accomplishment allowing him to face death. He did so by combining technical training with practice of yoga/meditation and *mantra* thereby achieving superior self-control, mental calm, single-point concentration and access to powers in the use of combat weapons. As we shall see in Chapters 3–8, this antique pattern of training toward accomplishment is assumed in traditional kalarippayattu practice.

KALARIPPAYATTU IN MEDIEVAL KERALA

Historians agree that by the end of the twelfth century, with the disintegration of the Cera empire and its fragmentation into numerous principalities, brahman socio-economic dominance was consolidated through control of extensive areas of gifted lands, ritual dominance by means of hierarchically ordered relationships, and an intricate pattern of marital relationships with ksatriyas and high-ranking Nayars (Narayanan 1972: 455–6; A.K.B. Pillai 1987: 67–8ff). One of the most important developments during this transition period was the emergence of the Nayars from among the indigenous Dravidian peoples as 'a group of service personnel comprised of many subcastes and status groups constituting nearly a quarter of the population of Kerala'. (ibid.: 82; Narayanan 1972: 457–62).[37] As a distinct term 'Nayar' first appeared only in the ninth century at Thrikkodithanam Temple at Changanacherry, but by the eleventh century was appearing with great frequency (E.K. Pillai 1970: 191, 204).[38]

Although by birth sudra, royal lineages developed among the Nayars such as the Zamorins of Kozhikode or chieftains of smaller localized districts who functioned as ksatriyas (Figure 2.1); however, the numerical majority of the lower-ranking Nayars provided military, personal or managerial services for Namboodiri Brahmans, ksatriyas or higher-ranking Nayars (Pillai 1987: 83). Some served as district chieftains or military commanders, village chieftains and soldiers in service to a ruler, military trainers for royal families or at the village level, managers and/or supervisors of estates, palanquin bearers, oil extractors, washermen or barbers (A.K.B. Pillai 1987: 99–109; K.V.K. Ayyar 1938: 43).[39]

Figure 2.1: An early woodblock print showing Nayar soldiers wielding the sword and shield, and use of bow and arrow. Both wear the kacca *wrapped tightly around the hips to provide firm support to the abdominal region.*

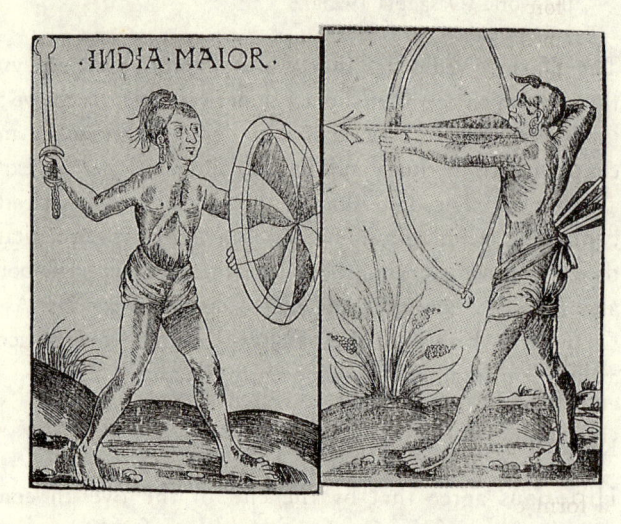

Although between the twelfth century and the beginning of British rule in 1792 Nayar males constituted the largest group possessing the right to bear arms in service to a leader, as noted earlier Cattar (or Yatra) brahmans, as well as significant numbers of Christians, Muslims and a special subgroup among the Ilava (Tiyya) community also learned, taught and practised all aspects of kalarippayattu.[40] Among at least some Nayar and Ilava families, for whom it was traditional to practise the art, young girls also received preliminary training up until the onset of menses. We also know from the *vattakan pattukal*[41] that at least a few women of noted Nayar and Ilava masters continued to practise and achieved a high degree of expertise.[42] Like their Nayar counterparts, Muslims and Christians were also pledged in service to their respective rulers; however, the Ilava practitioners served the special role of fighting duels to the death to solve disputes and schisms among higher caste extended families.

Each of these numerous small states was governed by its own ruler who wielded widely different degrees of influence and power. The ruler of each kingdom aspired to expansion as part of an implicit understanding of kingship as ritual sacrifice. As Chris Fuller explains:

> . . . the ideal Hindu kingdom is coextensive with India, the world, and the universe, and every Hindu king should strive to expand his kingdom's boundaries to the uttermost frontier. This ideal, which necessitates expansive conquest, is evoked in the classical rite of 'crossing the limit' . . . [I]t is the king's duty to make war to expand his kingdom, principally by forcing other rulers to submit to his suzerainty, rather than by annexing their territories as such. Because it brings the kingdom closer to its ideal form, military expansionism is a harbinger of prosperity for the realm, which engenders a more perfect order, not the opposite. Furthermore, because war is classically conceptualized as sacrifice . . . military confrontation can be seen as a religiously sanctioned act necessary for the sustainment of the world. Consistent with this, to fall in battle is to die a glorious hero who is likely to be deified. Thus warfare itself is a reiteration of the idea that an ordered cosmos is created by sacrificial destruction (1992: 124–5).

Anthropologist John R. Freeman explains that this form of kingship does not follow the commonplace 'conception of a single individual, occupying the unique structural center of a political organization', but rather is an example of '"little kingdoms" which are segmentary', and therefore exemplify a form of political authority which is 'multiplex and contestatory' (1991: 715). In this system the

> center (or centers) exhibit . . . an ideal sovereignty that is primarily ritual; but actual executive authority is distributed at many lower sites of the structure, where there are multiple, scaled down replicas of the king . . . [I]n Kerala, even a minor chieftain might be called the 'Pre-eminent King' (Rajadhiraja) in the context of his own little domain (ibid.).

The four most powerful among the larger kingdoms were the Kolathiri of Kolathunatu and Zamorin of Kozhikode in the north, the ruler of Kochi in central Kerala and the Travancore Raja in the south. Each state was divided into a number of districts (*nadu*), which in turn were divided into counties (*desam*) within which were numerous villages (*amsa*). Each district was governed by a *nadu vali* whose rights included criminal and civil jurisdiction and 'the right to claim military service from the Nayars under him' (Panikkar 1918: 257–8). Next in authority were the *desa vali* ruling the counties, who were in charge of maintenance and training of local kalari where training in the martial arts was given. At each segmentary level of organization, a mini-'kingdom' or locus of power and authority existed.

The right to hold land was only in the possession of the highest ranking non-polluting castes (Puthenkalam 1977: 14)—Namboodiri brahmans, the royal lineages (a few ksatriya groups and the highest-ranking title-holding Nayars, often called Samanthan), lesser-ranking Nayars who were local rulers (*nadu vali*), heads of villages (*desa vali*), and temples. Those with the right to hold land did so by birthright (*janmam*). Those working the land did so by tenure (*kanam*), in service to landholders (Moore 1983: 28ff; Gough and Schneider 1961: 308–9).

The basic unit, 'house and land', was a royal model ideally intended to be a self-sufficient microcosm,

> designed to contain a more or less complete set of the beings inhabiting the universe and the entire set of life-cycle events of persons who are its members . . . [T]he rest of society seems to remain solitary by means of a set of ritual relationships defined relative to it (Moore 1982: 26).

This ideal microcosm was only realized by those at the very top of the hierarchy, Namboodiri brahmans, the aristocratic or ruling lineages, or large temples dedicated to pan-Indian puranic deities. Each house and its land provided for

> not merely subsistence, but the conduct of cultural activities (temple maintenance, festivals); and was not satisfied merely with things, but required persons of all kinds (i.e. *jatis*) who were either granted along with the land (e.g. the Cerumans) or encouraged to settle on it (e.g. the Ilavas and artisans) (ibid.: 142).

Each basic unit, house and its land, ideally supported and thereby patronized all rituals and cultural activities associated with the necessities of maintaining both socio-economic and cosmological equilibrium, from the sponsorship of the ritual life and annual temple festival to training men-at-arms ready to defend the unit.[43]

Therefore, many, if not most, villages had their own kalari where youth from families whose duty was to provide military service went for training under a gurukkal or asan who also led them in combat when necessary.[44] Royal lineages had their own kalari for training royal offspring.[45] Some masters trace their lineage of practice back generations to the era when a special title (Panikkar or Kurup) and commission to teach was given by a ruler. K. Sankara Narayana Menon of Chavakkad was trained by his father, Vira Sree Mudavannattil Sankunni Panikkar of Tirur, who in turn was trained by his uncle, Mudavangattil Krishna Panikkar Asan, who learned under his uncle, etc.[46] As recorded in the family's palm-leaf text, the Mundavannadu family was given the title 'Anchaimakaimal' by the Vettattu Raja in recognition of its exclusive responsibility both for training those who would fight on the Raja's behalf and bearing 'responsibility for destroying evil forces' in their region. Christian master Thomas T. Muttothu Gurukkal traces his family tradition back to Thoma Pannikkar who held the rank of commander-in-chief (*commandandi*) for the Christian soldiers serving the Chempakasserry Raja until his fall in 1754.[47]

After completing his advanced training in the weapon to which he was suited, a youth might be pledged to military service at the local or district level, or serve a ruler directly as part of a rajah's retinue (*akampadi*) by taking a vow of service-to-death on his behalf, a tradition and organization dating from at least the period of Cera rule. As early as the Cera kingdom at Makotai the various districts or states under the rule of the Cera king had attached to them bodies of trained fighters known as the three hundred, the five hundred, or the seven hundred. The Cera king had in his service one such group known as 'the thousand' which accompanied him in public.[48] By the twelfth century these groups of retainers were popularly known as *caver*, and later *amoucous* by the Portuguese, i.e. those bound to die in service to their master (Zacharia 1994: 54–5).

Serving the 'King': Professional Rites of Passage

Soon after the arrival of Vasco da Gama at the close of the fifteenth century, Europeans began to comment upon the martial spirit and practices, especially among the Nayars. Jonathan Duncan, who served more than once a Commissioner of Bengal and later as Governor of Bombay, visited Malabar in 1792–3 and noted how a Nayar walked

> holding up his naked sword with the same kind of unconcern as travellers in other countries carry in their hands a cane or walking staff. I have observed others of them have it fastened to their back, the hilt being stuck in their waist band, and the blade rising up and glittering between their shoulders (Logan 1951: 139).[49]

When they arrived home, the weapons were left near the entrance so they were close at hand if needed.

Especially important are the detailed observations of Duarte Barbosa who was fluent in Malayalam and lived in northern Kerala for an extended period. Barbosa records the ideal pattern of martial service to the local ruler, as well as its practical realities:

> When these Nayres accept service with the King or with any other person by whom they are to be paid they bind themselves to die for him, and this rule is kept by most of them; some do not fulfil it, but it is a general obligation. Thus if in any way their Lord is killed and they are present, they do all they can even unto death; and if they are not at that place, even if they come from their homes they go in search of the slayer of the King who sent him forth to slay, and how many soever may be their enemies yet everyone of them does his utmost until they kill him . . . (Barbosa 1921: vol. II: 48).

Barbosa records how kalarippayattu-trained youth underwent a special 'knighthood' ritual which bound him to his master to death. Observed in Kannur, northern Kerala, Barbosa provides a wealth of detail about this essential rite of passage for the martial practitioner:

> The youth who wishes to become a knight, calls together those of his kinsmen who are already knights, that they may come to do him honour, and thus many join them to him, and take him honourably to the palace, having had a time appointed for this by the King. When he is come to the King's palace he commands him to enter with as many as are with him, whereupon he lays before the King on a leaf three small coins . . . The King then asks him if he will maintain the customs and rules of the other Nayres, and he and his kinsmen respond 'Yes'. Then the King commands him to gird on his right side a sword with a red sheath, and when it is girt on he causes him to approach near to himself and lays his right hand on his head, saying therewith certain words which none may hear, seemingly a prayer, and then embraces him saying 'Paje Bugramarca', that is to say 'Protect cows and Bramenes'; and when this ceremony is ended, a writer attends who forthwith asks him in the King's presence in a high voice, so that all may hear, to declare his name and lineage, and they all repeat it that it may be yet more known. Then the scribe enters it thus in the pay-book, that he may draw then his first stipend. His kinsmen then lead him with great respect to the house of the Panical who taught him, and they go through many ceremonies. Then he springs to his feet.

Then they conduct him to his house and give him a banquet in accordance with his quality; and thus he remains for a little while that he may be able to serve the King, go to the wars, or challenge any man at his pleasure (ibid.: 45–7).[50]

Undergoing this initiatory rite, Nayars pledged-to-death in service to their 'lord' participated in the symbolic and literal actualization of his power and authority as a 'divine king' protecting the social order ('brahmans and cows'). This power was symbolized by the ruler's sword, but was won through their own whenever they 'sacrificed' themselves in battle on his behalf.

Although at a political level the Nayar's pledge theoretically circumscribed his right to exercise violence against anyone above him in the social/caste hierarchy, as Barbosa's comment ('challenge any man at his pleasure') makes clear, his coming-into-manhood simultaneously sanctioned his right to exercise violence virtually as he pleased on those equal to or lower than him in the social hierarchy.

Warfare erupted for a variety of issues, from caste differences to pure and simple aggression.[51] Shaykh Zaynu'd-Din's *Tuhfat-al-Mujahidin* (*c.* 1558–80) encouraged an armed Muslim response to the incursion of the Portuguese. His account discusses the intricate relationships between the numerous rulers of the period, and the common code of conduct of interstate warfare which ideally governed combat (1941–42: 1–112). One typical example of interstate warfare, and exemplifying the ideal bond Nayars took to die for their rulers is the well-documented dispute between the Zamorin of Calicut and the Raja of Valluvanadu over which ruler was to serve as convenor and protector of the *Mamakam* festival. Held every twelve years, this 'great' festival celebrated the descent of the goddess Ganga into the Bharatappula river in Tirunavayi, north Malabar, which by her miraculous presence made the Bharatappulha as holy as the sacred Ganges itself. Until the thirteenth century when the dispute probably arose, the ruler of Valluvanadu possessed the traditional right of inaugurating and conducting the festival. The Zamorin set out to usurp this right. After a protracted conflict, the Zamorin wrested power by killing two Vellatri princes. The event created a permanent schism between the kingdoms. At each subsequent festival until its discontinuation in 1766 following the Mysorean invasion, some among the Valluvanadu fighters pledged to death-in-service (*caver*) to the royal house attended the Mamakam to avenge the honour of the fallen princes by fighting to the death against the Zamorin's massed forces (Pallath 1976, passim; K.V.K. Ayyar 1928–32, passim).

Legislating Death: Duels (ankam) and the Chekors

Kalarippayattu was used not only for interstate warfare among petty principalities, but also as a legal means of last resort for solving disputes within a *taravadu* through a special form of duel (*ankam*). The special subcaste of Ilava practitioners called chekors[52] played a unique role in northern Kerala—they were engaged to solve disputes between higher caste opposing parties by fighting to the death in public duels (ankam). Permission to settle a dispute by ankam was decided only by a *nadu vali* as a legal means of last resort when all other methods of conflict resolution had been exhausted. Once permission to hold an ankam was given, each party to the dispute sought out a chekor to fight on his behalf, paying the combatant a large duel-fighting fee. Even though the holding of an ankam resulted in the death of a lower-ranking chekor, it served as a legal means of preventing permanent schism within higher-ranking extended families which might lead to loss of life or a partitioning of family property. For the *nadu vali*, resolution of disputes through ankam meant that the lives of Nayars in his service would not be lost.

One cycle of the northern ballads revolves around the famous Aromar Chekavar and his family. Aromar was hired by one of two Nayar brothers to settle a dispute over inheritance since both claimed to be the elder brother, and therefore claimed right to serve as head of the extended family. When Aromar goes to inform his brother (the youngest in their line of chekors) of the impending duel and to seek his official permission to fight, the balladeer uses the opportunity to further delineate and celebrate the chekor ideal of heroism. Aromar tells his brother:

> Grain or wealth we can buy or borrow,
> But honour we cannot beg or borrow. When father went for combats
> How much younger was I than you now are.
> Father asked my consent,
> Which I readily gave;
> Even so do I ask of you.
> Our forefathers came here
> Adorned as professional combatants . . .
> When one is born a *Chekavan*
> The *Chekor* has to earn his bread at the point of his sword.
> If anybody comes for *ankam*
> He cannot refuse to go . . .
> Better to die with honour
> Than to die a plain death . . .
> Have you not heard of the four states?

> *Ankam* fighting alone makes a *Chekor*,
> As girding the sword makes a Nayar,
> And the sacred thread makes a Namboodiri,
> And wearing the *tali* makes a woman (Raghavan 1932: 111–15).

He recounts the numerous honours and rights given to their Ilava ancestors by ruling lineages including headship, full household rights, 'the *ankam* fighting platform', and 'the rank and status of *Chekors*'; and likewise the gifts given to their own household (Putturam) by the local ruler (*tampuran*) including both their house and kalari (ibid.: 112–15). He instructs his sister that if she has a son, 'he should be well trained in physical and fencing exercises, and if anyone should ask for his services in *ankam* fighting, don't you stand in the way of his going . . . Let not the prestige of the land suffer, nor the *kalari* be dishonoured or its name and fame allowed to suffer . . .' (ibid.: 152).

As represented in the northern ballads, once the two champions have been selected by the contending parties and the fighting fee set, each chekor began a period of intense preparation for combat including 'devotion and prayer to his deity to crown his efforts with success' (Raghavan 1929: 146). The ankam itself was a highly ceremonial occasion from the building of the duel platform, to the elaborate procession to the place of duel, to the announcement of the dispute to be settled, to the proclamation of victory at the termination of the fight when one of the combatants had been killed or vanquished.

In addition to ankam, kalarippayattu was also used in two other forms of duel—to resolve blood feuds (*kutipakka*) between households and to resolve interpersonal disputes through duel (*poyttu*) without having to inform local authorities (Devi, 1975, passim). It was in these non-legislated forms of conflict that more unconstrained forms of violence could be exercised as a means of social protest. Freeman analyses the story of the god Urpalacci, propitiated as a *teyyam,* who gained his power through the exercise of an extraordinarily self-serving, 'clearly sociopathic and criminal' form of violence by initiating blood-feuds 'with sixty-four different lineages through murder', eventually gaining 'enough notoriety to be recognized by the various regional powers as a chieftain deserving of investment with the curika sword and an entitlement' (1991: 592–5).

The inherent instability within the socio-political order is evidenced as well in the stories of the infamous hero of the northern ballads, Tacholi Otenan. From a Nayar family said to have lost much of its previous wealth, Otenan's exercise of power should have been circumscribed by the authority of the local ruler in whose service his exercise of kalarippayattu would have been pledged. However, Tacholi Otenan's great powers and prowess are constantly negotiated and contested within each specific context to quite different ends. In some ballads he challenges and defeats a figure of authority, as when he avenges the treatment of his younger brother, Kunjan, by the Ariarkovil Tampuran ('lord') by beheading him. In another story Tacholi is deputed by a local ruler to collect three years' back rent from a landholding family in the Kodumala area where the powerful young woman of the Kunki family was holding sway and refusing to pay. Tacholi uses his expertise in attacking the body's vital spots (Chapter 6) to subdue her with a cattle prod, and sexually take control of her as well. In this case, Tacholi tames and controls this malcontent ostensibly on behalf of the 'legitimate' local authority. Tacholi's celebrated exercise of extraordinary power is decidedly ambivalent in relation to the social and political hierarchy—he is something of a 'joker' in the ideal deck.

Following Weber, Freeman calls this expression of power (sakti) 'charismatic, for it defines itself individualistically within and against a traditional and established authority' (1991: 718). Urpalacci and Otenan, both of whom are propitiated as teyyam, exemplify the ambivalent and contested nature of socio-political power in medieval Kerala.

THE PLAY OF POWERS IN ANTIQUITY

What is implicit in these Dravidian, Sanskritic, as well as medieval Kerala sources and histories is the view that combat was not simply a test of strength and/or will between two human beings like modern sport boxing, but rather a contest between a host of complex contingent, unstable and immanent powers to which each combatant gains access through divine gifts, magico-ritual means and/or by attaining accomplishment in some aspect of power through practice/training. The first two of these modes of gaining access to power are religio-sacred, and the third is more 'rational' in that accomplishment comes through entrainment. Other realms of practised knowledge in South Asian antiquity reflect a similar symbiotic relationship and interaction between the divine and the 'scientifically' explainable, such as Ayurvedic medicine. The antique medical authority, Susruta, early articulated the existence of both rationally understood causes for systemic imbalance in the body's humours, as well as the possibility of divine and/or magical sources of imbalance and/or cure. Therefore, Susruta identified one of seven kinds of disease as 'the providential type which includes diseases that are the embodiments of curses, divine wrath or displeasure, or are brought about through the mystic potencies of charms and spells' (*Cikitsasthana* XXIV, 10. Bhisagratna, 1963: 231).

Likewise, the agency and power of the martial artist in Indian antiquity must be understood as a complex set of interactions between humanly acquired techniques of virtuosity (the microcosm) and the divine macrocosm. Unlike our modern biomedical and/or scientifically based notions of power and agency which assume that any type of power (electricity, gravity, etc.) is totally rational, stable, and therefore measurable and quantifiable, 'power'—*ananku* or sakti—in Dravidian antiquity and at least through the medieval period in South India was, as we have seen, considered unstable, capricious and locally immanent.

The Sanskrit epic literature reflects this complex interplay between divinely gifted and humanly acquired powers for the martial practitioners of antiquity. One example is the playwright Bhasa's version of Karna's story, *Karnabhara*, which illustrates the divine gift of power (sakti) which requires no attainment from the practitioner. When a messenger gives Karna Indra's gift of an 'unfailing weapon whose *sakti* is named Vimala to slay one among the Pandavas' (102), he asks, 'when shall I gain its power (sakti)?' The messenger responds, 'when you take it in [your] mind, you will [immediately] gain its power' (trans. Gautam Dasgupta 1993b: 105–6). Unlike other powers to which a martial artist gains access through exercise and/or austerities, Karna simply 'take[s] [the weapon] in mind' for its full power to be realized.

A more complex set of circumstances are at play in the story of Arjuna and the Pasupata, and his attainment of this weapon requires more of him than simply accepting the weapon as a gift.[53] Yudhisthira knows that should combat come, the Kauravas have gained access to 'the entire art of archery' including 'Brahmic, Divine, and Demoniac use of all types of arrows, along with practices and cures'. The 'entire earth is subject to Duryodhana' due to this extraordinary accumulation of powers. Therefore, Yudhisthira calls upon Arjuna to gain access to still higher powers.

Yudhisthira prepares to send him to Indra who possesses 'all the weapons of the gods'. But to gain access to Indra, Yudhisthira must teach Arjuna the 'secret knowledge' which he learned from Dvaipayana which will make the entire universe visible to him. After Arjuna is ritually purified to win divine protection, and once 'controlled in word, body, and thought', he meets Indra in the form of a blazing ascetic who attempts to dissuade him from his task. But he is not 'moved from his resolve' and requests that he learn from Indra 'all the weapons that exist'. Indra sends Arjuna on a quest—he can receive such knowledge only after he has found 'the Lord of Beings, three-eyes, trident-bearing Siva'.

Setting out on his journey 'with a steady mind', Arjuna travels to the peaks of the Himalayas where he settles to practise 'awesome austerities'. Eventually, Siva comes to test him in the form of a hunter. After a prolonged fight with bows, swords, trees and rocks and fists, Siva-the-hunter subdues Arjuna when he 'loses control of his body'. Siva then reveals his true form to Arjuna, who prostrates himself before the god. Siva recognizes that 'no mortal is your equal' and offers to give him a boon of his desire. Arjuna requests the Pasupata, the divine weapon. Siva agrees to give him a weapon so great that 'no one in all the three worlds [the Brahmic, Divine, and Demonic] . . . is invulnerable to it'.

To gain access to the weapon's power Arjuna must undergo ritual purification, prostrate himself in devotion before Siva, embrace his feet and learn its special techniques. Siva instructs him in the specific techniques of the Pasupata, and having become accomplished in these techniques Arjuna also learns 'the secrets of its return'.

As illustrated in this and other stories, Arjuna is the perfect royal sage (stoller Miller 1984: 8–9), possessing the ideal combination of martial and ascetic skills, and able to marshal the various powers at his command as and when necessary. Arjuna is the model of the 'royal sage' because his 'spiritual power is equal to his martial strength and moral superiority. He is a sage (*rsi*) by virtue of his discipline (*yoga*), austerity (*tapas*), and knowledge of sacred law (*dharma*) . . . The ideal royal sage is a figure of enormous physical strength and energy who also has the power to control his senses' (ibid.). Arjuna is able to attain the awesome power of the divine Pasupata weapon because of his extraordinary 'steadiness of mind', his superior skills at archery and his ability to undergo 'awesome' austerities.

In contrast to the subtleties of the paradigm of the royal sage embodied in Arjuna, there is the contrasting paradigm of practice and power embodied by his brother, Bhima. Bhima is associated with the raw power of physical/muscular strength (*balam*), exemplified in his use of wrestling and grappling techniques—the 'lowest' forms of fighting.[54]

Although Arjuna's skills and accomplishments appear super-human, the process of attainment of powers is a pattern followed by some traditional masters in the ethnographic present: ritual purification, superior devotion, practice of techniques to gain accomplishment and/or strength, achieving access to higher powers through austerities or special meditational practice attaining secrets of practice, and use of magical means to access a specific power.

Practitioners who had pledged themselves to death on behalf of their rulers or their patrons in a duel were obliged to develop both the mental power and combat skills which would allow them to fulfil their pledge of a sacrificial death. This pattern of sacrificial death fits a religious and socio-political ideology in which 'battle serves as a dominant metaphor for conceptualizing relations of spiritual and socio-political power' (Freeman 1991: 588).

Implicit in this unstable setting is the early Dravidian notion of *ananku* as capricious and immanent where the 'locus of divine power is not primarily, or at least usefully, transcendent, but immanent, and located in human persons and their ritual objects' (ibid.: 130). Anthropologist Saskia Kersenboom points to the sociological results of this unstable and ambivalent notion of power:

> the concept of being or eternity as a process of cyclically repeated evolution and involution, of a divine that is immanent, composite, ambivalent and even dangerous, expressing itself incessantly in the dynamic tension of creation and destruction, of balance and imbalance, of auspicious and inauspicious, gave rise to the need for efficient specialists who could control any critical accumulation or eruption of dynamic force. Throughout history, the ambivalent dynamism of the divine has been felt and, although man could not construct an exact pattern of dynamic change, he distinguished diagnostic features (*laksanas*) of the basic oppositions at play and sought to regulate their cause and effects for the benefit of mankind (1990: 48).

Eruptions of this unstable dynamic power were witnessed 'in illness, drought, diseases among cattle, barrenness and madness', and most often in South India were attributed to some form of the goddess (ibid.). Historically, a variety of ritual specialists arose each of whom had the task of attempting to devise a means 'to control this danger from *within*'—some were the female ritualist specialists (*devadasi*) attached to major temples 'whose individual female powers (sakti) were ritually merged with those of the great goddess (Sakti)' (ibid.: 49; see also Kersenboom-Story 1987).

In Kerala a variety of specialists developed, each of whom also attempted to find a means of controlling this inherently unstable power (sakti) in specific contexts from teyyam ritual specialists (Freeman 1991, passim), to performers who propitiate the goddess as Kali in *mudiyettu* ritual performances (Caldwell 1995, passim), to kalarippayattu martial practitioners. Each of these specialists developed means of psycho-physiologically embodying and actualizing techniques of controlling this divine power in specific contexts.

As we shall see in Chapters 3–7, like his epic counterparts, the kalarippayattu martial practitioner attempted to find a variety of means of gaining access to sakti, and as many means as possible of accumulating specific powers through any/all means at his disposal; therefore, he depended not only on his own humanly acquired skills achieved under the guidance of his teacher(s), but also on the acquisition of powers through a variety of magico-religious techniques such as attaining particular powers through repetition of mantra.

Although this pattern of attainment is still assumed by some masters in the ethnographic present, since the *necessity* of gaining access to powers when confronting death in combat has become largely a moot point, the hitherto capricious, unstable, immanent and local nature of power(s) has been pacified today—a subject to which I shall return later.

CULTURAL PERFORMANCES OF POWER AND PRACTICE

So important was kalarippayattu in medieval Kerala that both its heroic demeanour and its practical techniques were constantly on display whether in 'actual' combat such as interstate warfare or duel, or in forms of cultural performance from mock combats or displays of martial skills at public festivals to dances and dance-dramas where the heroic was virtually displayed as heroes vanquished the forces of evil. Mock combats were presented as part of local and regional festivals including the harvest festival of Onam celebrating the return of Kerala's important mythological figure Mahabali,[55] and at Navaratri, the festival of nine nights which celebrates new beginnings as well as marks 'the ritual representation of kingship, especially the relationship between human king and royal deity' (Fuller 1991: 108).[56] Along with other festive, educational, or instructional items martial techniques were displayed in paired fights. In notes on the letters of Jacobus Canter Visscher, Chaplain at Kochi 1717–23, K.P. Padmanabha Menon described one scene:

> Every year during the Onam festival, sham fights were arranged throughout the country, when the adult members of the community arranged themselves into two parties under their respective leaders, and tried their strength in the open field. Large crowds used to gather to witness the combat, even Nayar ladies, attired in gay apparel and decked with jewels, graced the occasion . . . (1982 (1924): 470).

Sir Thomas Munro noted as late as 1817 that these mock fights often became real and few 'terminated without the loss of a few lives' (ibid.: 471–2).[57]

Martial techniques were also demonstrated for village audiences at the annual completion of a season of training in each local kalari (*cuvadumakam*). The public demonstration of skill served as an entertainment, a test of a student's progress and an opportunity to display 'heroic' spirit.

Other cultural performances include ritual propitiation (teyyam) of deified ancestor/heroes (Figure 2.2) who practised kalarippayattu and which are the legacy of early Sangam age deification of warriors; folk dances (stick play or *kolkali*); sword and shield dances (*paricamuttumkali* and *velakali*); a spectacular mass enactment of an important historical battle performed as part of an annual temple festival (*Oacchirakali*); a brahman variety entertainment (*yatrakali*) which included kalarippayattu demonstrations as one item in its repertory; an elaborate all-night multi-day Christian form of dance-drama (*cavittu natakam*) enacting the stories of St George and the Dragon and King Charlemagne, among others; and Kerala's closely related devotional and dance-dramas, Krsnattam and Kathakali.[58] The range and breadth of these genres involved virtually all religions (Hindu, Christian and Muslim) and castes (from low-caste Hindu ritual specialist performers through yatra brahmans), and provided numerous festive opportunities for performers to embody, display, represent and negotiate particular interpretations of an 'heroic' demeanour (*utsaha bhava*), the 'fury' (*raudra*) of battle, as well as the power(s) attained by these heroes. Chapter 7 continues this discussion with one reading of how Kathakali dramatic actors and kalarippayattu social actors negotiate states of heroism and fury to achieve an ideal state of 'mental power'.

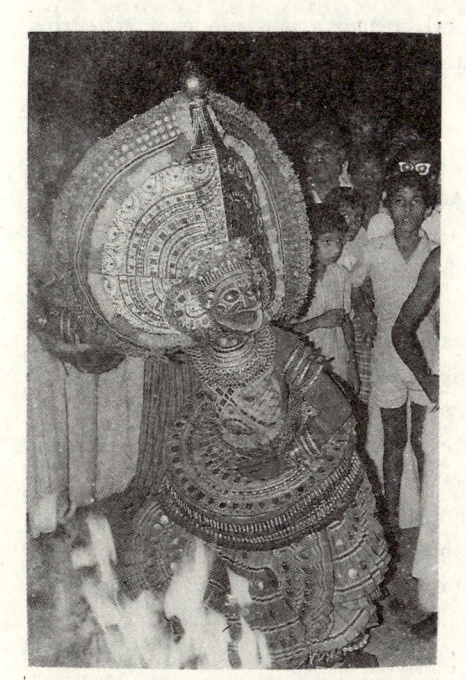

Figure 2.2: Kuttysasthan—one of many 'hero' teyyam *in which deified ancestor/heroes are propitiated in the north Malabar region of Kerala. Most infamous among these is Tacoli Otenan.*

Colonial Chaos and Transition

The arrival of Vasco da Gama and the Portuguese at the end of the fifteenth century introduced colonial influence in Kerala as well as increased use of firearms in warfare. European traders, missionaries and soldiers brought intrigue and heightened bellicosity as they played one ruler against another. The machinations of the Portuguese and later colonial powers (Dutch, French and British) intensified the jealousies and strife which already characterized interstate relations. Swiftly changing allegiances and alliances constantly altered the precise configuration of powers fighting one another even if it did not at first substantively alter daily social, economic and cultural life.

For several centuries no single power emerged dominant. However, a series of factors combined to produce fundamental changes in the socio-economic order by the turn of the nineteenth century. By 1750 Martanda Varma Maharaja (1729–58), the king of Venad, conquered the surrounding kingdoms in southern Kerala and created a new mode of governing Travancore. He organized his fighting forces as a standing army, and created a set of governmental departments with divisions for employees. These changes brought unprecedented power into the hands of a single Kerala ruler, checked only by Tipu Sultan's successful invasion of Kerala from Mysore in 1790. When Rama Varma Maharaja formed an alliance with the dispossessed rulers of Malabar and Cochin, and sought the help of the British in 1792, this alliance brought further erosion of Nayar influence, especially in southern Kerala.

More European modes of organizing police, armies and governmental institutions, and the increasing use of firearms, gradually eroded the need for traditional martial training associated with caste-specific duties. Like some other traditional occupations, the majority of families practising kalarippayattu eventually had to fend for themselves in the emerging marketplace economy.[59] Some families abandoned their traditional practice of kalarippayattu. For others kalarippayattu necessarily became an avocation rather than a vocation. In southern Kerala where there was active suppression of the Nayars, by the mid 1950s Chirakkal T. Sreedharan Nayar notes, the unique southern *dronampalli* style was virtually non-existent (1963: 11).[60] In northern Malabar in particular, and to a lesser degree in central Kerala, kalarippayattu continued to be practised, and some masters continued to make a subsistence living by maintaining their medical practice (Chapters 4–6) and teaching local children.[61] For the majority of masters who continued to practise kalarippayattu, it became increasingly divorced from practical use as a fighting art; therefore, masters often stopped teaching meditation and secret practices used to gain access to 'higher' and more dangerous powers in combat or duel (Chapters 5–6).

KALARIPPAYATTU, HISTORY AND THE 'KERALA HERITAGE'

It was in Tellicherry that the resurgance of public interest in kalarippayattu began during the 1920s as part of the wave of rediscovery of the traditional arts throughout south India which characterized the growing reaction against British colonial rule.[62] The revival was led by C.V. Narayanan Nayar (1905–44) and his teacher, Kottakkal Karnaran Gurukkal (1850–1935) (Figure 2.3).[63] Together they created a 'composite system of training' from the techniques and styles of many masters, and organized these techniques into a set of theatrical techniques for public performances (Kunhappa 1984: 8). Included in the performance repertory were the fluid and gymnastic preliminary body exercises, paired fights with long staff, short stick, otta (curved wooden stick), dagger, sword and shield, spear versus spear, spear versus sword and shield, empty-handed defence against knife attack, defence against knife attack with a shoulder cloth and urumi.[64] To enhance public appeal, many innovations were made. Combining his natural abilities with a flair for the theatrical, Narayanan Nayar's son, Govindankutty Nayar, told me how his father

Figure 2.3: Kottakkal Karnaran Gurukkal (1850–1935) (seated, right) with his student C.V. Narayanan Nayar (1905–44) (seated, left), and students at their kalari—probably during the early 1930s.

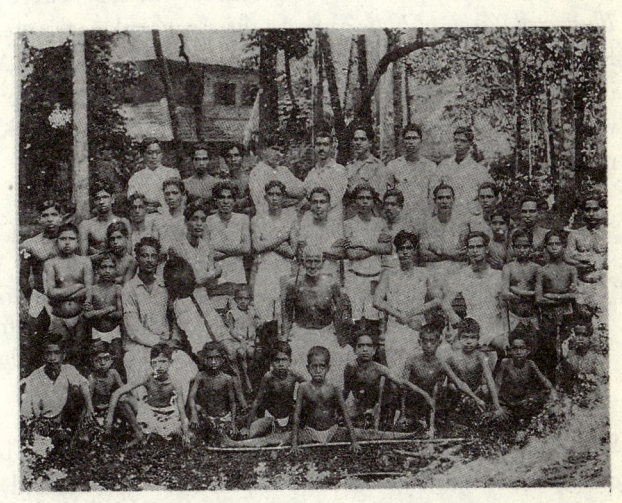

improved on the techniques of the jumping kick and introduced use of the volley ball or a bunch of bananas for greater stage effect. With the dagger too . . . he made changes for audience presentation. Each time he made a presentation there were modifications.[65]

Narayanan Nayar's group began to participate in public art festivals like the Kala-kayika Mela in Kozhikode where they took first prize in a kalarippayattu competition. As Narayanan Nayar's reputation for excellence and showmanship developed, invitations for demonstrations came from many places, including a performance for the Kochi royal family and guests at Thrippunithara Palace. Radhakrishnan and Chempad report that the Amma Maharani of the royal family was so impressed that she told Narayanan Nayar: 'You are equal to the great heroes of history. From now on you will be called by the name, "Virashri" C.V. Narayanan Nayar' (1984: 46). The Maharani's granting of a title to Narayanan Nayar re-enacts the traditional pattern of kingly authority over their Nayar subjects, and the right of ruling families to confer appropriate titles on their subjects.

Just as significant as the conferring of the title is the Maharani's linking of Narayanan Nayar with the 'great heroes of history'. In this and other forms of public discourse between the 1930s and 1960s what had been implicit became explicit—a narrative emerged at demonstrations or in photographic images of the art of kalarippayattu as an encapsulation of Kerala's valorous, heroic, mytho-historical heritage embodied in medieval heroes like Aromar Chekavar, Tacholi Otenan and Kandar Menon. The 29 January 1956 *Illustrated Weekly of India* carried a three-page colour feature, 'Kalari Payattu: Kerala's Ancient Martial Art', with photographs of the C.V.N. team taken in Bombay. Witnessing a demonstration portrayed in the present, audiences were 'transported' to the glorious medieval period in which Malayali heroes reigned:

> Excited crowds gather from the coconut groves and rice-fields and form a ring. Among them are women holding palm-leaf umbrellas and aged men retelling old tales of heroism to intently-listening youngsters. Then for a moment all is silence as two young men enter the arena from opposite directions, their eyes glinting, their bronzed bodies glistening in the sun . . . Now the clash begins . . .

Similarly, the voice-over for the 1952 Burmah-Shell black-and-white documentary film, *Martial Dances of Malabar*—prominently featuring Balan Nayar, Govindankutty Nayar and others in the C.V.N. group and filmed on location in the Tellicherry area—reifies the spirit of the 'warlike past' within the quaint, tranquil images of Kerala's backwaters beauty:

> Often the quiet harbours rang with the clash of arms. Warfare became a rule of life. A man's worth lay in his strength and skill at arms . . . The code of courage hardened in the fires of war. The warrior tradition strengthened through centuries and still lives today . . . Kalarippayattu [is a strong] survival of the warlike past . . . The memories live on: the long past, the times of war, the bravery of heroes are not forgotten. In their dances and war-like games the people of Malabar remember the stirring days of their long history.[66]

The reification of the martial spirit of old, projecting this idealized image of Malayali manhood, also became commonplace at public demonstrations, such as in the narrative read before performances by K. Narayanan Nayar (a student of C.V. Narayanan Nayar) and his students during the 1960s and 1970s:

> There is no country in the world which has not got its own arts and fine arts which portray the genius of the nation. Kerala, the land said to have been re-claimed from the sea by the sage warrior Parasurama, the progenitor for this art is proud of two. They are kathakali and kalarippayattu . . . Kalarippayattu . . . may be said to have got its equal [sic] any where in the world . . .
>
> In the days when Man's ingenuity had not invented the deadly poison gas [sic], when bombs and machine guns had not replaced hands and the sword, when personal prowess had more to do in deciding a battle than destructive engines the power of Malayali manhood had its military training in the Kalari of Malabar. Every year it sent out of its portals hundreds of youthful warriors who fought and conquered or died, but never yielded.
>
> Such were the brilliant Aromar Chekavar, the great Ilava leader who flourished in the 12th century AD and the immortal Otenan who is acknowledged on all hands to have been the greatest exponent of this ancient art (K Narayanan Nayar 1983).

This particular discursive formation of kalarippayattu as an encapsulation of Kerala's mytho-historical heritage and Malayali manhood emerged simultaneously with the writing of now-standard versions of Kerala history;

the increasing circulation of printed versions of the oral northern ballads and the popularization of those ballads through comic books (Figure 2.4), Malayalam films, as well as drama; the spread of mass education which includes representations of Kerala's past; and the increased popularity of harvest festival celebrations supported by private enterprise and government sponsorship of Onam celebrations where live kalarippayattu demonstrations are common. These cultural performances helped establish a common Malayali identity and past, symbolized by kalarippayattu.

Especially important in this process has been the Onam celebration commemorating the return of the mythical Mahabali (emperor of the Asuras, son of

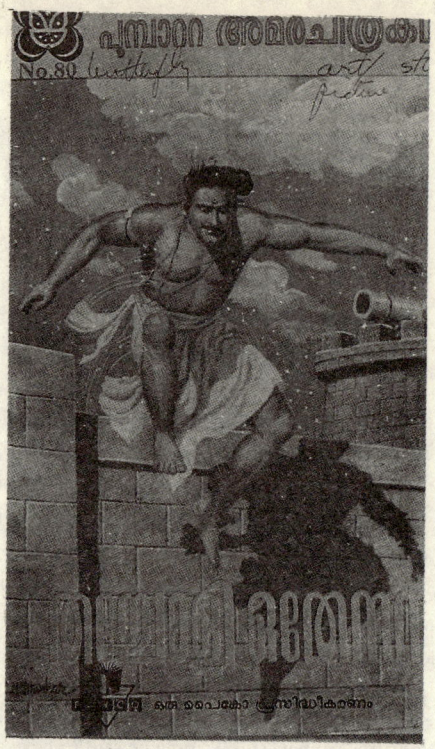

Figure 2.4: Tacholi Otenan's story in comic-book form.

Virocana and grandson of Prahlada) to Kerala where he ruled before his expulsion. According to the *puranas*, Mahabali was expelled from his throne by Vamana, the dwarf incarnation of Visnu. The period of his reign in Kerala is depicted as a golden era of happiness, peace and prosperity where there was neither falsehood nor dishonesty. This golden era came to an end when Mahabali was expelled from his kingdom by Vamana. However, his subjects

> demanded that their former ruler should be permitted to return to his country once a year. This request was granted. The time for his visit was fixed in the first Malayalam month Sravana (August–September), and this occasion became one of jubilation throughout the length and breadth of the land, reminiscent of the prosperous times of Mahabali (S.P.N.K. Pillai 1966: 5).

The celebration was originally a Hindu ritual set to begin on the lunar asterism, *attham*, ten days before the asterism, *tiruvonam*, and it required the ritual involvement of local rulers. However, under increasing colonial influence, the active participation of Kerala's ruling families lessened until Onam became 'a people's concern' (ibid.: 9). As a local festival, Onam is a time for family members to return home; for special cleaning of houses; for preparing flower designs before houses (*athappovu*); for feasts and gift giving; for wearing new clothes and playing games; and for celebrating the return of prosperity for the new year, symbolized by placing clay cones in front of the house to receive Mahabali on his return.[67] During Onam film distributors re-release popular ballad films which often include spectacular scenes of traditional festivals; songs, music, and dance; stories featuring heroism, personal valour, and the overcoming of evil treachery; secondary love themes; comic characters providing comic subplots and comic relief; and numerous fight scenes using a variety of weapons from the kalarippayattu repertory, especially sword and shield and/or flexible sword.

Especially during Onam kalarippayattu is a primary symbol through which a unified Malayali identity is established. It is simultaneously a narrative of 'nationhood' in which Malayali social identity and history are figured as unique. My use of 'nation' is equivalent to what is usually called a 'region' within the nation-state. Indeed, Kerala is a distinctive example of the region whose 'socio-cultural homogeneity . . . is supposed to make the region a more appropriate foundation of political organization than the nation-state precisely because it connotes a common historical experience, perspective and purposes' (R. Roy 1985: 277).[68] Nevertheless, Kerala state is, like the nation,

> . . . a thing without a past. It is radically modern. It can only look for subterfuges of antiquity. It fears to face and admit its own terrible modernity, because to admit modernity, is to make itself vulnerable (Kaviraj 1993: 13).

The invention of this narrative of 'nationhood' during the 1940s and 1950s coincides with the creation of the modern state of Kerala, 'unified' by its common language and cultural heritage.

Although Indian independence was won in 1947, it was not until 1956, with the passage of the States Reorganization Act, that the modern state of Kerala united Malayali speakers in a Malayali Kerala. One of the explicit goals of the Kerala branch of the Communist Party of India was to establish an appreciation for and preservation of 'a purely Malayali Kerala' (Nossiter 1982: 94–5). For then state-less Malayalis, whether living in Kerala *or* as part of the new middle and upper middle class groups of expatriates dispersed throughout India's cosmopolitan cities, there was a collective need to assert one's Malayali identity.

As a celebration of collective identity and prosperity, Kerala state's patronage of Onam helped it become what Benedict Anderson calls a newly 'imagined political community' (1983: passim). After Indian independence in 1947 and the founding of the republic in 1950, 'the awakening of national consciousness has been responsible for resuscitating Onam and making it as much a national [i.e., state] celebration as a people's festival' (S.P.N.K. Pillai 1966: 9). Except for periods of drought or during government emergencies, since 1961 the Kerala state government has sponsored state-wide celebrations of the traditional Onam festival, in the capital city, and in major regional zones. Each year the state-sponsored celebrations include an eclectic variety of events and cultural programmes, among which there are always kalarippayattu demonstrations. Kerala's mytho-historical heritage is displayed on floats in government-sponsored parades in which weapons are readily recognizable signs of that past, such as the 1962 parade in which numerous floats represented moments of Kerala's mythical heritage complete with kalarippayattu-associated symbolism, sometimes with performances. The sword and shield are always present since the sword represents not only the prowess of the martial practitioner, but is also the vehicle of divine power and kingship.

Kalarippayattu was an ideal symbolic vehicle for this narrative of Malayali statehood since it was practised across many (if not all) caste, religious, as well as gender boundaries—it could encompass the 'unity within diversity' required of the modern Indian 'nation'-state. Consequently, it could stand for a 'deep horizontal comradeship'—part of the pluralism which ideally supplants traditional social hierarchies in a contemporary egalitarian state. Once Kerala became a state, kalarippayattu, its martial heroes, and their stories could help assert a unified pan-Kerala Malayali identity, especially during Onam celebrations which represented, through Mahabali, the nostalgia for a lost past—a period of idealized wealth, prosperity and well-being associated with the 'old' social order.

Part of that 'old' social order was the central role that kingship played in the maintenance of a sense of political and cosmic order. Although 565 kingdoms or 'princely states' were still in existence at the time of independence in 1947, all of them disappeared within a year or two. As Chris Fuller asserts,

> Despite this history, kingship retains a central importance in Hinduism and Indian society. In the traditional Hindu worldview, as expounded

most clearly in textual sources, kingship is seen as a vital institution; a
society without a king is unviable and anarchic . . . [A]ll sources agree
that the king's first responsibility is to protect his kingdom and subjects,
by guaranteeing their safety, prosperity, and well-being . . . [T]he order of
the kingdom is itself part of the sociocosmic order or *dharma*, and it is
ultimately preserved by king and deity together, rather than the king alone
(1992: 106).

Because kalarippayattu-trained soldiers were pledged to fight to the death on behalf of their rulers, for Malayalis kalarippayattu became a powerful performative assertion of the past.

When figured as symbols of this past, these versions of kingship and kalarippayattu gloss the segmentary divisiveness of both past and present—a past in which, as already noted, rulers and their retainers lived in a state of virtually constant antagonism and warfare. Heroes like Aromar Chekavar and Tacholi Otenan were exclusively local heroes whose exploits were sung and propitiated within specific spheres of influence and power. Today they have become pan-Kerala/Malayali 'heroes' of a 'unified' Malayali consciousness and identity—Tacholi Otenan has become the Malayali 'Robin Hood'. As Kaviraj asserts, 'in a society still knowing only one legitimizing criterion—tradition—it must seek to find past disguises for the wholly modern proposals' (1993: 13).

The Modern Organization of Kalarippayattu

The modern history of kalarippayattu has also included its organization into a modern institution—a phenomenon which in part disguises the reconstitution of kalarippayattu as a 'modern proposal'. On 26 September 1958, two years after the founding of a united, Malayalam speaking Kerala state government in 1956, the first modern association, the Kerala Kalarippayat [*sic*] Association, was founded under the leadership of Govindankutty Nayar with fifteen member kalari. The new Association was one among seventeen members of the Kerala State Sports Council. With jurisdiction extending over the entire state of Kerala,[69] its goals were to 'encourage, promote, control and popularize' kalarippayattu, conduct annual inter-district and state championships, set standards for practice and construction of kalari, accredit and affiliate member kalari, oversee teachers through publication of a common syllabus of traditional techniques, supervise annual competitions of student practitioners and disburse funds from the Sports Council to subsidize purchase of kalari equipment (weapons) and travel to annual competitions.[70]

When founded in 1958, the Association included under one banner the two previously separate, although closely related martial arts, kalarippayattu and varma ati. Of the original fifteen member kalari, twelve practised kalarippayattu and three varma ati. In setting up this institutional framework, kalarippayattu became known as 'northern' kalarippayattu and varma ati as 'southern' kalarippayattu in spite of differences in history and techniques outlined earlier. Standard rules governing kalari were revised at the 1961 Palakkad meeting, while those for varma ati clubs were drafted in 1967.[71] In keeping with the labels 'northern' and 'southern', the geographical distribution of kalari in 1985 shows that 34 of the 68 active northern kalari were located in Kozhikode and Kannur districts—the area of north Malabar traditionally associated with kalarippayattu practice. Of the other 34 northern kalari, 23 were located in central Kerala, and of these 18 were in Trissur district. The other 11 northern kalari were located in southern Kerala. Of these 11, 8 were in Kottayam district and only 2 in the southernmost Thiruvananthapuram district. Of the 32 southern varma ati clubs, 25 were in Thiruvananthapuram district, and only one in central Ernakulam district north of the southern Kerala region. In 1990 the 'central' Kerala style was formally recognized, although the number of kalari teaching this style are relatively few.

Although kalarippayattu and varma ati were institutionally joined under the common label 'kalarippayattu', their organizational history shows that the two were originally perceived as, and have remained, separate but equal, i.e. their techniques, rules, competition items, place of training, etc., have all remained distinct and separate.[72] Not surprisingly, the Association has been strained at times because of the differing and sometimes conflicting needs and opinions of masters of the related arts. Not unlike the fractious factionalism characteristic of Kerala's modern political life and segmentary history, at times these differences have boiled over into public disputes and debates taken to the highest levels of the Sports Council for resolution.

When founded, the Kerala Kalarippayat Association established a set of rules and regulations for kalarippayattu which clearly reflected a view of the art as 'traditional' and 'customary'. It assumed that legitimate practice could take place only in a kalari *per se,* i.e. a traditional space for practice where students would learn a common core of 'traditional' techniques. As stated in the 1961 revised guidelines for members, 'in accordance with the traditional customs a *kalari* should necessarily' teach a common set of preliminary exercises and weapons, and that 'no exercise systems should be taught in *kalari* other than the arts in the *kalarippayattu* system'. It also established minimal requirements for teachers, meant to guard against untrained individuals from opening schools: 'only those who have learned kalarippayattu for at least six years under a guru in a *kalari* will be eligible to be a *kalari* guru and run a *kalari*. The gurukkal of a *kalari* should be equanimous and highly refined in nature so as to be a good model to his students.'⁷³ If for the majority of Association members its rules seemed fair, some practitioners perceived the regulations as exclusionary. Some poor masters were unable to join because they could not afford a kalari. Others objected because they practised a style and techniques not in the official syllabus. Others wanted an association of teachers and not kalari. Consequently, the Kerala State Kayikabhyasa Kalari Sangham was founded in 1982 to rival the original Kerala Kalarippayat Association, with an original membership of 133 teachers, and by 1983 162 members.

Considerable conflict between the two associations ensued until 1993, when the Kayikabhyasa Kalari Sangham disbanded and most members joined the Kerala Kalarippayat Association, which now numbers over 600.

Kalarippayattu as a Traditional Art

The above discursive and institutional formations emphasize kalarippayattu as a traditional art and carrier of the Kerala heritage more than its practical use in fighting. At yearly Association competitions, a panel of senior gurukkal judge students on the basis of aesthetic form and style in execution of the traditional techniques. In pamphlets advertising practice at the C.V.N. Kalari in Thiruvananthapuram, programmes for public demonstrations and in the 1994 publication of P. Balakrishnan's book (in Malayalam), *Kalarippayattu: Keralattile Prachina Ayodana Mura*, this version of kalarippayattu emphasizes the ancient or traditional (*prachina*) aspects of the art, and the laws (*mura*) pertaining to its traditional techniques of practice.⁷⁴ The jacket cover of the 1994 Malayalam edition displays key symbols of the Kerala heritage and kalarippayattu's place in it—the sword and shield being the paramount weapons and symbols of Nayar identity as martial practitioners and protectors of the established order of dharma, a palm-leaf manuscript indicating the antiquity of the art and its 'laws' of practice, the traditionally crafted Kerala wooden box in which texts and/or other valuables would be kept, and the bronze lamp whose flame symbolizes and actualizes the daily renewal of the relationship to the past as it is lit each day to begin training.

A second way in which kalarippayattu has come to represent the customary past and tradition itself is when it is included in government-sponsored national tours—as representations of India's cultural heritage, especially at the Festivals of India in Russia, Great Britain and the United States during the 1980s.⁷⁵ On such occasions the discourse of tradition or the 'authentic' becomes a powerful tool as it places this discourse of antiquity on state, national and transnational levels. In both these examples, the implicit discourse of authenticity assumes a construction of India's past, encapsulating an eternal Indian wisdom. Discourses of tradition, the authentic and the classical highlight particular versions of the distinctively local and particular—those that point to continuity and commonality. A particular version of the past and, therefore, of practice is represented as authoritative. This particular discursive formation is by no means uncontested. After examining some of the assumptions about the body, practice, power and agency that inform 'traditional' kalarippayattu techniques in Chapters 3–7, in Chapter 8 I will discuss other discourses and paradigms of practice which reposition the body, practice and power in alternative ways today.

Chapter

3

The Ritual Life of the Kalari and its Deities:
Protecting and Empowering the Body-in-Practice

Kalarippayattu training traditionally revolves around two closely interrelated systems of practice—the daily process of training *per se*, which is understood to transform the practitioner's physical body (*sthula sarira*) as well as his internal subtle body (*suksma sarira*), and the daily, seasonal and calendrical rituals which circumscribe every activity in the place of training (kalari) and provide access to the powers of the deities. Both the rituals and the practice of exercises are understood to 'do' something. The rituals make the kalari safe and protect students from inadvertent injury, help develop a devotional attitude, and contribute to a student's interior transformation. Correct practice of the exercises eventually affects and transforms the practitioner. Training and rituals together allow the practitioner to gain access to powers for practice.

This chapter focuses on the kalari, its deities and the ritual life of the kalari which circumscribes practice within. Chapters 4, 5 and 6 follow the progression of the practitioner as he moves from neophyte to a state of accomplished mastery. Chapter 4 focuses on assumptions about the physical body based on Ayurveda, the process of daily practice in the kalari, and how the practice of exercises is understood to have a healthful effect on the body of humours and saps. Chapter 5 goes on to examine the effect of practice on the more esoteric, internal, subtle body of practice. Chapter 6 focuses on the effects of practice on the person, and how some masters practise to enhance both their devotional lives and access to powers by practising special forms of meditation.

THE TRADITIONAL KALARI AND ITS CONSTRUCTION

The place of martial training is known as a kalari.[76] In the Malabar region of Kerala, the kalari is a single, simple, rectangular room—ideally a sunken 'pit' (kuli) dug out of the earth (Figure 1.3)—or a ground-level room in locations where high ground water makes digging a pit impossible. In a pit-kalari mud is piled up around the perimeter to form walls. Inside, deities are installed around the perimeter and worshipped. Training takes place in the centre. With its thatched, steeply pitched roof, the sunken, cocoon-like kalari is designed to remain cool and protect practitioners from four potential causes of disequilibrium among the body's humours (wind, phlegm and fire): wetness of monsoon rains, the heat of direct rays of the sun, drafty winds and skin disease caused by 'contact with worms and manure' (C.T.S. Nayar 1963: 3). The traditional Hindu kalari is a temple where the deities are worshipped, a place to practise exercises and weapons, and a clinic where treatment is administered.

Although all kalari are as much temples as places of training, some kalari were traditionally constructed as parts of the temples of the goddess (Bhadrakali on Bhagavati). One such temple is the Mukkannur Kuttala Bhagavati Temple of north Kothakulangara; the devi of the temple was the titular deity of the Cherampilly karthas who were 'great gymnasts and once the chiefs of the locality. This temple was constructed by the karthas for teaching the art of fencing to the local inhabitants and also for worshipping Devi'. (*Fairs and Festivals* 1966: 247–8; Caldwell 1995: 238–9). Many of these temple kalari no longer exist.

Creating an appropriate atmosphere and actualizing the protection and well-being of all who enter a kalari begin from the moment of site selection and continue through construction and inauguration. Like traditional methods of house construction, strict guidelines should be followed in selecting the plot, locating the kalari on the plot and building according to auspicious dimensions. The kalari gurukkal consults a local specialist in the construction of buildings and idols—an *asari*, a relatively high-ranking expert in *taccusastram* (the science of architecture)—thereby ensuring the future safety of practice within the kalari.

On a well-suited site a kalari is built in the south-west corner of the plot. Like a house, a kalari should 'face toward' the auspicious east. The length of a practice kalari is ideally forty-two foot lengths and that of the duel kalari is sixty-four foot lengths (Figure 3.1). The width of both is one-half their length.[77] The kalari is created by digging down into the ground approximately one *kol* (thirty inches). The earth dug out is used to build up the surrounding walls another thirty inches above the ground, thus creating the 'pit'. From the sunken floor to the top, the walls rise to approximately five feet. The only opening is the thirty-inch wide set of steps in the centre of the eastern side of the kalari, also dug out of the earth. Finally, the steeply sloped roof of the kalari, reaching a height that equals the width, is made of plaited coconut palm leaves supported by a frame of poles and wooden slats.

Since the specific dimensions and proportions (twice length as width) (Figure 3.1), and the optimal location (south-west or north-west) are understood to ward off evil and dangers, the gurukkal himself oversees construction of a kalari. He ensures that the asari's precise measurements

Figure 3.1: Measurements for construction of a kalari.

Traditional forms of measurement include the *padam* or 'foot measure' from the tip of the toes to the heel; angulam, the distance from the tip of the thumb nail to the first joint of the thumb; and *chan* or 'span', the distance between the outstretched thumb and second finger of the hand.

1 padam	= a 'foot measure' from the tip of the toes to the heel
1 angulam	= distance from the tip of the thumb nail to the first joint of the thumb
1 chan	= a 'span', the distance between the outstretched thumb and the second finger of the hand
1 padam	= 8 angulam
1 cottachan*	= a special type of chan equal to 8 angulam
1 padam	= 1 cottachan
3 padam or 3 cottachan	= 1 kol

Conversion to approximate English equivalent measures

1 padam	= approximately 10 inches
1 kol	= approximately 30 inches
payattu kalari	
42 padam	= 14 kol = 35 feet (length)
21 padam	= 7 kol = 17 1/2 feet (width)
angakalari	
64 padam	= 53 1/3 feet (length)
32 padam	= 26 2/3 feet (width)

* A cottachan is also a deadly weapon which, because of its small size, may be easily concealed. It is used to attack the marmmam (vital spots) of the body (Chapter 6).

for length, width and height are followed. Kalari masters recognize that the locations and measurements in their manuscripts are ideal and 'must be adjusted according to the asari's understanding of the situation'. The precise location, depth of the pit, orientation, etc., are based on the asari's reading of the site's signs or marks (*laksana*) and his ability to make the necessary adjustments to optimal location and dimensions. As Gurukkal Govindankutty Nayar explained to me, he reads the marks to avoid *mrtyogam*, the 'tendencies or predilections of the form (site) reacting to bring about accidents or death'. When Chandrashekaran Gurukkal wanted to construct a kalari on his family property in Kannur district in 1984, the local asari determined that it could not be constructed in the south-west corner of the property since it was bounded by a stream flowing in an inauspicious direction. The kalari had to be built far from the stream to compensate for its inauspicious flow. Therefore, it was built closer to the house than ideal. Anthropologist Linda Moore says of traditional Kerala house construction: 'To be guided by these rules of location is to be assured of harmony and compatability among the house, its surrounds, and the people living (or practising) within it' (1983: 220); the same is true for a kalari.

In addition to the traditional one-room kalari, some masters have constructed multipurpose kalari of concrete, plaster and tile with modern designs. Some include separate spaces for training, treatment and living. Built in 1976, the C.V.N. Kalari, Thiruvananthapuram, is a two-storey modern structure (Figure 1.4) which houses a pit kalari and a separate massage area on the lower level; a spectators' gallery, bathing facilities for students, and a waiting room, an office, a treatment room and a medicinal preparation kitchen on the ground level; and an apartment and long-term live-in patient bedrooms on the second storey. Although of modern design on the outside, the dimensions and location of the kalari were determined by an asari.

Whether modern or traditional in design, the degree of success or failure of the ritual preparation of a kalari is tested when practice begins. If a site's negative signs have been ignored or misread, or if any step in the ritual process of construction and purification is incomplete, it could lead to injury.

THE KALARI DEITIES AND THEIR INSTALLATION

Before a Hindu kalari can be used to hold classes, its deities must be appropriately installed and invoked. Preston has noted that all Hindu images of divinity are '"lifeless" until ceremonies of installation are performed.

Thereafter the image *is* the deity, *not* merely a symbol of it' (1985: 9; Babb 1975: 184ff). The actions and objects (ceremonies) which bring life into the mounds/images are not 'symbols of' the infusion of life—they actually infuse that life-force into the mound/image.

One of two sets of rituals are used for installation depending on whether the deities are to be 'temporarily' or 'permanently' installed. Temporary installation is most common and is conducted by the kalari gurukkal himself. Permanent installation is less common, and must be performed by a brahman *tantri*.

The gurukkal is empowered to effect temporary installation in a pit kalari. He prepares places for each of the kalari deities. With the earth dug out to make the pit, he shapes each place (*sangalppam*) where a deity will be lodged, beginning in the south-west corner with the most important *puttara*, usually a seven-tiered platform for the guardian deity of the kalari (Figure 3.2), and continuing around the perimeter of the kalari. Beginning with the puttara in the south-west corner of the kalari, the master invokes the guardian deity. He faces the puttara and recites a specific mantra which 'brings the power (sakti) of the deity' into the puttara (Govindankutty Nayar, interview). While reciting the mantra he holds fresh flowers in his right hand. Simultaneously, he closes one nostril with the fingers of his left hand and breathes in. On exhalation through the opposite nostril he circles his head with his right hand, still holding the flowers. On this exhalation the sakti of the deity is breathed into the mound. The gurukkal's vital energy (*prana vayu*) is the vehicle for infusing the power of the deity into the mound.

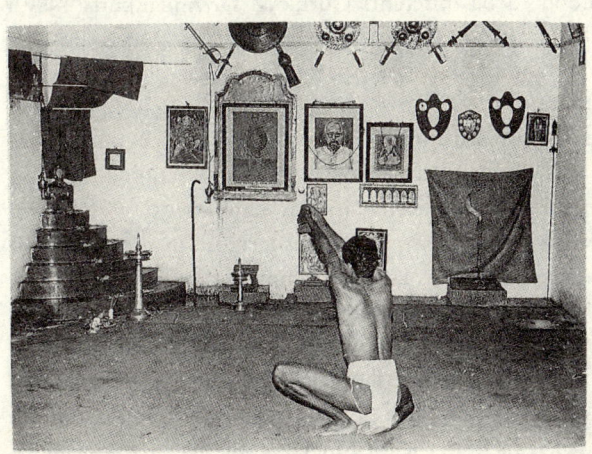

Figure 3.2: Krishnadass, son of C. Sankaranarayana Menon Gurukkal (S.N.G.S. Vallabhata Kalari, Chavakkad) executes part of the puttar tol—worshipping the goddess with his bodymind, and activating the joining of Siva/Sakti.

The same invocation and actions are repeated at each mound where a deity is to be lodged. Once the power (sakti) of each deity has been invoked, the deities are present and reside in their respective places in the kalari until dismissed. One master explained how the ritual installation 'brings the deity and puts it on (*avahikkunnatu matrameyullu*) each mud mound he has fashioned.

Most kalari are ritually temporary in that the deities need be present only during the training season. At the end of each season after monsoon, the master dismisses the deities through a simple ritual. With no one else present, in front of each mound he takes a flower in his right hand and, circling his head, throws off the flower. During the months in which there is no training, it is not necessary to worship the kalari deities since they are no longer present; but neither may anyone enter the kalari until the master again invokes the deities on the opening day of the next season of training.

In contrast to the 'temporary' installation of the deities of most kalari, some are 'permanently' installed. Permanent installation (*pradistha*) is only performed once. When installed, the deities require daily worship even when there is no training in the kalari. Rather than mud mounds, the *puttara* and other places where deities permanently reside are made of stone (*bimbam*). For the installation, the gurukkal calls a brahman tantri since he himself does not possess the requisite purity, expertise or power to install deities permanently. Only a brahman can 'bring the life of the deity permanently to the image' (Govindankutty Nayar, interview).

Although power (sakti) and presence (*sanniddhyam*) are actualized in both modes of installation, the qualitative and temporal nature of that presence is understood to be different. Gurukkal Govindankutty Nayar explained that in the temporary kalari the presence of the god is felt only during the course of training, but in the permanent kalari the presence of the gods is always there.

Once permanently installed, propitiation of kalari deities continues in perpetuity. Even in kalari where there has been no martial training for years, the landholder must continue daily and/or calendrical worship of permanently installed deities. Like serpent deities installed in a serpent grove (Neff 1987), these kalari deities require continuous ritual propitiation for the well-being of the property and the family residing there; otherwise, as Kalarikkal Velu Panikkar explained, 'grave consequences would have to be borne by the family'.[78] Even though the Velayattu kalari in Malappuram district is said to have been established 683 years ago (as of 1996) and not used for three hundred years from the time of Tipu Sultan's reign in Mysore, the Madhavan Panikkar family carries out their ritual responsibility by performing simple morning and evening puja by lighting lamps daily before each of the deities inside the shell of the old kalari.

Unlike major high-caste Kerala temples where the deities are located at the centre of a series of enclosures and where physical access is restricted to the brahman tantri considered pure enough to be in the presence of the deity, the deities of a kalari are located around the outer perimeter of the space, and all who enter have direct access (Figure 3.3). The protection and powers of the deities are spatially actualized in different ways. The deities are located in one of the corners of the half-directions (south-west, north-west, north-east or south-east), along the western wall facing the auspicious east, or are assumed to be present (but unrepresented by a mound) in the centre of the kalari floor. Surrounding and suffusing the space with their power they protect the practitioners training within.

The kalari deities usually number from seven to twenty-seven, and include one or more forms of the goddess, Siva, Siva-Sakti combined, Ganapati (Ganesh) and past gurus. Other deities sometimes include Hanuman, Ayyappan and local ancestors or heroes. As Govindankutty Nayar explained, whatever the deities, what is most important is that

> you follow your own tradition. Different kalari may have their own deities, explanations and theories. But if you change the form (of your belief or practice) you won't have its sakti (power). If you simply believe (what you practise), it will have its power.

At the C.V.N. Kalari, Thiruvananthapuram, Gurukkal Govindankutty Nayar installed the deities according to instructions in a manuscript in his possession (Figure 3.3):

> In the four corners of the kalari, deities should be erected and consecrated (*pradistha*). In the south-west corner (*kanni mula*) *kalari parambara devada* are dwelling. Siva and Sakti should be made to inhabit or settle on the seventh step of the seven-tiered royal chamber (*maniara*) as Kalabhairavan and Kalabhairavi and be worshipped. On the left side below, god Ganapadi and Nagabhagavati should be consecrated. On the north-western corner known as *dhanu mula*, Andimahakalan, also known as Andhiviran, should be consecrated. On the north-eastern corner known as *minakkon*, Bhadrakali, and on the south-east corner a hunting deity known as Vettakkorumakan should be consecrated respectively, and worshipped. On the west part the three times seven (twenty-one) Gurukkanmar (past gurus) should be assumed to be present and worshipped.

68 • *When the Body Becomes All Eyes*

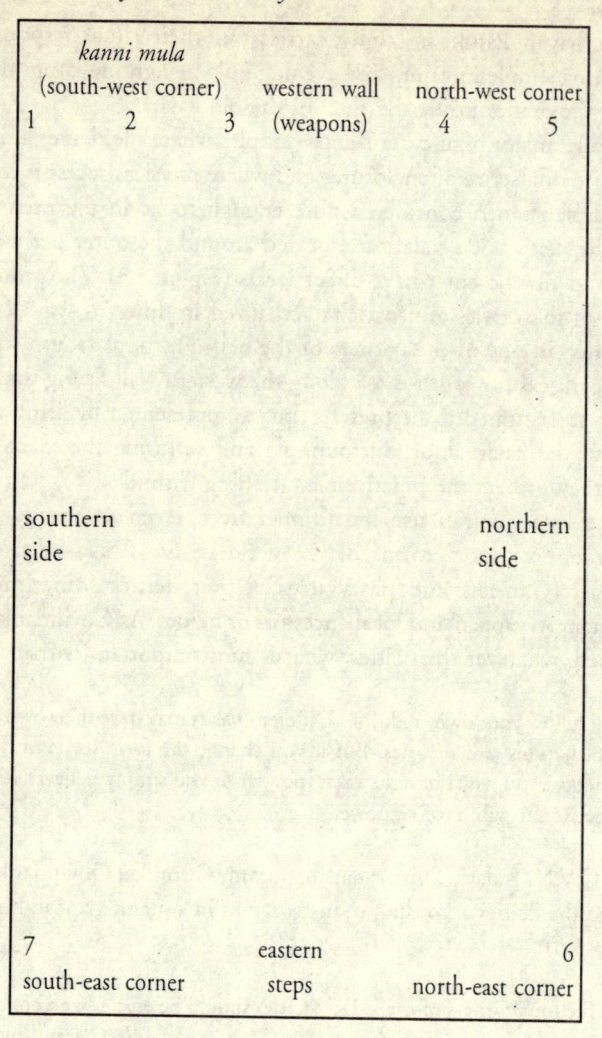

```
           kanni mula
      (south-west corner)    western wall    north-west corner
    1      2         3       (weapons)       4        5




southern                                              northern
side                                                  side










    7                        eastern                          6
south-east corner             steps                  north-east corner
```

Key:
1 = puttara where Kalabhairavan and Kalabhairavi are lodged
2 = Nagabhagavati
3 = Ganapadi or Vigneswara
4 = pitham or tripod where past gurus 'sit' (Figure 3.5)
5 = Andimahakalan
6 = Bhadrakali
7 = Vettaykuramakam

Figure 3.3: The location of the deities of C.V.N. Kalari, Thiruvananthapuram.

In all Hindu kalari, most important is the guardian deity, either a form of the goddess (Bhagavati, Bhadrakali, Chamundi or Durga), or a combination of Siva-Sakti such as Kalabhairavan and Kalabhairavi. The goddess takes various forms and her names are virtually interchangeable. She is best known as Bhagavati. As Bhagavati she encompasses 'a wide range of divine personalities ranging from the benign to the ferocious . . . (and is) associated with both the Sanskritic goddesses of the greater pan-Indian Hindu tradition, and with local village goddesses associated with fever diseases' (Caldwell 1995: 17). Bhagavati is 'conceived of as primarily benevolent and powerful, simultaneously a chaste virgin and a care-giving mother' (ibid.). When propitiated by Kurup ritual specialists, she is conceived in elaborate multi-coloured floor drawings as 'an even more intense form of the *urga* class of fierce deities' notable for her 'energized eyes', and with an expression evoking 'the rasa of vira or valour, supported by raudra or fury' (C.R. Jones 1981: 73).

Bhadrakali is her violent form. She is the goddess of war and weapons and is popularly known as that form of Kali which possesses boundless powers of destruction.[79] Bhadrakali is depicted in popular religious art as holding a sword representing her destructive power. As Bhadrakali she is the goddess 'of the hot months' (Meenam) who in Kerala 'never marries, is never tamed', remains 'independent and unfulfilled' and whose 'sexual desire can be quenched only by violence and . . . by incestuous union with her father, Siva' (Caldwell 1995: 328). In a few kalari she also appears as Chamundi, a ferocious local form of Kali, said to be a combination of Siva and Sakti, or as Durga.

Bhagavati is central to all aspects of Nayar life. She assumes 'paramount importance among household deities' where it is typical for her to be installed in a room on the western side of a Nayar house or a niche where household deities are maintained (Moore 1983: 242). Bhagavati also played a central role in realizing the aspirations to kingship of each of the local rulers of medieval Kerala. As Caldwell notes:

> each king had his own local installation of the goddess, who was considered to be a tutelary matrilineal ancestor and protectress of his family's personal political interests . . . Propitiation of one's own local Bhagavati ensured the power and success of the kingdom and its dependants (1995: 34).

For the goddess as well as other deities, 'the most significant insignia of the god's power, and the essential prop . . . of all forms of worship in this region, are weapons' (Freeman 1991: 242). Weapons do not simply represent or symbolize a deity's power: they are invested with and animate the deity's power since the weapons themselves are often installed, propitiated and then utilized for the literal transfer of the deity's power to his medium—at Bhagavati temples the oracle known as a *veliccappatu* (see Caldwell 1995: 19ff; also Freeman 1991: 244–6). Weapons in general, and the sword in particular are the vehicle through which divine power is manifest in the human spatio-temporal domain. Royal power is invested in rulers and royal lineages symbolized by the sword. That power is literally actualized through the martial-warrior whose hands wield power through their swords (and other weapons).[80] Freeman notes that ritual weapons are indexical icons:

> ritual weapons, through being icons of those used in battle, are believed to actually index that charismatically divine capacity to kill; in other words, the capacity and drive to kill are perceived as instantiated in the symbols that signify them (1991: 299).

As detailed in Chapter 5, the weapons wielded by the martial artist are also indexical icons since they too instantiate the divine through inner actualization of sakti.

Masters associate the goddess with Sakti, the divine embodiment of the active principle of power/energy. As Sakti, the goddess embodies the dangerous, unstable feminine energy and is associated with the generation of a powerful, 'furious', heated condition, and, therefore, inspires terror. As Caldwell notes, 'the colour worn by Bhadrakali in *mudiyettu* is brilliant red, which generally symbolizes feminine energy in south Indian ritual' (1995: 324)—the colour of blood associated with animal sacrifices for the goddess, as well as the sacrifice of war, and the colour often worn by kalarippayattu practitioners in the past when they tied the traditional *kacca* (a long cloth wrapped around the abdominal/hip region to support the 'vital energy' of the practitioner). P.K. Balan Gurukkal explained, 'Devi *is* sakti (power); she is a force, energy, and she is dangerous. Through practice you are seeking to control this force within you so that you can use it in practice.'[81] Consequently, traditional training is a means of literally embodying, harnessing and, to the degree possible, controlling the inherently unstable and potentially dangerous 'power' of the goddess as Sakti. Like the goddess herself, embodying sakti allows the practitioner to utilize these powers either beneficently for healing and saving lives, or for destruction by killing.

The goddess also appears as a combination of Siva and his consort, Parvati or Sakti. Gurukkal Govindankutty Nayar explained,

> Kalari Bhagavati *is* Siva-Sakti or Siva-Parvati. This Siva-Sakti has the *raudra bhava* (furious aspect). In the kalari tradition, Siva and Sakti are there in

the puttara in the form of *ayudha* (weapons), Bhairava and Bhairavi. These are their specific forms in our kalari.

Bhairava and Bhairavi are local names for Siva and Sakti. Bhairava as Siva in his destructive or raudra aspect, represents the fearful destroyer who takes pleasure in destruction or the wrathful one, and is often called Ayudha Bhairava Murti or the god of weapons, war and destruction.[82] Bhairavi means the 'terrible' or the fearful goddess, the power of death and the night of death or the time of the fearful (*kala-bhairava*).

Whatever form it takes, the guardian deity is brought to the top step of the puttara in the south-west corner by ritual installation. The puttara is a seven- or six-stepped platform (*manittara*) made of mud or stone, topped with a flower- or bud-shaped mound. It is given different interpretations. As detailed in Chapter 5, the steps of the puttara are often interpreted as corresponding to the wheels or centres (*cakra*) of the subtle body. Although most interpretations centre around the association of the puttara with Sakti, Siva or Siva-Sakti combined, P.K. Balan Gurukkal from central Kerala offered the following elaborate interpretation of the seven steps and their relationship to practice:

> The seven steps of the puttara are the seven presiding deities of the kalari. A man who knows perfectly all these seven, and imbibes them, will be able to have voice and seeing power.
>
> First is Vignesha or Ganapadi at the base of the puttara who gives initiating power.
>
> On the second step is Candika, or Bhumi of the Bhumi Sakti or Parvati (Earth power) who gives the power of patience of the earth.
>
> On the third step is Vishnu who gives Agnisakti or commanding power. Vishnu has the chakra as his weapon and its rotation in the atmosphere destroys all enemies. You get the power of rotation from Vishnu.
>
> On the fourth step is Vadukisca or lightning. The weapon in itself has no lightning power. It is only the action with the weapon that gives the power associated with speed and quickness (Ayudhaprabhasakti).
>
> On the fifth step are the power and blessings of the guru (gurusakti).
>
> And on the sixth step is Kali in her raudra aspect. Here you get this special power of fury.
>
> Finally, at the seventh is Vagastapuruso where you get the power of voice/sound. By making certain noises you can terrify your opponent like an animal.

Only the man who knows these will be able to have superior manasakti. The mental power will only be acquired by a person who realizes the above-mentioned seven powers and keeps his mind always concentrated.

Like other interpretations, P.K. Balan's stresses the role each deity plays in actualizing a specific power for combat.

Although many masters explain the directional significance of the south-west corner of the kalari with the formulaic expression, 'it is the best' or 'it is according to sastra', the south-west–north-east axis within the kalari is extraordinarily important in practice. In classic texts the south-west is associated with Nirrta (Misery), Surya (the Sun), or as Sakti and the female destructive power of the goddess, especially as opposed to the north-east—the direction strongly associated with Siva.[83] As detailed in Chapter 5, the Sakti (south-west)—Siva (north-east) axis within the kalari is used for special body exercise sequences through which the goddess as sakti is internally awakened and brought to actualization within the practitioner.

Next to the puttara in the south-west corner at the C.V.N. Kalari, Thiruvananthapuram, along the western wall is Nagabhagavati, Bhagavati or Siva's 'pet serpent or ornament' (Gurukkal Govindankutty Nayar, interview). Nagabhagavati is located next to the puttara since serpents are often worn as ornaments around Bhagavati or Siva's neck.[84] Next to Nagabhagavati is Siva and Parvati's son, Ganapadi, remover of obstacles, dispeller of handicaps and failures, also known as Vigneswaran. He is most important as that deity to which respects must be paid before beginning daily practice or taking up any weapon.

Along the western wall is a place where past masters sit, preside over practice, and are worshipped. The line of masters begins with the present master's own teacher, and stretches back in time to the mythical Parasurama, founder of Kerala and transmitter of the art to his twenty-one disciples, and is said to stretch back even to Drona, teacher of the Pandavas of *Mahabharata* lore. The gurukkal himself is the living embodiment of past gurus; therefore, Hindu masters are usually called by the plural gurukkal, rather than the singular guru or asan.[85] The guru does not just represent god or a line of teachers, he is the living embodiment of the lineage. His practice, behaviour, and powers should manifest his superior mental powers (*manasakti*) of accomplishment. K. Narayanan Nayar explained: 'In the word guru, "gu" represents darkness and "ru" represents light. One who gives light from darkness and knowledge from ignorance is known as a "guru". According to tradition, you should give respect to your mother, father, guru and god.'

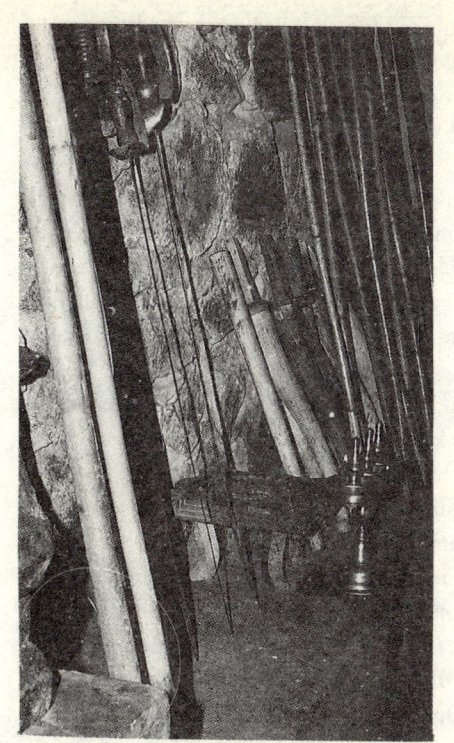

Figure 3.4: The pitham *(seat, pedestal or tripod) represents past gurus at the C.V.N. Kalari, Thiruvananthapuram. Located on the western side of the kalari facing the auspicious east, arrayed on either side of the pitham are weapons used in training.*

In most kalari the gurukkal and his lineage are lodged in a simple mud mound called the *guruttara*. In other kalari including the Thiruvananthapuram C.V.N. Kalari past masters are lodged in the wooden pitham (seat, pedestal, tripod or throne; Figure 3.4). The pitham is the seat through which power is made manifest not only in the kalari gurukkal, but in many forms of ritual performance including *ayappan tiyatta, pampin tullal, mudiyettu,* and teyyam where the ritual performer who sits on the pitham embodies the god's power (sakti) and is the vehicle for his visitation. As Freeman argues, the term is of Dravidian origin, and reflects 'the Dravidian cultural configuration of deifing the king' since in the seat there is a convergence of both kingly and divine powers (1991: 225).

Some kalari also have small idols representing local deified kalari heroes. This is a legacy of the deification of fallen heroes and ancestors in the early Sangam period, and parallels the continued propitiation of such historical kalarippayattu fighters as the infamous Tacholi Otenan and other hero teyyam in their yearly propitiation at their ancestral villages. Worshipping these local heroes allows practitioners in these kalari to gain access to the special power gained through their death and deification.

The other deities in the corners of the C.V.N. Kalari are various manifestations of some aspect of Siva, Siva-Sakti or the goddess. Gurukkal Govindankutty Nayar explained that Antimahalan is 'one aspect of Siva'. Bhadrakali's countenance in the north-east corner possesses the raudra or furious aspect of the fierce goddess who represents war. Govindankutty Nayar added that 'All the god's powers combined together and produced Bhadrakali. She is the destructive power created out of the third eye of Siva to kill all *asura*.' Vettaykkorumakan is the forest offspring of Siva and Parvati. The god of the hunt, he is represented by his popular depiction with bow and arrow.

Hanuman, son of the Wind, is traditionally associated with wrestling, physical exercise and yoga and is important in all the gymnasia (*akhara*) of the Banaras region (Alter 1992). He is also very important in the practice of southern Kerala's varma ati. Hanuman is worshipped in some kalari like the Sree Narayana Guru Sangham (S.N.G.S.) Vallabhatta Kalari. If not present in the form of an image or mound, Hanuman is said 'to be worshipped in the mind' of the practitioner or as the master's personal deity.

The deities at the S.N.G.S. Kalari in Chavakkad near Guruvayur differ slightly from the C.V.N. Kalari, Thiruvananthapuram. This kalari (Figures 3.2, 3.5) has Candika Devi in the puttara, Narasimham, Vettaykkorumakan, Kiratan and Nagas next to the puttara, Ganapadi (assumed to be in the lamp), a wooden pitham representing Sankunni Panikkar (the present master's father), Siva, Sakti, Bhumi Devi (mother earth), Bhadrakali, Kshetrapalam, past gurus, Ayyappan, Vanadurga (forest Durga), Hanuman and Garuda. Like P.K. Balan's interpretation of the specific powers of each of the seven steps of the puttara, K. Sankara Narayana Menon Gurukkal's interpretation of his kalari deities stresses the particular power each brings to the practitioner:

> Vettakkaran and Kiratan are meant to stop the weapon of an opponent. Virabhadran and Narasimhamurthi are meant to destroy one's enemies. Candika Devi is meant to give prosperity. Garudan is for pranasakti (the power of vital energy/breath). Hanuman is meant for strength (balam), Vignesvaran (Ganapadi) to remove obstacles and give mental power, and the Gurukanmar (past masters) for hereditary power.

The panoply of kalari deities and the specific power each manifests reflects the inherent instability of traditional assumptions about power (sakti) noted in Chapter 2. Belief in these many powers was ubiquitous in the past, and as detailed in Chapter 5, the special powers associated with particular kalari deities were brought to realization not only through daily exercise, but also by inner actualization through the repetition of mantra. The *interpretations* of both P.K. Balan Gurukkal and K. Sankara Narayana Menon Gurukkal agree that one crucial 'power' to be attained is 'mental power'—a subject to which we shall return in Chapter 8.

Although the deities are worshipped daily in Hindu kalari, most of

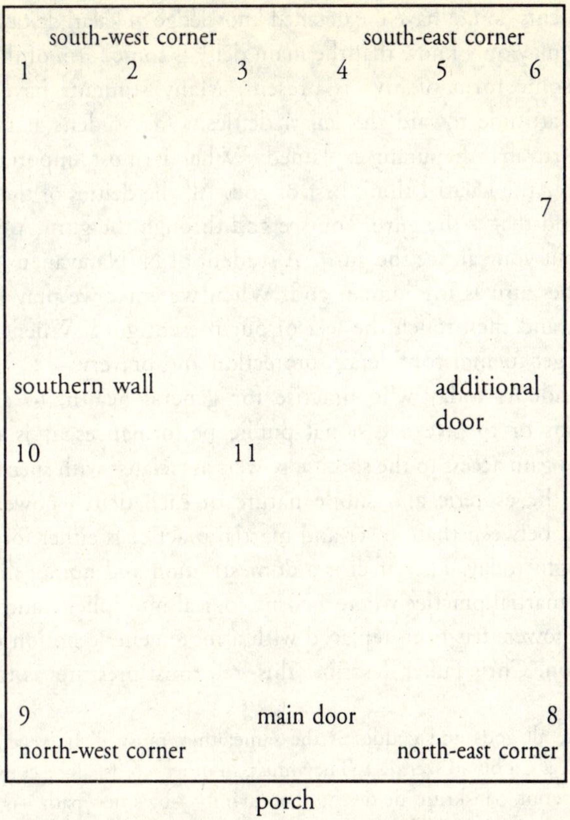

The Ritual Life of the Kalari and its Deities • 75

```
                south-west corner              south-east corner
           1        2         3        4         5         6


                                                                 7




             southern wall                    additional
                                                 door
          10                  11




           9                  main door                   8
        north-west corner                        north-east corner
                               porch
```

Key:
1 = puttara where Candika Devi is lodged
 [next to the puttara are assumed to be Narasimham,
 Vattaykkommalcan, Kiratan, and Nagas]
2 = lamp representing Ganapadi
3 = wooden pitham representing Sankunni Panikkar, the present master's father
4 = low wooden platform where Siva is lodged
5 = low wooden platform where Sakti or Parvati is lodged
6 = red cloth with sickle sword of Bhavaneswari or Bhumi Devi (mother earth)
7 = low wooden platform where Bhadrakali is lodged
8 = mound for Kshetrapalam or the 'god of the kalari'
9 = mound for the 21 past gurus and Ayyappan
10 = place (no image or mound) where Vanadurga or the Forest Durga resides
11 = the centre of the kalari where Hanuman, Durga, and Garuda reside
 Due to very high ground water, this kalari was constructed as a raised kalari.

Figure 3.5: Deities of the Sree Narayana Guru Kalari

today's students do not have the detailed knowledge of kalari deities explained here. They may only know that the main deity is some form of the goddess, and that some form of Siva is present. Many students have a simple devotional attitude toward the kalari deities. One student at the C.V.N. Kalari, Thiruvananthapuram explained: 'What is most important is that when I enter the kalari I think first of god. All the deities of the kalari are one god, and that is the guru. You see god through the guru. You can't see the gods, but you can see the guru.' A student of N. Narayanan Nayar told me that 'the guru is the human god. When we enter we pray to the old gurus first, and then touch the feet of our present guru. When I think of the guru I get mental confidence, protection and bravery.'

For students today who practise for general health, to enter state competitions or to give occasional public performances, it is no longer necessary to gain access to the specific powers associated with specific deities. Therefore, the esoteric and subtle nature of each deity's power and the relationship between that power and martial practice is either forgotten, or seldom taught today. The effect is a domestication and homogenization of traditional martial practice where a cosmological multiplicity and hierarchy of specific powers has been replaced with a more generic notion of 'power' and devotion. Chris Fuller describes this 'reformist pressure' as tending

> to make all gods and goddesses the same; they must all be vegetarians who never get blood sacrifices. They must, in other words, all be converted into superior 'Sanskritic' deities, so that divinity—by a new path—is made uniform and substantial, rather than variable and relational (1992: 103).

THE RITUAL LIFE OF THE KALARI

At most kalari, practice is open to students of any religion. Christians and Muslims studying in a Hindu kalari are expected to observe all the rituals of the kalari, but are free to 'imagine who they like in each mound. For the Christian that may be Christ; for the Muslim, Allah' (Madhavan Panikkar Gurukkal, interview). A Catholic Christian makes the sign of the cross as he enters the kalari and pays respects to each of the deities. Christian and Muslim kalari usually have no place for iconic representation of deities, although the presence of Allah or the triune God is assumed. Here also students are free to 'believe according to his own religion'. Some include a pitham representing past teachers in one corner of the kalari. In Thomas T. Muttothu Gurukkal's kalari, the Christian fighting saints, St George and St Sebastian, are assumed to be present.

Once a kalari has been inaugurated and the deities installed or the divine presence assumed, training is circumscribed by various rituals: (1) Hindu deities are treated as guests with suitable daily or special offerings and worship (puja) prepared according to their nature and mode of installation; (2) special rituals punctuate the process of training; and (3) all entrances to and exits from the kalari are ritually marked. These rituals are performed 'in order to make the classes and treatment held in the kalari not inauspicious' (Gurukkal Govindankutty Nayar, interview). Like a house, 'if these rituals and ritual behaviour are neglected, the prosperity of the house (or the kalari) itself can change' (Moore 1983: 470).

The simplest ritual act is stepping into the kalari with the right foot first, and touching the floor, forehead and chest with the right hand. Through ritual entry the student 'asks the forgiveness of Bhumi Devi (mother earth) for exercising on her'. Ideally, it separates the outside world from that inside the kalari, and prompts the practitioner to clear his mind of distractions. Once inside, the student crosses to the south-west corner to 'pay respects' (by touching the base of the mound or image, and in turn one's forehead and chest) to the guardian deity of the kalari at the puttara. More elaborate forms of ritual entry which exercise the entire body are practised in some kalari. Here, as the student steps into the kalari with his right foot, he executes an elaborate and gymnastic set of steps, jumps and turns so that he ends up touching the base of the puttara, and receives the blessing of the guardian deity. The student then proceeds around the kalari and pays respects to each of the other deities. At the puttara and each mound or image, one 'takes the god in his mind' or 'prays to the god'—internal acts of communing with each deity (Gurukkal Govindankutty Nayar, interview).

Collectively, these entry rituals should both ritually protect practitioners from harm and help them to focus the mind for practice by clearing away any mental or emotional obstacles in the way of practice. However, the degree to which students actualize such focus varies greatly. Many students enter the kalari and perform these simple ritual acts perfunctorily; few enter mindfully.

At the end of training in the simplest mode of exit, the student pays final respects to each of the kalari deities, circumambulating the interior beginning with the guardian deity in the south-west corner. Still facing the puttara, the student steps backward on to the first step with the left foot, and touches the floor, forehead and chest with the right hand, turns, and exits up the steps.

Each day of practice in a temporary pit kalari concludes when the gurukkal, the last to leave, performs a special ritual of exit, *taccumayakkal* or *cuvadumayakkal*, literally 'wiping out the steps'. In one version, the master takes a weapon, often a short stick (*ceruvadi*), and sits before the brass lamp in front of the puttara in a specific pose (often the 'cat', Figure 3.2). In this pose he repeats a mantram 'handing over the kalari to the goddess' or guardian deity. He strikes the stick three times with his right hand on the floor. Standing, he drags the stick along the floor as he steps backward across the kalari, still facing the south-west corner. When he reaches the stairway exit, he turns once to his right, throws the stick high into the air, and steps up and out with his right foot before the stick touches the floor. 'Erasing the steps' removes all the human impurities of the day's activities, and leaves the kalari purified for the deities of the kalari who will enjoy and protect the space until the next day of training.

The installed deities must be appropriately worshipped with daily and special offerings according to their nature and mode of installation. Whatever the occasion, kalari puja are considered 'simple rituals' sufficient to please kalari deities. They are usually thought of as 'middling' in degree of purity and substance when compared to a brahman tantri's 'high' rituals, or the 'low' rituals of blood sacrifice which 'control evil spirits'.

At dawn each day the kalari is cleaned. Anything remaining from the previous day's offerings is removed. The puttara is purified with water, and the kalari floor is swept. The basic elements for kalari puja include five types of offerings corresponding to the five elements of the universe: water for atma or soul; incense for bhumi or earth; flowers for akasam or space; smoke of fire for vayus or souls; and light for agni's soul.[86] At dusk fresh wicks are lit and offered to the deities.

The gurukkal's engagement in the puja process should not be perfunctory. One master's manuscript records the following method of daily worship:

> During puja in your mind you must meditate on all the Gurudevada which dwell in the forty-two by twenty-one kalari, and also the twenty-one masters, the eight sages, and the eight *murtikkal* (aspects or forms) of Brahma, Vishnu, Siva, the forty-three crores of devas, four sampradaya (lineages) which are meant for kalari practice, the sampradaya which are used in Tulunadu, the famous past kalari gurus of the four Namboodiri households known as *ugram velli*, *dronam velli*, *ghoram velli*, and *ullutturuttiyattu*, the eight devas connected with the kalari, and the *murti* positions connected with kalari practice.

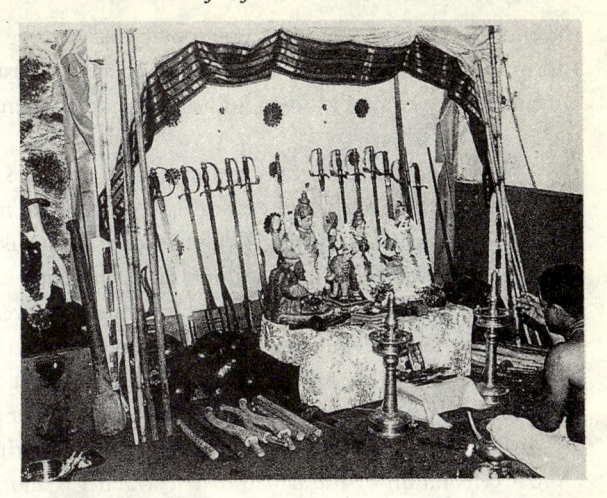

Figure 3.6: Celebrations of Navaratri Mahotsavam at the C.V.N. Kalari (Thiruvananthapuran). A local brahman pujari performs weapons puja facing Saraswati, Durga and Mahalakshmi.

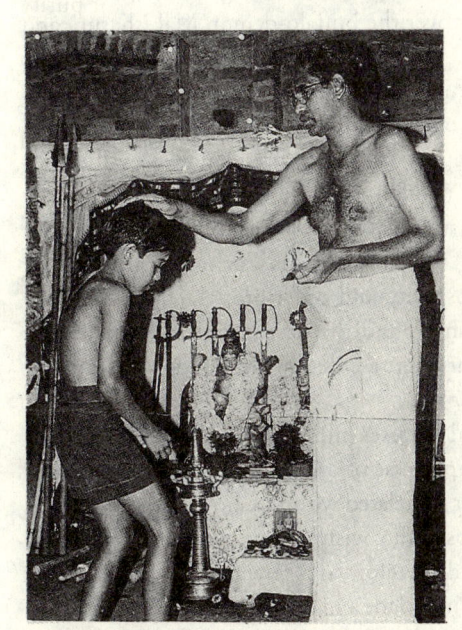

Figure 3.7: Gurukkal Govindankutty Nayar blesses a new student.

The master's full concentration is required when making each offering. Therefore, conducting puja is ideally an important part of the master's ongoing, life-long process of attaining accomplishment in developing higher devotional and mental powers.

In addition to inauguration, more elaborate special puja may be conducted on ritually important occasions like the annual celebration of a kalari's inaugural date or the pan-Indian annual celebration of new beginnings, Navaratri Mahotsavam (Figures 3.6–3.7). Special puja may also be done to mark a student's progression to a major new stage of training or as part of the closing ceremonies (*cuvatumakam*) at the end of a training season in a temporary kalari. Like inauguration, ritual and practice are knit closely together on all such occasions—new students are either received into training and/or advanced students progress to a new stage.

When puja are specifically performed to mark a student's progress to more advanced lessons, the occasion is considered a 'new beginning' or a 'turning point in the training of the student', (Gurukkal Govindankutty Nayar, interview). What is most important is marking each first lesson such as learning a new weapon; the teacher's side of a weapon; massage; the location of the vital spots; or special meditation practices. Puja clears the path of obstacles in the way of successful completion of the lessons to follow and therefore ideally leads to a state of accomplishment.

In some kalari today, one of the most important ritual occasions is the annual celebration of the pan-Indian Navaratri Mahotsavam—the festival of new beginnings and for 'weapons (ayudha) puja' lasting nine nights, in October/November. Also known as Durga Puja in Bengal, Navaratri enacts the celebration of Durga's victory over the buffalo-demon Mahishasura and his forces which 'enables the gods to regain their kingdom and so restore universal *dharma* predicated on rule by a rightful king' (Fuller 1992: 109). 'Often described as *the* festival (*utsava*) of kings and Kshatriyas', in its royal form, Navaratri celebrates 'a new universal order, presided over by the gods under their king', which recreates 'a kingly order' (ibid.: 108, 111), especially evident in the celebration of the articulation between the king's power (in the sword) and divine power sanctioning his authority to rule. It simultaneously celebrates the prosperity and order brought by this victory associated with the goddess Lakshmi, and the new beginning signalled by this defeat of the demonic order and represented by the goddess of learning, Saraswati.

In Kerala today the festival focuses more on the new beginnings associated with Saraswati and the promise of order and prosperity associated with fulfilment in the coming year associated with Lakshmi, than on Durga's victory.[87] It is celebrated by those who wish to honour their traditional source and way of knowledge, and therefore as a ceremonial beginning of a new season of practice/training in a trade, art or discipline (Ayrookuzhiel 1983: 61–4). Along with the goddess Saraswati, the tools, texts and teachers of one's trade or art are honoured and worshipped directly—for the dancer the cymbals that keep time, for the mechanic the tools he uses for repairs, for the martial artist his weapons.

Among kalarippayattu masters who celebrate Navaratri, Gurukkal

Govindankutty Nair of the C.V.N. Kalari, Thiruvananthapuram, gives particular care and importance to the annual celebration organized on the eighth, ninth and tenth days of the festival. During the three days of preparation and celebration, regular training in the kalari is suspended. First, the kalari is cleaned and decorated. A special altar is set up on the western side of the kalari where Sarasvati, Durga and Mahalakshmi are temporarily installed within a decorative canopy (Figure 3.6), festooned with fresh palm leaves, plantain and lights. The pitham is placed in front of the three goddesses, and on it pictures of the gurukkal's father, and his father's teacher, Karnaran Gurukkal. All the kalari weapons are arranged within the canopy around the deities, and the master's texts are placed next to the pitham in front of the goddesses.

A brahman pujari is hired to perform the Navaratri pujas, beginning on the ninth night with the all-important worship of weapons (ayudhapuja) and the knowledge of the martial art—represented by the master's texts.[88] The pujari conducts the puja with the typical offerings given to the kalari deities, but concludes with an offering of *arat* or flame, which is then offered as *prasad* to the gurukkal and students.

On the tenth day of the festival, the brahman pujari conducts two more elaborate pujas—a Ganapadi *homam*, or fire sacrifice, completed before sunrise,[89] and in the evening a Durga or Bhagavati puja. For the Bhagavati puja, a special kalam (floor drawing) is created in front of Durga in red, white, black, green and yellow, and two simple kalams are also drawn for Saraswati and Mahalakshmi. Most important is the pujari's repetition of a special mantra to appease Bhagavati while offering fresh flowers and leaves.[90] When Bhagavati puja is complete, a special cultural programme is usually organized at this kalari—often a music concert.

The new season of lessons is now set to begin. Early next morning, the gurukkal himself conducts the usual simple puja to all the kalari deities with continuing students present. In a ceremony marking the beginning of all knowledge, the master sits in front of Saraswati where he writes a single letter—an *aksaram* which 'always exists, is the basis of all knowledge, and cannot be destroyed'. Beginning with the most senior student present, each student comes forward to write his own 'first letter', establishing his own new beginning. Each continuing student comes forward and gives traditional daksina to the master. In turn, the student receives the master's blessings for the new year. Students now begin a review of their old lessons. In groups students perform a sample of the kalari exercises (Chapter 4)—a review of the entire system of practice from the simplest to advanced techniques.

Now new lessons begin. As a day of new beginnings, this is *the* most auspicious day on which to begin any new course of study; therefore, a large number of new students—always an odd number—usually begin their training on this day. In groups they are taught to pay respects to the gurukkal and kalari deities, and then are initiated into training by the gurukkal when they give offerings (Figure 3.7) and perform their first exercise—*nerkal*, the 'straight leg' kick. Continuing students ready for new lessons in advanced techniques then begin these lessons. The day of new beginnings concludes as prasad from the morning offerings is passed around to everyone present. As another master fond of the rich ritual life of his kalari told me, 'worship is performed for the mental happiness and prosperity of the master and his pupils'.[91]

The rituals of construction, inauguration, and installation marking kalarippayattu create a set of ritual frames clearing away obstacles to safe and auspicious practice. Daily and seasonal rituals through simple or special puja please the kalari deities, assuring continued safe and auspicious practice, and at least in the past were understood to provide access to gaining special powers of the deities for combat. Daily puja marks each day's practice with an auspicious beginning, and the gurukkal's special ritual of exit marks the conclusion of practice in a temporary kalari. Long-term students participate in the ritual life of the kalari when they assist the gurukkal on special ritual occasions as well as perform simple daily tasks which knit them into the devotional life of the kalari.

Within the auspicious frames created by the gurukkal's daily rituals, each student's entry, practice and exit are marked by individual rituals of practice, i.e. paying respects to the kalari deities. These personal rituals frame each student's daily round of practice and optimally provide a means to internalizing devotion, further developing single-minded concentration and gaining access to the power of specific deities.

Individual rituals mark each student's progress. In addition to prostrations, prayers and circumambulations of the kalari marking each part of daily practice, special puja offered when a student advances to a new stage of practice publicly acknowledges and ritually marks the interior process of transformation and embodiment realized in a student's practice.

Kalarippayattu training is traditionally understood as an ongoing discipline of practice in which the student will gradually be 'transformed'; therefore, traditional training itself is a ritual process. As a discipline of practice, kalarippayattu is similar to other rites of passage in that it too refashions 'the very being of the neophyte' (V. Turner 1969: 103). Martial artists traditionally had to be transformed *for* combat, i.e. to be able to fulfil their dharma, they had to enter an arena in which they would fight to the death to uphold the social/moral order to which they had pledged themselves. In this sense, kalarippayattu practitioners in the past implicitly participated in the sacrificial paradigm of divine kingship (Fuller 1992: 83ff).

Chapter 4

'First the Outer Forms': The Physical Body and The First Fruits of Practice

Anthropologist John Blacking asserts that 'there is no such thing as "*the* human body", there are many kinds of body, which are fashioned by the different environments and expectations that societies have of their members' bodies' (1985: 66). As environments and expectations change, so do the kinds of bodies which societies produce. Today's martial practitioner assumes *a* body in his practice, but 'the body' he assumes is a palimpsest of both traditional assumptions about the body, practice and power, as well as more recent paradigms and discourses of the body-in-practice. In Chapters 4, 5 and 6, I examine the 'lived' (Leib) body-in-practice, as well as the representations and assumptions (Korper) about the bodies of practice through which power[s] are traditionally assumed to be actualized.

A traditional Muslim master told me, 'he who wants to become a master must possess complete knowledge of the body'.[92] Possessing 'complete knowledge of the body' traditionally meant gaining knowledge of three different 'bodies of practice'—(1) the fluid body of humours and saps, (2) the body composed of bones, muscles and the vulnerable vital junctures or spots (marmmam) of the body and (3) the subtle, interior body. The first two bodies are based on Ayurveda, and together constitute the *sthula-sarira*. The third—the *suksma-sarira*—is understood to be encased within the physical body. Each of these three bodies possesses its own conceptual and practical history encoded and transmitted from generation to generation both in texts and in embodied practice. The assumptions articulated here are *written in practice* and so commonplace that they traditionally would have needed no explanation.

Since the assumptions about these three bodies are reflected in classic Ayurvedic and yoga/tantra texts which explain the principles and concepts of each, I write between these classic texts and current practice to disclose some of the continuities as well as discontinuities about these primary conceptual frameworks which model ways of understanding the body-in-practice.[93]

'Complete knowledge of the body' begins with sthula-sarira as it is experienced through practice of exercises and receipt of massage. Together they are considered 'body preparation' (*meyyorukkam*). The exercises include a vast array of poses, steps, jumps, kicks and leg exercises performed in increasingly complex combinations back and forth across the kalari floor. Collectively, they are considered a *meiabhyasam*. Individual meippayattu are taught one by one, and every student masters simple forms before moving on to more complex and difficult sequences. Most important is mastery of basic poses (*vadivu*), named after animals, and comparable to basic asana of yoga; and mastery of steps (*cuvadu*) by which one moves to and from poses. Repetitive practice of these outer forms eventually renders the external body flexible (*meivalakkam*) and, as Gurukkal Govindankutty Nayar said, 'flowing (*olukku*) like a river'.

At first the exercises are 'that which is external', but as the forms 'come correct' students should begin to manifest physical, mental and behavioural *lakshana* indicating change. Like long-term practice of hatha yoga, the exercises become 'that which is internal' (*andarikamayatu*). One master explained the progression: 'first the outer forms; then the inner secrets'. At first the student must overcome the physical limitations of the gross body, stretching muscles to enable the body to assume difficult forms, removing mental distractions, and beginning to actualize one-point focus. Eventually, one begins to experience and reap the first 'fruits' (*phalam*) of practice, changes in the body of humours and saps.

THE BODY OF HUMOURS AND SAPS: CORRECTION AND THE FIRST FRUITS (PHALAM) OF PRACTICE

The first concept of the body that informs the martial body-in-practice is based on traditional humoral concepts (Zimmermann 1979). Ayurveda, the classic tradition of Hindu medicine, seeks to establish harmony with the environment by maintaining equilibrium in a process of constant fluid exchange. The art of medicine is meant to establish

> yoga or *samyoga*, 'junctions' or 'articulations' between man and his environment, through the prescription of appropriate diets and regimens

> ... Equality, balance and congruous articulations are meant for the conservation and restoration of these precious fluids ... By means of *brahmacarya* ... and various other psychosomatic disciplines, one should establish congruous junctions with the surrounding landscapes and seasons, and thus one should protect one's powers, one should husband one's vital fluids (Zimmermann 1983: 17–18).

Kalarippayattu is one such discipline, the daily practice of which is popularly believed to establish congruence among the three humours (*tridosa; tridhatu*): wind (*vata*), phlegm (*kapha*), and fire (*pitta*). The master's understanding of the benefits of training and his treatment of injuries are based on this fundamental notion of the body.[94]

The role of exercise and massage in maintaining inner fluidity and articulation among the humours was explained in antiquity in a medical text attributed to Susruta:

> The act born from the effort (*ayasa*) of the body is called exercise (*vyayama*). After doing it, one should shampoo (*viMRD*) the body on all sides until it gives a comfortable sensation.
>
> Growth of the body, radiance, harmonious proportions of the limbs, a kindled (digestive) fire, energy, firmness, lightness, purity (*mrja*), endurance to fatigue, weariness, thirst, hot and cold, etc., and even a perfect health: this is what is brought by physical exercise.
>
> Nothing comparable to it for reducing obesity. No enemy will attack a man (literally: a mortal, *martya*) who practices physical exercise, because they all fear his strength.
>
> Senility (or the decay of old age, *jara*) will not seize him abruptly. The muscles keep firm in one who practises physical exercise, that is, one whose body is sudated by physical exercise and who is massaged with the feet (*vyayamasvinnagatrasya padbhyam udvartitasya ca*) diseases fly from him, just as small beasts do on seeing a lion.
>
> Physical exercise makes good-looking even the person deprived of youth and beauty. Physical exercise, in one who does it assiduously, digests all food, even the most inappropriate, turned sour or still crude without provoking the humours. For, assiduous physical exercise is beneficial to a strong man who eats unctuous foods (*snigdhabhojin*).
>
> It is especially beneficial to him in the winter and spring. But in all seasons, every day, a man seeking his own good should take physical exercise only to the half limit of his strength, as otherwise it kills.

> When the *Vayu* hitherto properly located in the heart (*hrdi*) comes to the mouth of the man practicing physical exercise, it is the sign (*laksana*) of *balardha*, of his having used half of his strength.
>
> Age, strength, body, place, time, and food: It is only after duly considering these factors, that one should engage in physical exercise, as otherwise it may bring disease (Cikitsasthana xxiv, 38–49) (Zimmermann 1986).

Another antique authority, Vagbhata, wrote that a 'harmonious and solid condition of the body result from gymnastics' followed by massage (Vogel 1965: 90).

Benefiting health is a commonplace reason to study. One student at the C.V.N. Kalari explained:

> I practise kalarippayattu to maintain health of the body. I can enjoy when I practise. When I exercise and then take a bath, I feel very energetic at work and sleep well. There is a big difference in my body when I come (to practice in the kalari) and when I don't. After practising for three years, I have not had any fever or headache, or any other diseases. I think the practice of kalarippayattu helps us to have preventive action in our body. The body can resist these usual and typical diseases.

Practice is traditionally regulated by *rtucarya* or 'the art of adapting one's diet and conduct to the cycle of the seasons' (Zimmermann 1979: 13; 1980). The most intensive period of training is the rainy season from June through August which is 'neither too hot nor too cold'. In a discussion about training Gurukkal Govindankutty Nayar told me,

> During this season it is good for the body to have oil and sweat. This is also the best season for massage (*uliccil*). It provides protection for the body. If one were to exercise during the hot season (April–May), he would feel weak and lack energy.

Vigorous practice is appropriate to monsoon season because more energy is thought to be available at this time. In this cool season the heat produced by vigorous exercise and massage is counterbalanced by the seasonal accumulation of phlegm. By contrast, the hot summer season is characterized by accumulation of the wind humour and therefore exercise should be avoided. Exercise and massage also increase the circulation of the wind humour throughout the body, and this, too, counterbalances the accumulation of phlegm during monsoon.

Special restrictions and observances traditionally circumscribed training are similar to the restraints and positive ways of practising Patanjali's yoga. The following restraints were required in the past of all practitioners during the fourteen-day massage period, but are required today only by a few practitioners: (1) refraining from sexual intercourse, (2) not sleeping during the day, (3) not waking at night, (4) including milk and ghee in the diet, and (5) taking a laxative to purge the digestive system as part of the cleansing of the body during massage. These practices conserve balance among the three humours as the body is heated by vigorous exercise. For example, sexual activity would expend vital energy and increase vata which, when combined with vigorous exercise which also produces vata, would create a humoral imbalance.

Behavioural constraints are as important as dietary and health considerations. From the first day of training students participate in the devotional life of the kalari. They are also instructed to use kalarippayattu only to defend oneself, never to practise what they learn outside the kalari, and to be of good character (i.e. not to steal, lie, cheat, drink liquor or take drugs). As Eliade explains, none of these restraints produces a yogic state, but rather 'a "purified" human being . . . This purity is essential to the succeeding stages' (1975: 63).

Exercise should always be within the limits of one's age and basic constitution. Susruta's classic text cautioned that excessive physical exercise would bring about 'consumption, haemmorhage (*rakta-pitta*), thirst, phthisis, aversion to food, vomiting, illusiveness, weariness, fever, cough and asthma' (*Cikitsasthana* xxiv, 49–50) (Bhishagratna 1963: 487). Exertion beyond one's normal limits causes an imbalance which can become pathological. Training is traditionally a long-term process through which one's capacity for exercise could be enhanced; therefore, it is best to begin at the traditional age of about seven for both boys and girls. Today, many students do not begin training until they are in the teens, twenties, or even thirties or forties. Students come to the place of training (kalari) before dawn (5:00–6:00 a.m.) while it is dark, cool and auspicious; however, in some city kalari the training may not start until well after dawn. In some kalari classes are also held in the cool hours of dusk (5:30–7:30 p.m.).

The daily application of specially prepared oil is thought to add flexibility and strength to muscles, joints and ligaments. A special form of seasonal, full-body massage given by the gurukkal's feet (*kal uliccil*) (Figures 4.1–2) and restrictions on behaviour and diet during the fifteen-day massage period are also understood to enhance the ease and fluidity of movement.

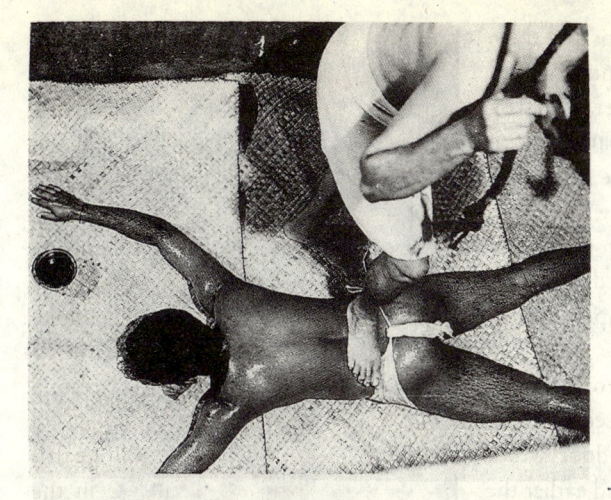

Figure 4.1: Gurukkal Govindankutty Nayar gives the first main stroke in foot massage (kal uliccil) *across the small of the back while holding on to ropes suspended from the ceiling.*

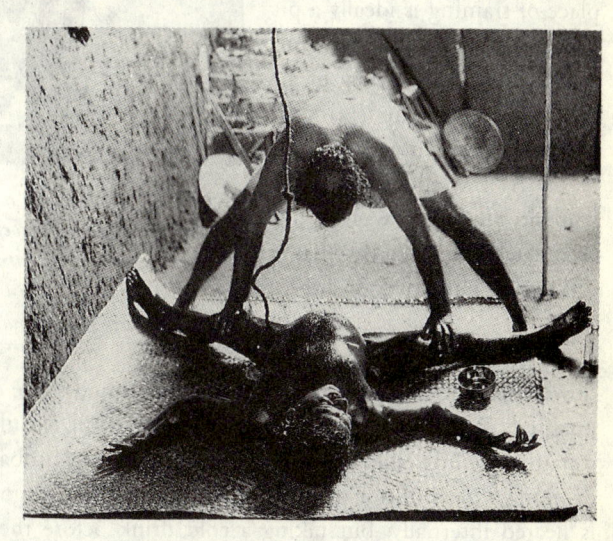

Figure 4.2: Sreejayan Gurukkal administers deep strokes to a student's thighs while keeping his legs open with his feet.

Oil is applied before exercise to produce sweat from internal body heat. The oil keeps the heat from dissipating and its medicinal properties seep into the body through pores opened by sweating. Were oil applied after exercise begins it would introduce a mixture of sweat and oil through the open pores, producing a cooling effect leading to a humoral imbalance. There are traditional recipes for oil to be used specifically for kalarippayattu training. One common name is *kalarimukutt* (meaning 'slippery'). One master's recipe calls for four parts of gingili oil, two parts castor oil, one part ghee, three herbs and three other dried ingredients decocted and applied after cooling (Figure 4.3). This particular oil is understood to give maximum flexibility to the body, combined with strength. Given the cost of traditionally prepared oils, most students use cheaper gingili (sesame) oil today.

The sweating oiled body should not be exposed to direct sunlight or to outdoor wind; therefore, as discussed earlier the place of training is ideally a pit protecting the practitioner from sun and wind. The flow of air remains above the trainees, keeping the building cool and fresh. At the end of practice students allow the sweat to dry completely, and then they bathe in a temple tank, river or shower stall.

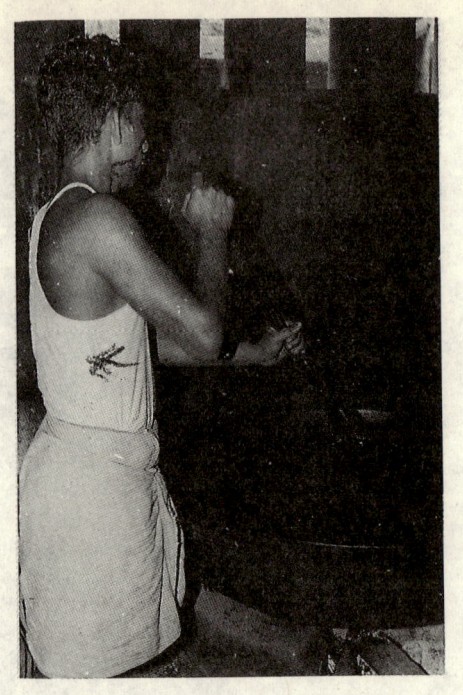

Figure 4.3: It takes days to prepare oils through cooking and decoction. Decoction results in a highly concentrated oil applied externally. Cooking oils in the kitchen at the C.V.N. Kalari, Thiruvananthapuram.

The body naturally 'cools down' after the heated exercise, and is understood to be cleansed as well as purified. Bathing while still wet with sweat/oil, would introduce cold unnaturally into the body and cause a humoral imbalance.[95] Similarly drinking a glass of hot tea after practice is considered good since the body is heated internally, but taking a cold drink before the body has cooled could cause an imbalance. Monsoonal colds are often understood to be caused by bathing 'before the sweat was dry'.

The special kalarippayattu massage (uliccil), traditionally administered to all students during the monsoon season, is only one of numerous massages in the repertory (Zarrilli 1995a). The full effect of the massage is only gradually realized as the novice's flexibility, balance and control improve when exercising.

The exercise, sweating and oil massage stimulate all forms of the wind humour to course through the body. Long-term practice enhances the ability to endure fatigue through balancing the three humours, and to acquire a characteristic internal and external ease of movement, and body fluidity. The accomplished practitioner's movements 'flow' (*olukku*), thereby clearing up 'the channels' centred in the abdomen since the navel is the point from which the channels branch out, and 'nourish the body fluids and tissues' (Zimmermann 1983: 19).

THE PHYSICAL BODY OF BONES AND MUSCLES, AND 'CORRECT' PRACTICE

The fluid humoral body is supported by the body as a frame of bones, muscles, ligaments, vessels, joints, as well as their junctures and vital spots. Making the body 'flow' and positively affecting both the fluid body of humours and saps and the subtle, interior body occurs only as the student learns to assume the 'correct' position of the basic forms and techniques of practice. But what constitutes 'correct practice'?

Kallada Balakrishnan shared one commonplace used to discuss correct practice: 'Each movement, step and pose (and weapon) has its own 'inner life' (*bhava*) which must be exhibited when practising kalarippayattu'. Bhava is a term commonly used to refer to the actor's psychophysiological embodiment of a character's emotions in the popular Kathakali dance-drama of Kerala (Zarrilli 1984b; Namboodiri 1983). Gurukkal Govindankutty Nayar compared the process of the martial artist's process of 'becoming one' with the 'original qualities' of the forms of practice with that of the Kathakali actor 'becoming' his role. He gave an example: 'Take the role of Duryodhana. He lives that part by becoming it'. For the Kathakali actor 'becoming the character' (*natan kathapathravumayi tadatmyam prapikanam*) is a process in which the actor controls and circulates his inner energy (prana vayu) into and through the stylized and codified forms he has come to embody and thereby uses to create the character. Just as the actor 'becomes' the character by embodying the various bhava required by the dramatic context of the play, so does the martial artist 'become' by embodying the bhava appropriate to each form he practises.

Govindankutty Nayar clarified the concept when he told me that one attains correct form by 'becoming one with the original qualities' (*tanmayatvam prapikkuka*) of a pose or movement. The 'inner life' of each movement is assumed to be present as the seed of the form, implanted by the master during each first lesson. 'In due time', training and careful correction nurtures this seed, helps it sprout and grow. The student slowly discovers the correct form, and its application. The practitioner himself does not create the benefits or powers which are eventually realized through practice of a discipline; rather, practice is a means of bringing such powers 'to their maximum efficiency' (Varenne 1976: 134).

This gradual discovery of a form and its application reflects the general cultural assumption that long-term practice of a body-discipline should lead the practitioner to such discoveries. Discussing what one learns through yoga practice, the *Bhagavad-Gita* (4.38) tells us, 'he who attains perfection through the practice of yoga *discovers of his own accord, with time*, the brahman present in his soul' (Varenne 1976: 58, italics mine). Varenne cites the *Amritabindu Upanisad* as further illustration of the idea that knowledge in a discipline of practice is assumed to be 'already there', hidden, waiting to be discovered:

> And knowledge is hidden in the depth of each individual just as in milk the butter we cannot see is hidden; this is why the wise practitioner must carry out a churning operation within himself, employing his own mind without respite as the churning agent (ibid.: 59).

By becoming accomplished in a form, one thereby actualizes its hitherto 'hidden' bhava in practice, realizing its full potential benefits to one's health through the body of humours and saps, to power through the eventual awakening of the subtle body within, and thereby to martial application.

Govindankutty Nayar continued his explanation by comparing kalarippayattu to other arts:

> All the arts have their prescribed forms, and they should be done according to those forms, like a fine carving which should be made of one piece of wood according to the dimensions recorded in the sastras. Or, for an ivory carving, to have its 'life force' it can only be taken from a live elephant to have that life force necessary for use in puja. If you take the ivory from a dead animal, it cannot be used. It will not have its life force (prana-vayu).

Likewise, each form and weapon in martial practice is assumed to have its ideal dimensions and dynamic mode of fulfilment. The master himself, having become accomplished in his practice, embodies this ideal. Although he possesses texts which record all the basic kalarippayattu techniques which are worshipped as sources of knowledge and authority (Appendix I), it is the gurukkal's body which possesses the authority of a sastra. The *vayttari*, recited by the master as students exercise, and copied in his texts are iconically written into *his* body. In the master's practice the student witnesses the 'inner life' of each form enlivened by the engagement of the master's 'life force' (prana vayu). In his practice is manifest the requisite power, energy and 'inner life' which iconically embodies the ideal state of accomplishment and form toward which the student should aspire in his own practice.

Like yoga asanas, becoming one with the inner life of a *vadivu* also means that the practitioner embodies the qualities of the animal for which each pose is named, and manifests this quality in his practice. The 'life' of the animal is assumed to be there in the form. To have attained the pose through repetition and correction is to 'become one with its original qualities'. If one is unable to achieve such oneness, then the martial form 'becomes nothing' or 'loses its actuality' (*onnumilataipokuka*). The potential of a form to manifest power (sakti) or to be of practical use in combat is never awakened or realized.

But the specific form of any pose, as well as its qualitative dimensions are open to interpretation. The specifics of what is or is not considered correct differ widely from master to master and style to style. Even among masters who had the same teacher and are from the same lineage of practice, differences are common. Each master believes that his own intepretation, practice and style, are the correct way of performing a form, or the correct method of application.

Whatever the particular master's interpretation, he reads the *laksana* in each student's external body of bones and muscles as being more or less 'correct' or 'incorrect', and gives corrections, examples and instructions based on his reading of the signs. The presence of such signs is assumed in all Indian disciplines of practice. They are most evident in yoga texts where the signs of long-term accomplished practice are described, as seen in the following passage from the *Siva Samhita* (III.28–9):

> Certain signs are perceived in the body of the Yogi whose *nadi* (channels of the subtle body) have been purified. I shall describe, in brief, all these various signs (III.28). The body of the person practising the regulation of breath becomes harmoniously developed, emits sweet scent, and looks beautiful and lovely (Vasu 1975: 28).

The process of teaching is a complex, interactive exchange in which the master continuously reads and re-reads the signs of a student's progress in each exercise and each form (Figure 4.4). Simultaneously, the student should also be observing, watching and reading what is iconically embodied in the master's accomplished practice.

BODY TECHNIQUES: KALA-RIPPAYATTU 'STYLES' AND 'LINEAGES' OF PRACTICE

Although the Kerala Kalarippayat Association officially recognizes three 'styles' of kalarippayattu according to the geographical region in which each originated, i.e. 'northern', 'central' and 'southern' styles, following Sreedharan Nayar, I have argued here that the dronampalli style of kalarippayattu that was at one time practised in southern Kerala became extinct by the twentieth century. What is called 'southern' kalarippayattu today is more appropriately known by its traditional names of varma ati or ati murai.

The term traditionally used to identify lineages of practice is sampradayam—a Sanskrit term

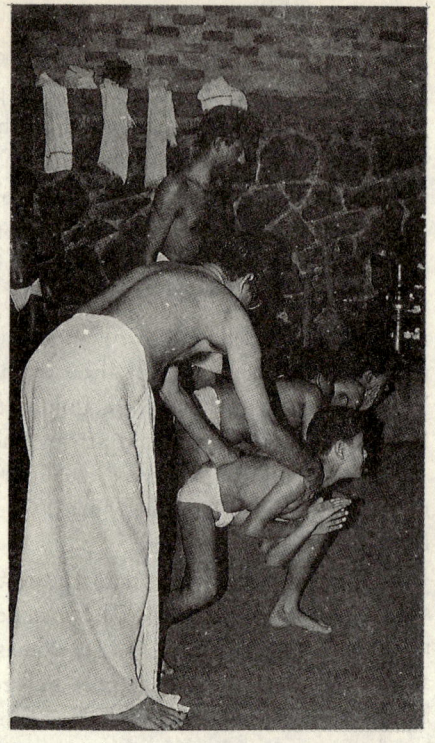

Figure 4.4: Gurukkal Govindankutty Nayar corrects a young student learning the 'lion pose' as part of the first body exercise sequence by attemping to get the student to lengthen and straighten his spine–part of a process that leads to correct spinal alignment, 'centering', and activation of the internal energy.

which does not necessarily refer to a geographical area, but rather to the teaching lineage in which an individual has been trained and which is easily recognizable to other practitioners as a style associated with a particular group of practitioners. As discussed earlier, kalarippayattu practitioners trace their mythological heritage to Parasurama and the Dhanur Vedic tradition, and all share practice of preliminary body exercises taught with verbal commands, massage and forms of advanced weapons training, culminating in sword and shield. Differences in sampradayam indicate differences within a common tradition of practice. Occasionally a sampradayam had its own peculiar techniques which are distinctive to that lineage of practice. Some of these distinctive sampradayam still exist and are especially evident in the north Malabar region. For example, P.P. Narayanan Gurukkal of Payannur, Kannur district, is one of the few masters still teaching the quite distinctive vattantirippu sampradayam which, as reflected in its name, is filled with highly gymnastic turns, body flips, and constant circling of the body. Masters in the Badagara region primarily practise pillatanni sampradayam which is distinctive for its percussive and strong stamps as the feet strike the earth while punctuating steps when performing body exercise sequences. Also, it is likely that some weapons, such as the otta and pondi, were specific to particular sampradayam and were not universally practised in all kalari. Velayudhan Asan was one of the few masters I met whose lineage of practice focused particularly on use of the spear.

What has made the question of distinctive kalarippayattu styles even more confusing is that historically, when Karnaran Gurukkal and C.V. Narayanan Nayar developed their 'composite' style of practice during the 1920s and 1930s which drew techniques from a variety of traditional sampradayam all located in the 'northern' Kerala region, they created what might be considered a 'new' style of their own which became standardized as a common syllabus shared by all C.V.N. kalari and teachers. Therefore, I identify what is practised in C.V.N. kalari as a distinctive and relatively 'new' sampradayam which, although it uses the same verbal commands as, for example, pillatanni sampradayam, performs those techniques in its own distinctive manner.

Given this complex history, I provide the most extensive description of 'northern' kalarippayattu techniques, drawing examples from several different lineages of practice while explaining the process of traditional training and correction. I then give shorter descriptions of the distinctive features of 'central' style kalarippayattu and varma ati ('southern' kalarippayattu).

PRELIMINARY TRAINING OF THE PHYSICAL BODY THROUGH 'NORTHERN STYLE' KALARIPPAYATTU TECHNIQUES

Training of the gross, physical body of muscles and bones begins with preliminary leg exercises (*kal etupp* or *kaluyarttal*) (Figure 1.5; Figure 4.5). As Gurukkal Govindankutty Nayar said, 'You are trying to make the leg as flexible as a (rubber) band. Anyone can kick their leg up, but superior balance is the key.' As early as the sixteenth century Duarte Barbosa described the exercises as tricks of nimbleness and dexterity . . . (in which) they teach them to dance and turn about and to twist on the ground, to take royal leaps and other leaps . . . and they become so loose jointed and supple that they make them turn their bodies contrary to nature (1921: 39–40).

In the C.V.N. style students practise eight basic leg exercises, each performed with right and left legs (Figure 4.6). Although not at first evident to young students when they begin training, some of the kicks also have offensive or defensive applications.

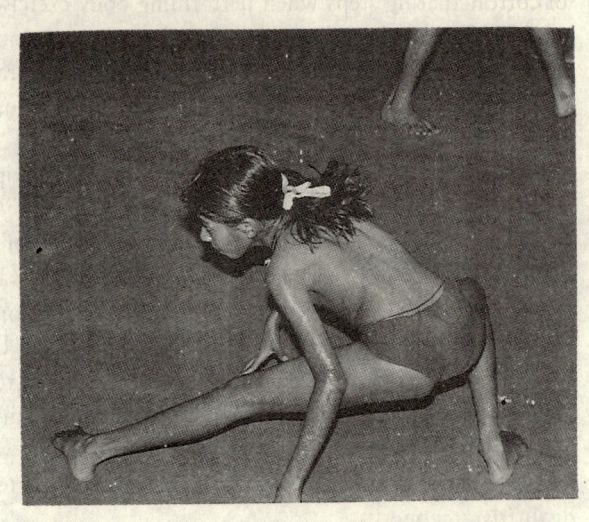

Figure 4.5: A young female student performs the 'sitting leg' (iruttikal) at the C.V.N. Kalari, Thiruvananthapuram.

Figure 4.6: The eight basic leg exercises of the C.V.N. Kalari, Thiruvananthapuram.

---

nerkal (straight leg, Figure 1.5): with the knee locked and the toes extended, the leg is kicked above the head.

tiriccukal (turning leg): two straight leg kicks in quick succession with a 180 degree pivot between.

vitukal (circling leg): the leg is circled in a high, swinging arc in front of the body.

konkal (angle leg): like the straight leg but performed at a 45 degree angle to the line of movement across the kalari.

iruttikal (sitting back leg, Figures 4.5): after a straight leg, the entire body weight is drawn back to the ground as the foot is placed behind the body.

akamkal (instep leg): an outside, sweeping kick.

puramkal (outside leg): a quick kick with the outside top of the foot.

catipuramkal (jumping outside leg): the quick kick with a jump.

One of the important dimensions of initial training with the kicks is direction of the student's visual focus. Students are told to 'look at a specific place' on the opposite side of the kalari while kicking. The instruction seems a nuisance to the young student trying to make the body kick the leg as high as the teacher or an advanced student. Those who stress focus do so because they understand this as the initial step in developing one-point focus (*ekagrata*) and an awakening of the subtle body. As master Achuthan Gurukkal told me, 'one-point focus is first developed by constant practice of correct form in exercises'. Once the external, physical eye is steadied, the student eventually begins to discover the 'inner eye' of practice—a state of inner connection to practice detailed in Chapter 5.

Once the student manifests a minimal level of balance and control, he is introduced to *meippayattu*. In the C.V.N. style, the sequences are dance-like in their gracious, undulating fluidity. Yet behind the fluid grace is the strength and power of movements which could, if necessary, be applied with lightning-fast speed and precision. In the Badagara style, the sequences are much more staccato and percussive, with strong steps/stamps. In all styles, often hidden, yet waiting, are potentially deadly blows, cuts or thrusts of the hands or feet.

The body exercise sequences (4.7–4.8) are linked combinations of basic *meitolil* including *vativu, cuvat, kal etupp,* a variety of jumps and turns, and coordinated hand/arm movements performed in increasingly swift succession back and forth across the kalari. Like the leg exercises, the body sequences at first develop flexibility, balance and control of the body; only much later are martial applications taught.

The number of body exercise sequences usually numbers from eight to fourteen. At the C.V.N. Kalari in Thiruvananthapuram, there are twelve regular and two special sequences. The first five regular sequences use various combinations of leg kicks to develop the lower half of the body. When the hips and legs have developed sufficient strength, flexibility and control, more advanced sequences are learned. The sixth and seventh give prominence to the hips and upper body, while the eighth through twelfth concentrate on hands, arms and upper body movements applicable in unarmed offence and defence.

As a student learns the first body exercise sequence, he is introduced to the poses, steps and jumps. Named after animals, they usually number eight. Styles differ considerably. Not only do the names of poses differ, masters also differ about application and interpretation. They are not static forms, but configurations of movements which embody both the external and internal essence of the animal after which they are named, and which are also used for offensive or defensive applications. For example, the C.V.N.

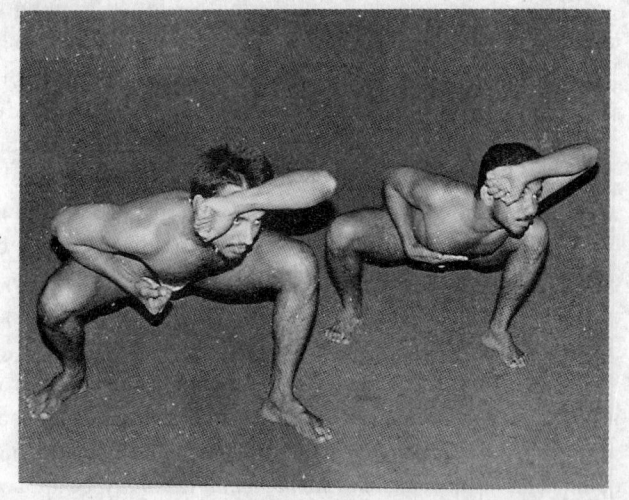

Figure 4.7

Figures 4.7– 4.8: Students of Sreejayan Gurukkal of Chembad performing the first section of a body exercise sequence which combines poses, steps, kicks and jumps in complex combinations performed back and forth across the kalari floor.

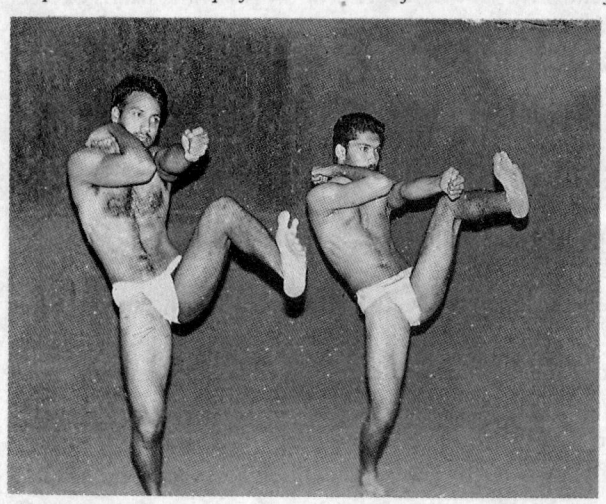

Figure 4.8

style 'serpent' allows for quick, low reversal of the body to defend against attack from the rear, or as a means of evading an oncoming attack. All masters emphasize the crucial importance of poses in a student's progression. As Gurukkal P.K. Balan explained, 'When any animal fights, it uses its whole body. This must also be true in kalarippayattu. Only a person who has learned these eight poses can perform the kalari law (*mura*), and go on to bare hand combat, weapons, massage, or applications to the vital spots (marmmam).'

Figure 4.9: The eight basic poses in two styles.

Gurukkal Govindankutty Nayar and the C.V.N. Style
gajavadivu–elephant pose *simhavadivu*–lion pose (Figure 0.1) *asvavadivu*—horse pose *varahavadivu*–wild boar pose *sarpavadivu*–serpent pose *marjaravadivu*–cat pose *kukkuvadivu*–cock pose *matsyavadivu*–fish pose
Gurukkal P.K. Balan
horse pose (Figure 4.10) peacock pose (*mayuravadivu*) (Figure 4.11) serpent pose (Figure 4.12) cock pose (Figure 4.13) elephant pose cat pose lion pose wild boar pose

Of the two versions, seven use the same names. Although the basic positions and movements are similar, except for the elephant and serpent, the names assigned the poses are different. What Govindankutty Nayar calls the lion, P.K. Balan identifies as the cock. P.K. Balan uses 'peacock' for the pose Govindankutty Nayar identifies as the 'fish'.

One of the most important sequences in the entire training process is one known as the puttara tol (Figure 3.2) or kalari *vanakkam/vandanam*. These sequences are an embodied mode of paying respects to the kalari's guardian deity, and therefore are crucial to both developing a sense of devotion, as well as one of the most important ways of awakening the subtle, interior body of practice.

The body sequences further develop flexibility, balance and control of the body when the training is rigorous. The oiled bodies begin to sweat, and by the conclusion of a class the student's entire body should be drenched in sweat. One day in class, Gurukkal Govindankutty Nayar told us, 'the sweat of the students should become the water washing the kalari floor.' Chirakkal T. Balakrishnan describes the results of such practice for one advanced sequence, *pakarcakkal* as being able to move like 'a bee circling a flower. While doing pakarcakkal a person first moves forward and back, and then again forward and back. It should be done like a spider weaving its web', (Sreebharath Kalari, interview). What is important are swift, light and facile changes of direction executed at the transition points between sets of movements, essential for combat where instantaneous changes of direction would have been necessary.

Behind the fluid grace of the gymnastic forms is the strength and power of movements which can, when necessary, be applied with lightning-fast speed and precision in potentially deadly attacks. 'Hidden' within all the preliminary exercises and basic poses are complex combinations of offensive and defensive applications which are eventually embodied by constant practice (see Figures 4.14–4.16). The body exercise sequences 'just look like exercises', but, as Gurukkal P.K. Balan explains, each pose has its own specific fighting applications:

> The horse is an animal which can concentrate all its powers centrally, and it can run fast by jumping up. The same pause, preparation for jumping and forward movement (that are in a horse) are in the *asvavadivu* (Figure 4.10).

> When a peacock is going to attack its enemies, it spreads its feathers and raises its neck, and dances by steadying itself on one leg. Then it shifts to the other leg, and attacks by jumping and flying. The capability of doing this attack is known as *mayuravadivu* (Figure 4.11).

> A snake attacks its enemy by standing up; however, its tail remains on the ground without movement. From this position, he can turn in any direction and bite a person. This ability

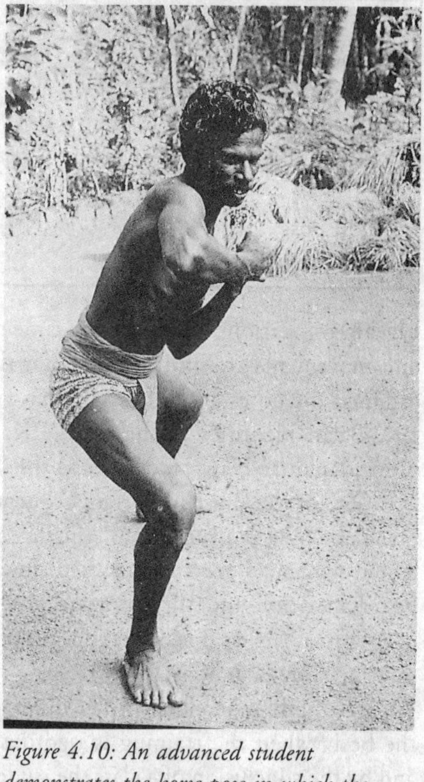

Figure 4.10: An advanced student demonstrates the horse pose in which the practitioner 'concentrates all [his] powers centrally' while jumping forward and thrusting with the elbow in an attack.

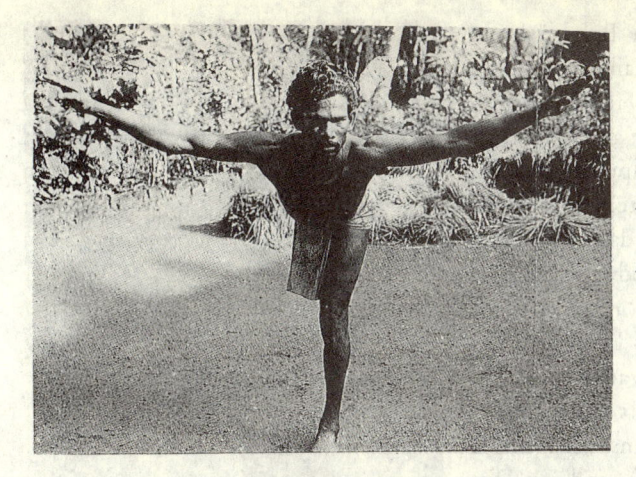

Figure 4.11: The peacock pose in which the practitioner, like the peacock, 'spreads its feathers and raises its neck, and dances by steadying itself on one leg'.

Figure 4.12: The serpent pose where the practitioner, like the serpent, always keeps its tail 'on the ground without movement' so that 'he can turn in any direction' to attack or defend.

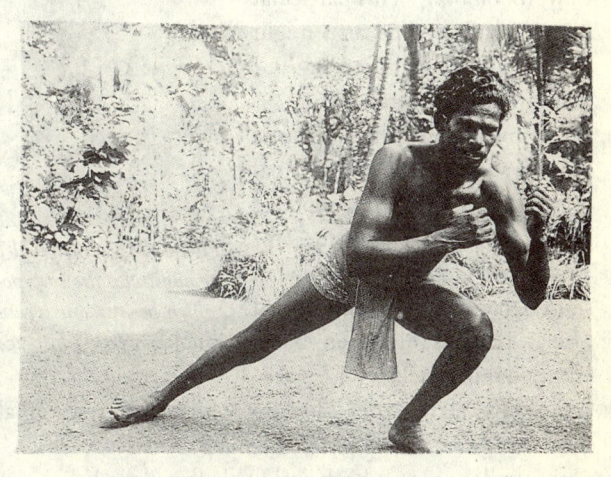

to turn in any direction and attack by rising up is known as *sarpavadivu* (Figure 4.12).

When a cock attacks he uses all parts of his body—wings, neck, legs, fingernails. He will lift one leg and shake his feather and neck, fix his gaze on the enemy, and attack. This is *kukkuvadivu* (Figure 4.13).

One advanced method of exercise is known as *kaikuttyppayattu*—literally 'putting the hands (on the floor) exercise'. Here the practitioner moves very deeply into the poses while keeping the spinal column and back in alignment, fully supported by the area between the small of the back and the navel region. Kallada Balakrishnan explained how 'kaikuttyppayattu develops the bladder region, correct breathing, and to increase flexibility and suppleness in the hip area. When practised repetitiously and daily it will give superior lower body strength and the foundation necessary for correct practice'. In some styles of kaikuttyppayattu technical names describe its fierce empty-hand applications: 'ten finger claw' (*dasa viral*), and 'one fist claw' (*ekamusthi*). This particular form of kaikuttyppayattu might be translated as 'piercing' or 'stabbing hand exercise'.[96]

Some masters who emphasize kalarippayattu as a practical martial art also teach a separate set of verumkai techniques for attack and defence of the vital spots (Chapter 6). C. Mohammed Sherif teaches eighteen basic empty-hand attacks (4.17–4.18)

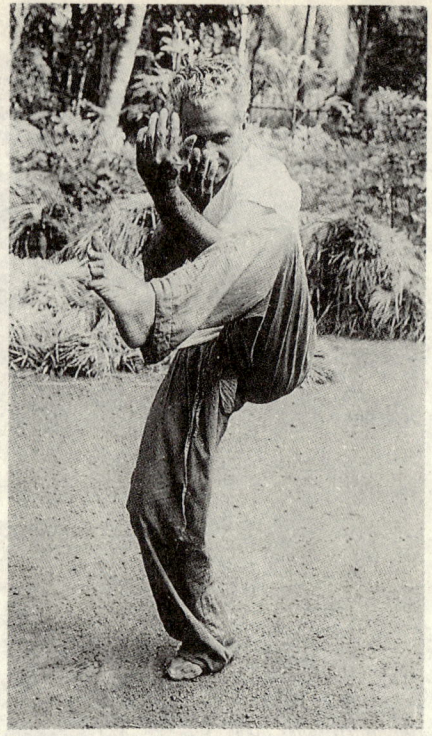

Figure 4.13: Gurukkal P.K. Balan demonstrates the cock pose—a position from which he lifts 'one leg and shakes his feathers and neck, fixing his gaze on the enemy and

and twelve methods of blocking which were traditionally part of at least some northern Kerala styles. Like leg exercises, each technique is practised as the student moves back and forth across the kalari. An advanced student should eventually improvise and move with fluid spontaneity in any direction, performing any combination of moves for offensive or defensive purposes. As Gurukkal Govindankutty Nayar explained, the student himself will begin to discover these applications 'in due time'.

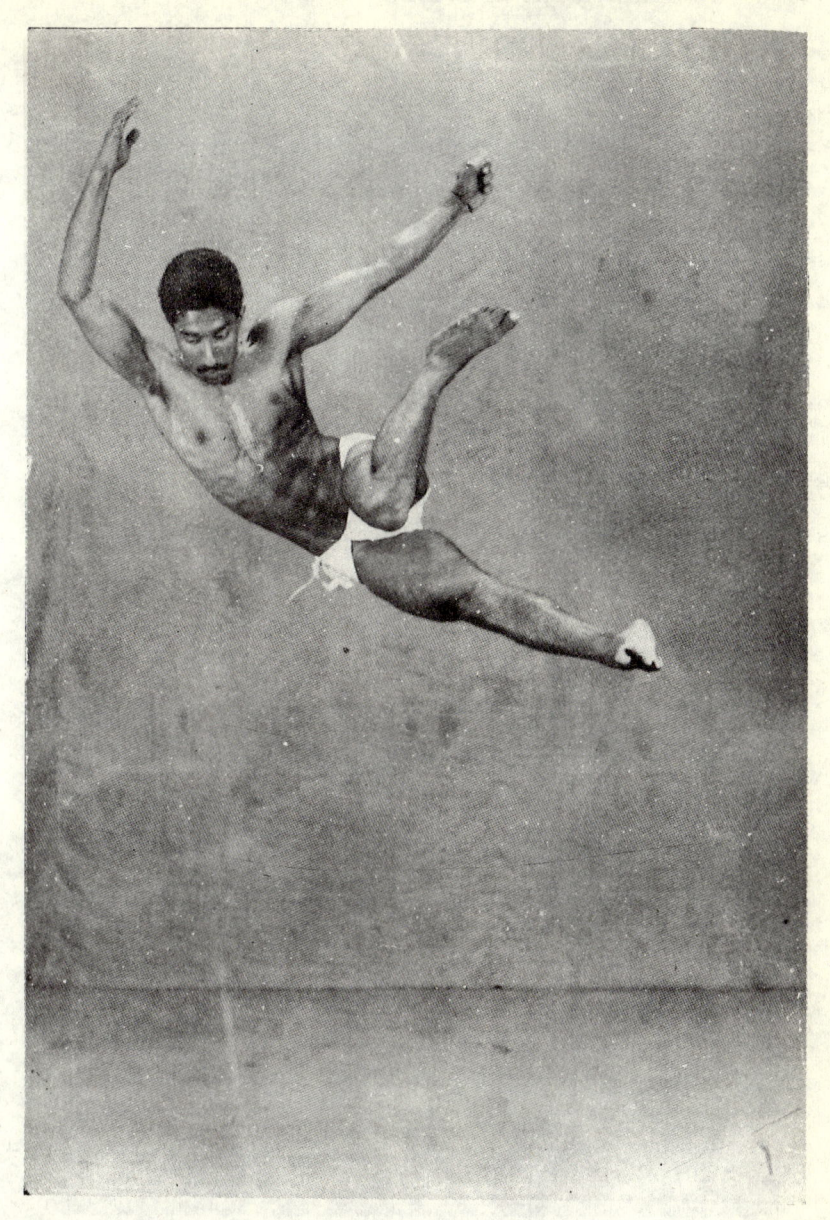

Figure 4.14: One of *kalarippayattu's* many jumps and body turns: As demonstrated by Sathyan Narayanan, in the *'turning jump'* when fully executed the body is extended in a straight line, horizontal to the floor. This same turning cut is later applied as a slashing sword cut with the sword. (Photograph courtesy of Sathyanarayanan Nayar.)

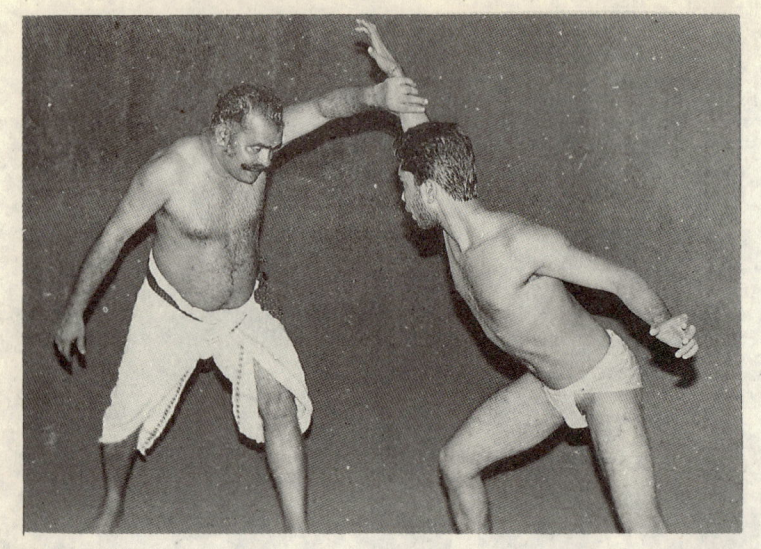

Figure 4.15

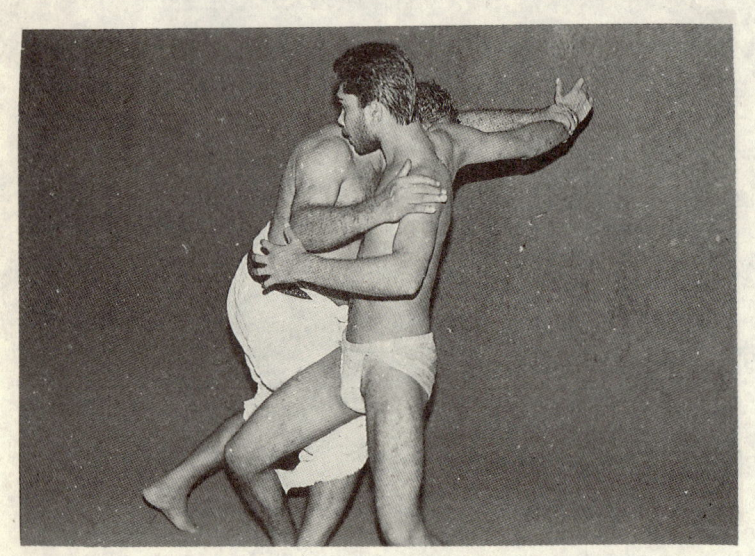

Figure 4.16

Figures 4.15–4.16: Sreejayan Gurukkal uses kalarippayattu's basic steps learned 'innocently' as part of the first body exercise to block an attack, enter his opponent and throw him to the ground.

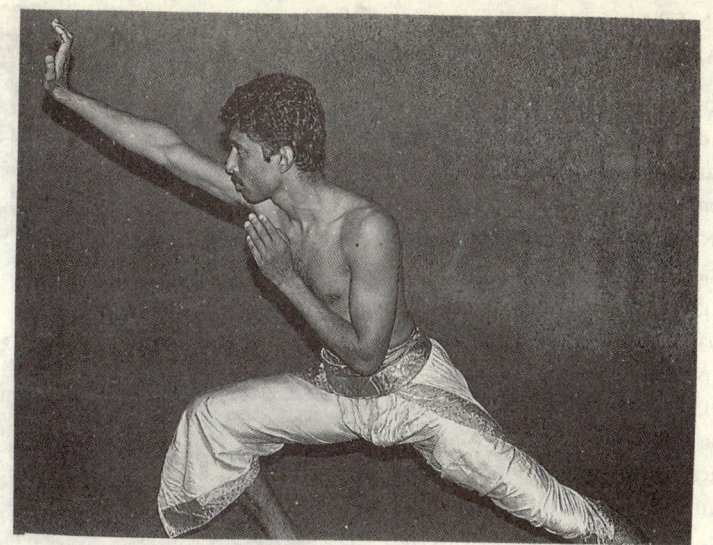

Figure 4.17: The seventh of eighteen empty-hand attacks practised by C. Mohammed Sherif, Kerala Kalarippayattu Academy, Kannur: literally 'right (palm or butt of the hand) to chin'.

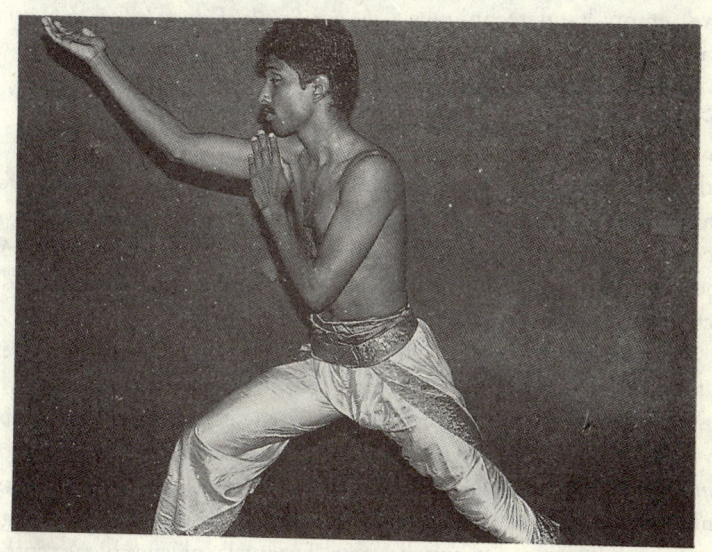

Figure 4.18: The fifteenth empty-hand attack—a 'right inside chop'.

CENTRAL STYLE KALARI-PPAYATTU

Although there are relatively few practitioners of central style kalarippayattu—'central' being a reference to the fact that it is practised in the central region of Kerala, i.e. Trissur, Malappuram, Palghat and certain parts of Ernakulam districts—I agree with C. Mohammed Sherif's observation that the central Kerala style is 'a composite' one which combines techniques and principles from both the 'northern' style and the Tamil-influenced southern styles. The central style includes practice of meippayattu preliminary exercises like those described above, empty-hand techniques and its own distinctive techniques.

Its distinctive techniques are performed within floor drawings known as kalam. Common in south India, they range from simple auspicious geometric patterns drawn each morning in front of the doorway to a house with white rice powder, to complex three-dimensional multi-coloured floor drawings of deities important in ritual performances. Kalam typically used in central style practice have two basic patterns: zigzags and triangles.

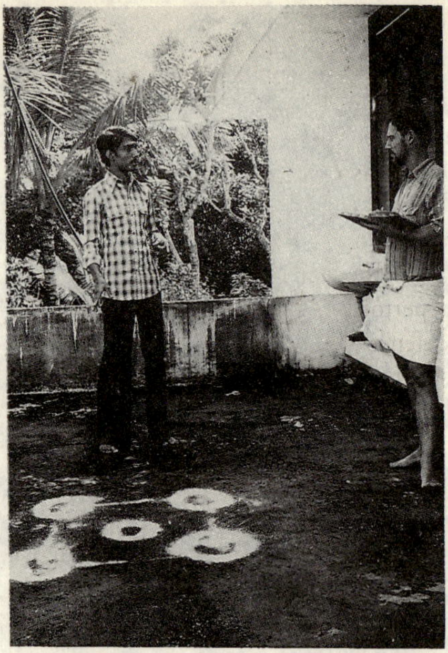

Figure 4.19: C. Mohammed Sherif explains the significance of a simple floor drawing of five circles used in central and southern style kalarippayattu practice. (Photo courtesy of Kerala Kalarippayattu Academy.)

As shown in Figure 4.19, when a spot is placed in the centre, there are the four corner points, and the central spot is the one to and from which steps are made as the practitioner steps between and among these five spots, moving in triangle or zigzag patterns. The teacher instructs students in basic *cuvatu* by making him place his feet in all the different possible combinations within, around and across the five circles. The emphasis is on developing the instinctive ability to step in any direction. Eventually practice blows, cuts and defensive moves are coordinated with the complex steps.

Over this same basic diagram can be laid a set of triangles, further complicating the possibilities for variation in the kalam. Thus the star of David is laid over a basic pattern of four. Rather than moving back and

'First the Outer Forms' • 107

forth across the floor, the direction of movement is constantly shifting and changing. The practitioner can easily move inside or outside, shifting and changing with each step, opening inward or opening outward. As with other kalam, in central kalarippayattu-style practice these geometric patterns are also often considered yantram, i.e. sacred diagrams for which esoteric interpretations abound. We shall return to a few of these more esoteric, subtle interpretations in Chapter 5.

P.K. Balan Gurukkal of Trissur district, central Kerala, includes in his repertoire of basic kalarippayattu techniques eighteen sequences of self-defence techniques known as *cumattadi* ('steps and hits', Figures 4.20–4.22).

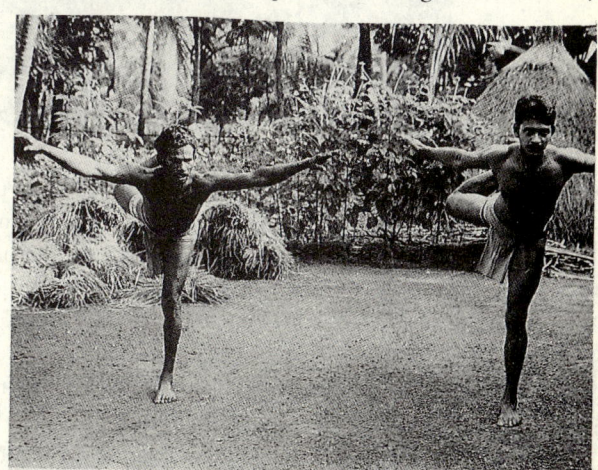

Figure 4.20

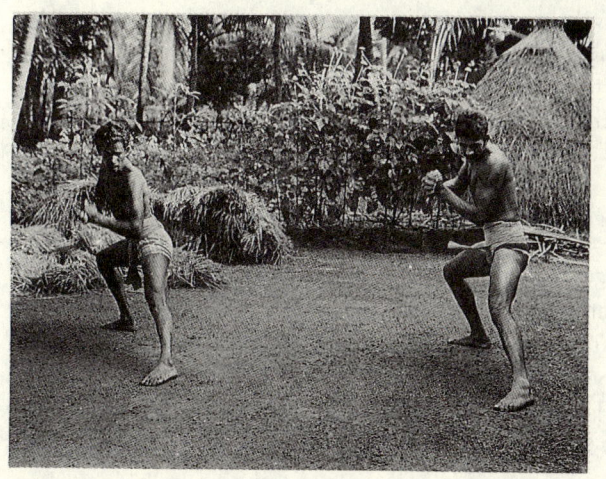

Figure 4.21

Figures 4.20–4.22 Part of the second, 'peacock' form of cumatadi as practised by P.K. Balan Gurukkal. In this part of the sequence, the students have moved into the peacock stance (4.20) from which they move quickly back into an extended leg position (4.21) from which a very strong, vigorous forward doubled-fisted thrust is made (4.22).

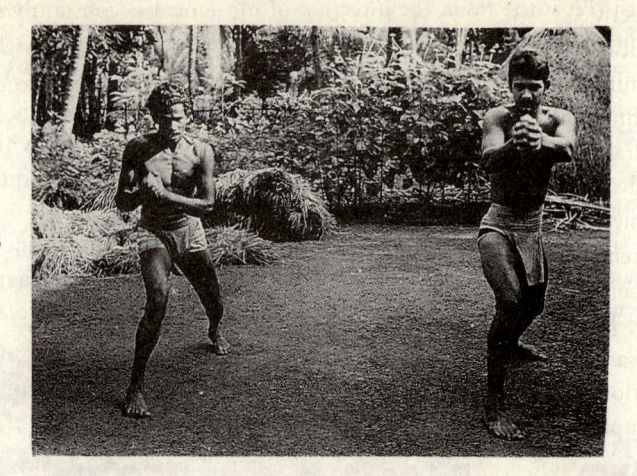

Figure 4.22

Each cumattadi is based on a particular kalarippayattu pose which, like body exercise sequences, are combined in increasingly difficult combinations. The first sequence is based on the horse, second on the peacock, third on the serpent, fourth on the horse again and fifth on the elephant. What is common to all is that each movement in a sequence has a specific and obvious fighting application. Unlike the graded body exercise sequences in which some movements are primarily for flexibility, balance and control, these techniques have direct martial application.

Another common feature of *cumattadi* is their directional orientation. While the body exercise sequences are primarily linear and performed back and forth across the kalari with 180-degree turns, like varma ati's basic techniques, cumattadi are performed in four directions, instilling in the student the ability to respond to attack from any direction. Like body-exercise sequences, these sequences also have verbal commands recorded in a master's palm leaf texts.

VARMA ATI ('SOUTHERN STYLE' KALARIPPAYATTU)

Although I have argued along with Sreedharan Nayar (1963: 9–11) that the distinctive dronampalli sampradayam practised at one time in southern Kerala is virtually extinct, there is no doubt that what is today identified as 'southern' kalarippayattu was more closely related to this particular style than to 'northern' kalarippayattu. I agree with C. Mohammed Sherif's opinion that unlike kalarippayattu with its preliminary body exercise and massage training, 'pure varma ati is a basic set of techniques which can be directly used for self-defence *or* for use with a variety of weapons'. The basic steps and body movements learned for self-defence are the basis for manipulation of all weapons in this system. There are three sets of basic techniques in varma ati: *otta cuvatu, kuttu cuvatu,* and *watta cuvatu.* What characterizes all these basic techniques is the emphasis not only on lower body control but attacks and defences with the hands/arms/elbows. As the name varma ati indicates, from the very beginning the student is learning a system of empty-hand attacks and defences of the body's vital spots (Tamil, varmam).

Training begins with 'salutation steps' (*vandana cuvatu,* Figure 4.23), i.e. a salutation to the four directions with one leg, usually the left, in a stationary position, and ending with salutations to the master. This is comparable to kalarippayattu's *puttara tol* or *kalari vandanam.*

Second in the system are otta cuvatu, or single foot steps. Some masters, like Raju Asan, draw a kalam of five circles on the floor within which the basic steps are taken (Figures 4.24–4.26). One foot, usually the left, remains stationary while the other foot moves in all four directions to defend and/or counter attack from the four basic directions. Included are a variety of kicks, blocks, hits and/or evasive moves. Such techniques are especially important for empty-hand fighting since it is assumed to be better *not* to enter directly into a counterattack, but to wait until one first determines whether the opponent has a weapon or not. By keeping one foot fixed in place, the practitioner can first block/evade, and only then attempt to enter for attack. Most masters teach twelve basic otta cuvatu

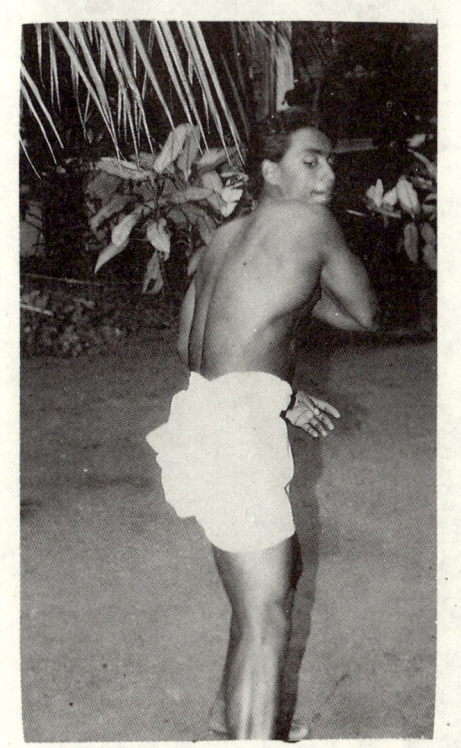

Figure 4.23: Vandana cuvattu—*Sadasivan Asan's son performs the salutation in four directions with his left foot stationary. Here he begins a right arm slashing cut from left to right.*

110 • *When the Body Becomes All Eyes*

sequences which form the preliminary body training of the student.

Vatta cuvatu are techniques performed with the same basic pattern as otta cuvatu, except for different steps. Here the practitioner can directly enter into a counter attack. Practitioners vary in the number of sequences practised between six and twelve.

Kutta cuvatu are combination steps which build in complexity of forms. Multiple steps with both feet are taken. These also include a variety of kicks, blocks, attacks and evasive

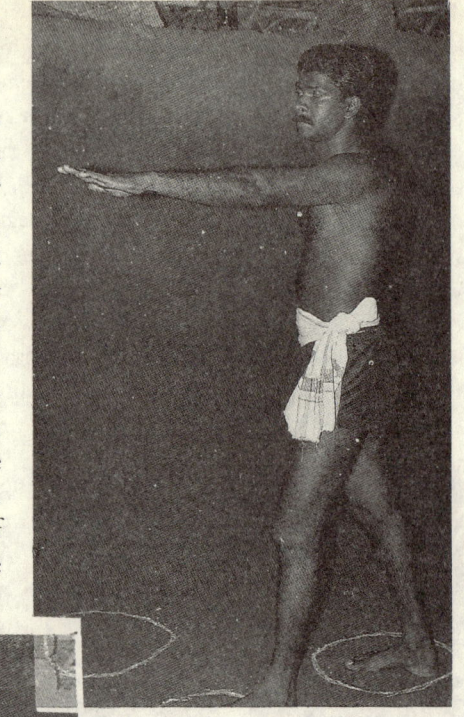

Figure 4.24

Figure 4.25

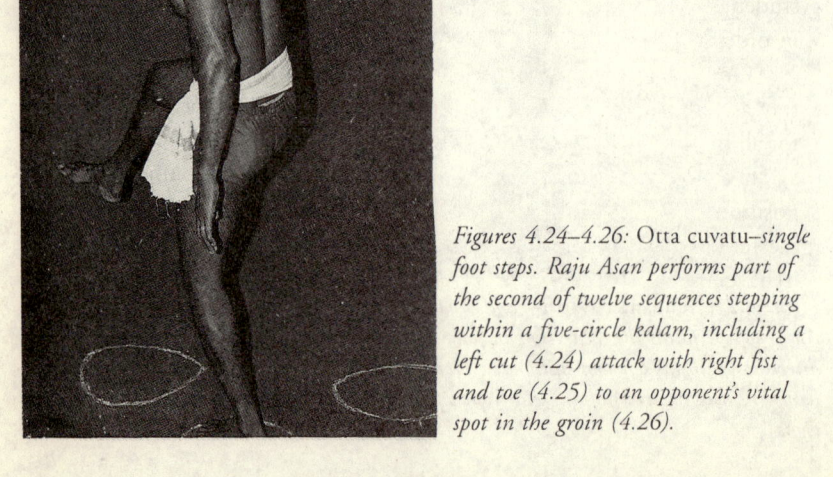

Figures 4.24–4.26: Otta cuvatu–*single foot steps. Raju Asan performs part of the second of twelve sequences stepping within a five-circle kalam, including a left cut (4.24) attack with right fist and toe (4.25) to an opponent's vital spot in the groin (4.26).*

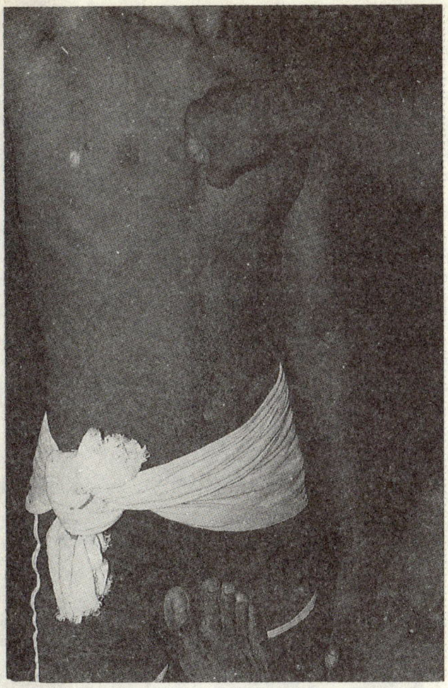

moves, and especially emphasized are complex combinations of simultaneous defences with attacks to the body's vital spots.

Given the primary importance of varma ati on attacking and defending the body's vital spots, its techniques include numerous locks and counterlocks—practical techniques to which we shall return in more detail in Chapter 6.

Advancing through the Preliminary Body Exercise System

Daily instruction is simple and practical. Few, if any, explanations are offered why something should be done. Consequently, students perform many repetitions of the same basic exercises and when the master or a senior student takes an interest, simple specific individual corrections are given like, 'place the foot here, not there', 'keep the hands above the head', or 'straighten the back'. As often as not, these corrections are accompanied by hands-on manipulation—the master or advanced student will literally put the student's foot where it belongs, or push on the small of the student's back in order to correct spinal alignment when assuming a pose.

One constant correction is to 'stay down in position (*amarnnu*)', i.e. to stay as low as possible in the pose being performed. The natural tendency for all but a few highly motivated students is to be lazy about getting down as far as necessary when assuming a pose, simply because the lower into position one gets the more difficult and exhausting it is to perform. The master knows that only when the student is fully in the correct position can it have its 'full' health and practical benefits for fighting. But such 'full benefits' are far from the young student's mind. He is usually more concerned about being the first one to get to the shower stall after practice than about getting into the correct position.

Figure 4.26

Another commonplace correction is, 'you're only moving the arm, use *the whole body!*' Mimicking only the external form of what they see advanced students doing, neophytes have yet to embody the internal process of coordinating the hand and leg movements by drawing both back simultaneously through the *nabhi*. They have not yet intuitively learned how to embody the ideal—performing each move with the entire body while keeping the central spinal column in its natural, firm alignment. Therefore, this type of correction may be greeted with confusion.

Specific correction is individual; however, body exercises are repeated in pairs or small groups organized by ability. The rhythm of each master's lineage of practice is unique, and is controlled by the gurukkal's vocalization of *vayttari*. Vayttari were traditionally kept secret and recorded in palm leaf manuscripts (Figure 4.27) passed on from generation to generation. Today many are available in cheap paperback books like Prasannan G. Mullassery's *Kalarippayattum Kayyamkaliyum* (1965, 1977)—available at railway or bus stand book stalls for Rs 2.50 (0.15) in 1980—Sreedharan Nayar's 1963 book, or Balakrishnan's most recent publication (1994, 1995). The verbal commands are in part descriptive, but practically function as verbal cues which, through repetition and familiarity, automatically trigger the appropriate movement. For example, the verbal commands repeated daily in class for the opening of the C.V.N. style body-exercise sequences begins,

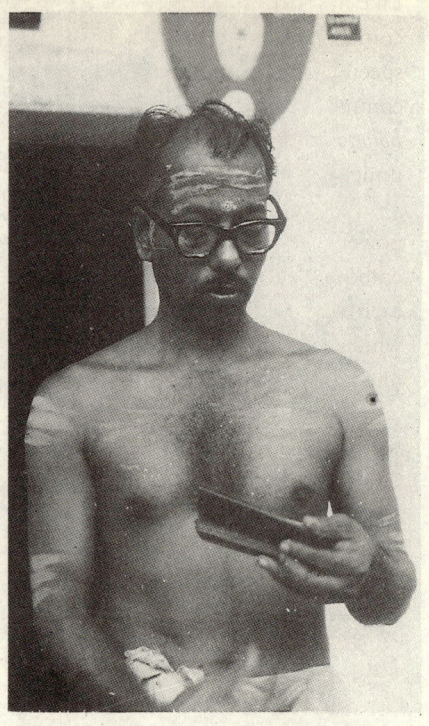

Figure 4.27: C. Sankaranarayana Menon consults one of his original family grandam.

Amarnnu, amarccayil itattu veccu valattu kondu cavutti, valattatu valiyottu mari itattatum kutti vanni amarnnu . . . (Take) position, from position left forward, put the right step forward, take the right back with the left into position . . .

Like military commands ('fall in'), the verbal commands encode a complete, complex set of movements—the student must intuitively embody all the specific movements assumed by each short-hand command. The verbal command, 'amarnnu', or '(take) position', tells the practitioner nothing about *how* to assume that position. The 'how' is learned only by repetitious practice under the watchful eye of the master.

When vocalized by a master with the appropriate vocal emphasis and power, the patterns of intonation and cadences should guide the student in embodying the correct form of each movement and the correct rhythm of each sequence. As C. Mohammed Sherif told me, 'Doing body exercises while listening to the verbal commands will make the mind concentrated; one naturally becomes fully involved (in the exercise).'

Once students have warmed up with the preliminary leg exercises, they are put through the body sequences in quick succession. Strict training is intentionally exhausting. Kallada Balakrishana explained the importance of stamina:

> The practitioner *had* to be able to fight for a long time, and therefore he *had* to have stamina and a strong will. You get stamina by just doing the body exercises over and over and over. In the old days, you might have had to fight for two or three hours, like the fights of Tacholi Otenan and Mathiru Gurukkal. But nowadays after two or three body sequences, students will be out of breath! To develop stamina every day of practice you should do *all* the body exercises and then do all the 'hands on the floor' sequences, and then do all the special sequences, and then do weapons, and finally run twelve kilometres. And after all this you should not feel tired. *Then* you will have developed stamina!

Although a few masters enforce a rigorous training regime on their students, at other kalari students may only perform a few preliminary exercises, and then perfunctorily perform one sequence before leaving for the day.

Where rigorous training *does* take place, and students are ensured of several months of sore muscles, progress through the kalarippayattu system can seem incredibly slow for many Malayali youth for whom karate classes are available around the corner. When they compare the one year spent doing kalarippayattu's initial psycho-physiological exercises which appear unrelated to self-defence, to karate classes in which they can begin the first day to learn self-defence, kalarippayattu's exercises can seem an anachronistic throw-back to an outmoded past.

Moreover, for those who begin training and wish to continue, but may have little opportunity of becoming 'professionals' making a living through teaching and giving treatment, the incentives to continue practising are few and the disincentives many. As family and work obligations increase, it becomes difficult if not impossible for students in their 20s or 30s to find the time or energy to continue training. Therefore, 'traditional' kalarippayattu training does not appeal to a large number of Malayali youth, and where the training *is* rigorous, it takes considerable perseverance and dedication to continue a discipline which will only grudgingly bring rewards. For any of a host of reasons, the vast majority of students who begin kalarippayattu training today only continue for a few weeks to a few years. For example, of twenty-two students who began training together at the Thiruvananthapuram C.V.N. Kalari in 1983, only one was still practising in 1988 when I returned.

The pace and tone of training and correction at any kalari depend on the personality of the master and are subject to changes in his moods. Some masters teach in what might be characterized as a rather quiet, low-key style; others are flamboyant and overtly vocal. At times instruction and correction are harsh and severe, and it is not unusual for teachers to become angry. A teacher may unexpectedly put a student through an extremely difficult body exercise sequence at an exhausting, break-neck pace, pushing the student to or beyond the point of exhaustion. If a correction has been given more than once, the student may feel a slap on an out-of-place foot, or hear, 'Don't you understand Malayalam!' Occasionally students may be held up to ridicule by being told to sit in a corner of the kalari with legs crossed and back straight in order to stretch wiry muscles, or by being told, 'Where is your mind!' A few students may be so harshly treated or embarrassed that they do not return.

The general cultural model and discourse assumed for training in traditional South Asia disciplines of practice is the *guru-sishya parampara* where a student, having sought out a teacher and been accepted for study, places his entire faith, trust, and future in the hands of his teacher. Duarte Barbosa also recorded the importance of the bond ideally developed between master and pupil during training:

> ... The masters who teach them are called Panicals (Panikkar), and are much honoured and esteemed among them, especially by their pupils, great and small, who worship them; and it is the law and custom to bow down before them whenever they meet them; even if the disciple is older than the master. And the Nayre are bound, howsoever olde they may be,

to go always in the winter (i.e., in the rainy season) to take their fencing lessons until they die (1921: Vol. II, 39–40).

According to this idealized discourse the student gives himself over totally to his master, usually by living with and doing service for him. The student is expected to have absolute trust in the master's intuitive wisdom and knowledge, never question a master's decisions, and accept the severity of his training. If a student perceives that the master is not pleased with his practice or behaviour, the student is expected to search out the fault. Students are supposed to assume that whatever the teacher does is done out of love for the art and the teacher's desire to instil that art in the student. Among some teacher-student relationships, such as that between Drona and Arjuna in the *Mahabharata*, this ideal is no doubt actualized, and the teacher-student relationship becomes closer than that of even father and son, or uncle and nephew; however, there is always the potential for abuse of power.[97]

Although kalarippayattu students probably never lived at their teacher's home during their initial period of training at the local village kalari, advanced students sought out masters for higher studies and undertook traditional service to them. In both cases, the idea that a bond of absolute trust and devotion should develop between master and student is implicit in kalarippayattu.

Students advance through the system individually. The teacher keeps a watchful eye on each student's progress, i.e. on how well he embodies the forms of practice, and on the student's general demeanour and behaviour. The teacher's discerning gaze does not simply look at a student's overt, physical progress, but includes 'looking within at the heart of the student'. Some masters say that they 'know (each student's) mind from the countenance of the face' (*mukhabhavattil ninnu manassilakkam*). Nothing overt is expressed, explained, or spoken; the master simply watches, observes, and 'reads' each student.

According to some masters, only when a master intuitively senses that a student is psycho-physiologically, morally and spiritually 'ready' to advance, should he be taught new, more difficult exercises. Ideally, each technique is given as a 'gift' (*upadesham*). The teacher should take joy in the act of giving, especially as the gifts become more advanced and therefore precious.

This ideal model of transmission, epitomized in the lifelong learning of the Pandavas and Kauravas under the master teacher Drona, implies that training takes place exclusively with one master. However, in kalarippayattu it is equally traditional for students to study with more than one master. One of many examples from the *vadakkan pattukal* is the story of how Allumkulangara Unichandror set out with his friends for Tulunadu, north of Kerala in Karnataka, to seek an expert master from whom to learn the highest feats in combat:

> They went to Tulunadu and also the house of the guru, and prostrated before him. Keeping his hands on their heads he blessed them. The guru asked, 'Children, why do you come here?' 'We want to learn more and so we have come to you. Please teach us *adavu* (forms) and our occupation', they said. Then the guru said, 'Alright, we can start from tomorrow morning' (Achutanandan 1973: 130. Trans. K.H. Devi).

Today it is commonplace for students to have had one or many teachers. C.V. Narayanan Nayar's teacher, Karnaran Gurukkal, learned from many masters before codifying the C.V.N. composite styled of practice. Like Karnaran Gurukkal, those who learn from multiple masters may either teach multiple sets of techniques, or develop their own unique style of practice. P.P. Narayanan Gurukkal of Kannur district teaches both vattantirippu and arappukkai style exercises and three different froms of massage learned from three different masters. Although speaking of other forms of traditional learning and initiation, Harvey Alper's observation that some practitioners even 'collect gurus the way some Americans collect baseball cards' applies equally to at least some kalarippayattu practitioners (1989: 2).

Although the ideal of the guru-disciple relationship still exists, there is considerable cynicism among some long-term teachers and students. As one teacher told me,

> I don't use the title guru for myself. Who can say if they are a guru? Someone may know something and go and open up a kalari and people will call him a guru. That is one reason why I stopped teaching myself. Kalarippayattu used to be popular because there were good masters who came through the gurukkula system. But today there are many who are charlatans! There are no rules or restrictions on who may be called a guru, or on the life of students today.

From the Body to Weapons as an Extension of the Body

Only when a student is physically, spiritually and ethically 'ready' is he supposed to be allowed to take up the first weapon. If the body and mind have been fully prepared (and therefore integrated), when the student takes up the first weapon it becomes an extension of the integration of the bodymind in action.

The student first learns wooden weapons: *kolttari*—first long staff (Figure 4.28), later short stick (Figure 4.29) and curved stick (otta) (Figures 4.30–31), and after several years combat weapons including dagger (Figure 4.32), spear (Figure 4.33), gada, sword and shield (Figure 1.6), double-edged sword (curika) versus sword (Figure 4.34), spear versus sword and shield (Figure 4.35) and flexible sword (Figure 4.36).[98] All weapons teach attack and defence of the body's vital spots (Chapter 6). The teacher's corrections are intended to make the weapon an extension of the body. Each weapon has one or more basic poses to and from which the practitioner moves, and through which the weapon becomes an extension of the body. For example, the staff is an extension of the natural line of the spinal column maintained as one moves to and from basic poses. The hands are kept in front of the body and the body weight is always kept forward, maximizing the length of the staff to keep the opponent at bay.

Practising with the curved stick (otta), with its deep, wave-like, flowing movements, is considered the culmination and epitome of psycho-physiological training because not only are its forms superb and beautiful, but these forms assist the internal awakening of the subtle body. When correct spinal alignment is kept, practice further develops the important region of the *nabhi mula*, hips and thighs (Chapter 5). Learning otta also initiates the student into verumkai, the most advanced part of total kalarippayattu training, which eventually culminates when the student learns the location of the body's vital spots. Unlike contemporary self-defence martial arts and similar to its Japanese counterpart—the traditional *bugei* or weapons forms in which use of weapons was historically the main purpose of practice—many empty-hand techniques are a means of disarming an armed opponent.

Correct practice of all weapons depends entirely on correct performance of preliminary body exercises. Weapons are never to be manipulated by using overt strength or physical force, i.e. trying to make a blow forceful. Gurukkal Govindankutty Nayar said, 'using overt force is the surest way for a blow to "become nothing" and "lose its actuality". Like the body exercises, each blow, thrust, cut or defensive movement must be performed *with the entire body* and not simply with the hand/arm/weapon.' While practising sword and shield, my teacher told me:

> A non-actualized cut originates from the shoulder itself, and does not bring the entire body into the execution of the cut, nor does it flow into the next cut in the sequence which follows.

Just as one movement should flow into the next when performing the body exercise sequence, so in weapons practice one blow merges naturally with the next as there is a continuous energy flow which should never be broken.

Exercises and weapons forms are repeated until the student has sufficiently embodied the inner life (*bhava*) of the sequence, i.e. until the correct form gets 'inside' the student's body. Once the exercise becomes 'effortless', as one performs the exercise one should naturally begin to experience the 'inner action' behind the external movement. It is to the more subtle, interior aspects of practice that we turn our attention in Chapter 5.

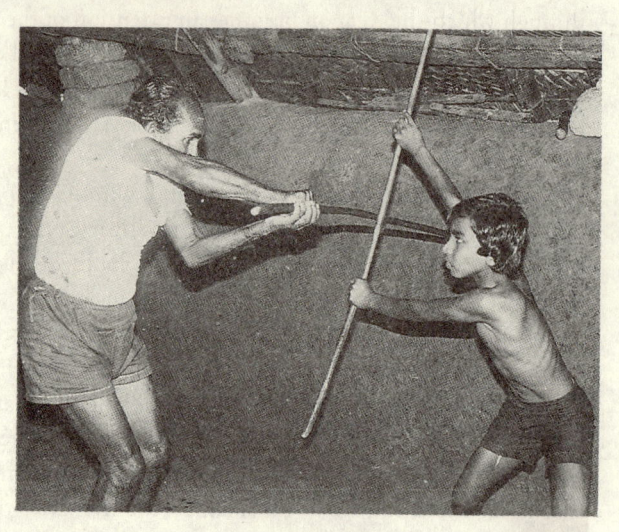

Figure 4.28: Training with long staff (kettukari). *Achuthan Gurukkal trains a young boy to defend his ribs with the long staff.*

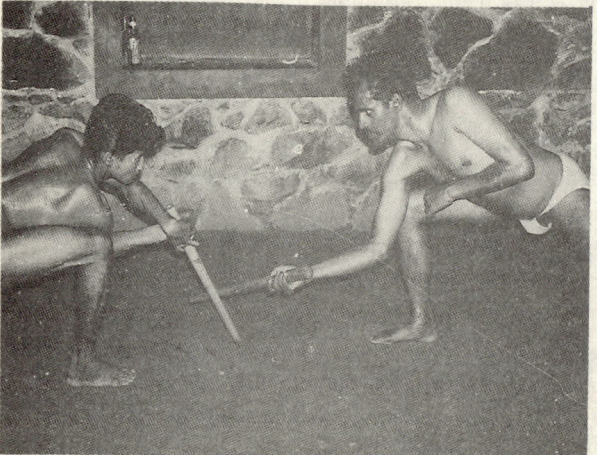

Figure 4.29: Basic techniques with short stick (ceruvadi) *usually include twelve basic sequences taught as codified forms. Rajashekharan Nayar and Aravindakshan Nayar practising attack to and defence of a blow to the ankle.*

'First the Outer Forms' • 119

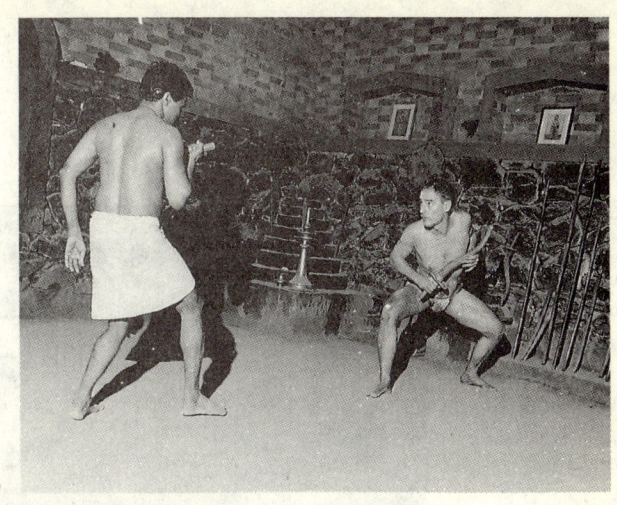

Figure 4.30

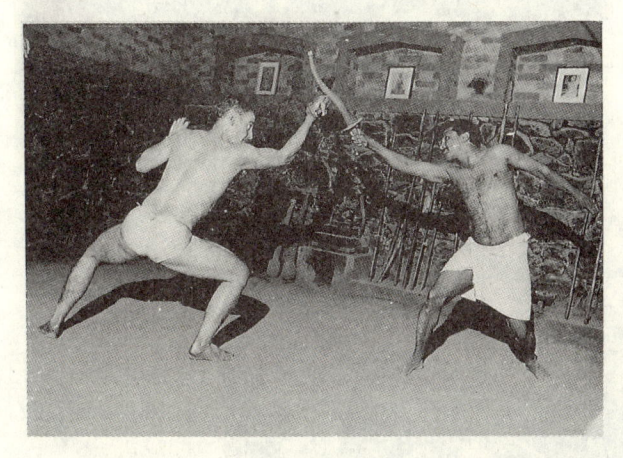

Figure 4.31

Figures 4.30–4.31: In otta practice the practitioner must keep spinal alignment while staying deep in position. The author (right) prepares to defend against an attack from Rajashekharan Nayar. The author (left) defends an attack from Rajashekharan Nayar (right). Otta requires the practitioner to keep spinal alignment while staying very deep in the position. (Photographs by Ed Heston.)

Figure 4.32: Practice with dagger: Sathyanarayanan Nayar (left) defends against a thrust from Hari at the C.V.N. Kalari, Thiruvananthapuram.

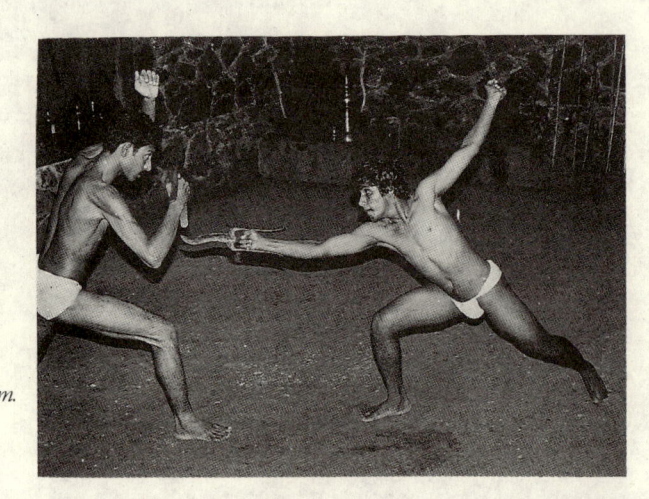

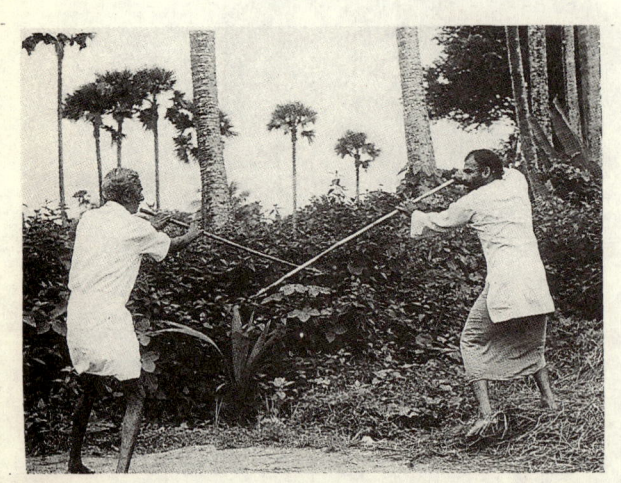

Figure 4.33: One of the few specialists in spear techniques, Velayudan Asan (left) attacks his student, Jayakumar (right).

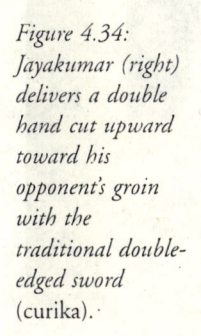

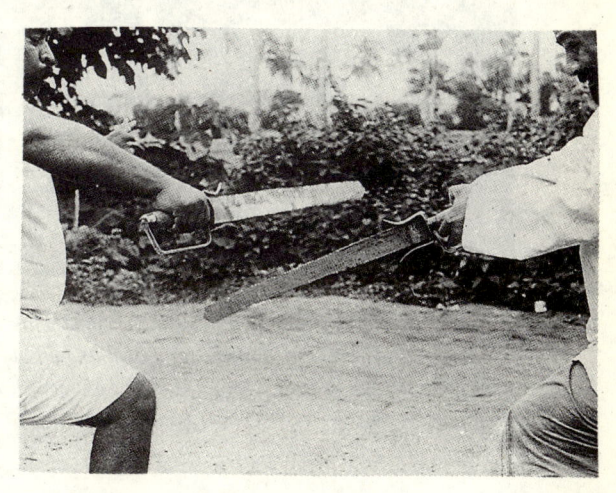

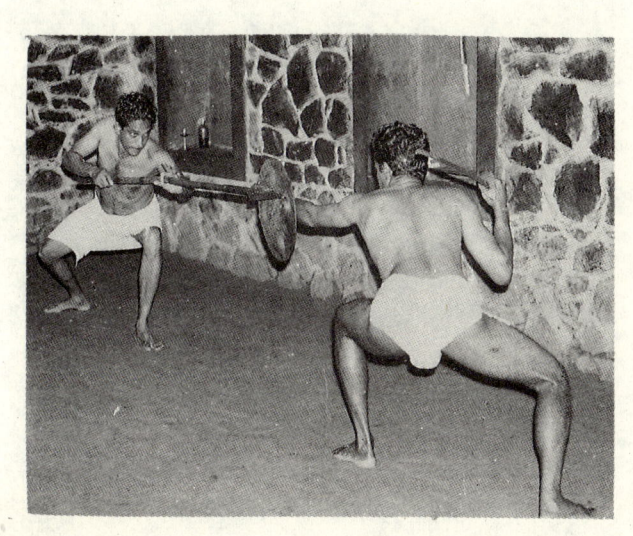

Figure 4.34: Jayakumar (right) delivers a double hand cut upward toward his opponent's groin with the traditional double-edged sword (curika).

Figure 4.35: Govindankutty Nayar thrusts with his spear as Aravindakshan Nayar defends with his shield.

122 • *When the Body Becomes All Eyes*

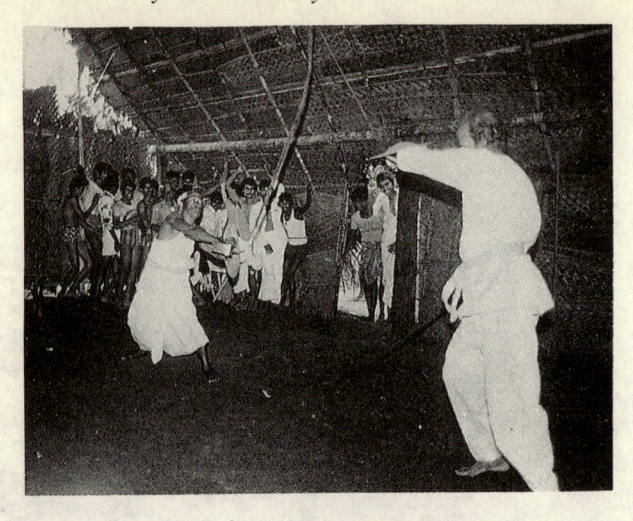

Figure 4.36: The flexible sword (urumi) *is swung with a slashing circling action around the head, warding off opponents from any direction or attacking an opponent also wielding an urumi. Here Gurukkal Madhavan Panikkar attacks Mohammedunni Gurukkal.*

Chapter 5

'Then the Inner Secrets': The Subtle Body *(Suksma Sarira)*, The Vital Energy *(Prana-Vayu)*, and Actualizing Power *(Sakti)*

Martial practice, like meditation, is understood to tame and purify the external *sthula-sarira*, as it quiets and balances the body's three humours. Eventually the practitioner should begin to discover the *suksma sarira* most often identified with Kundalini/Tantric yoga. For martial practitioners this discovery is essential for embodying power (sakti) to be used in combat or for healing.

The subtle body refers to the ideational construct used by many south Indians to identify and articulate the psycho-spiritual experiences of the yogi, martial artist and the pilgrim/devotee (Daniel 1984). It provides a map of an experiential landscape especially for those who practise psycho-physiological disciplines or *sadhana*. The map of this landscape allows the practitioner to 'make sense' of the psycho-physiological effects of practice on his bodymind as practice reshapes his experience.

The subtle body has been defined by others as 'mystical physiology' (Gupta et. al. 1979: 64), 'theoretical anatomy' (Filliozat 1964: 234) and an 'invisible *mandala* formed by a combination of symbolic (but also very real) geometric figures . . . (it is) a structure of reference, an image, a yantra' (Varenne 1976: 153–4). The subtle body is often depicted as a microcosm of the universe. As noted in one classic text, the *Siva Samhita* (II.4), 'All the beings that exist in the three worlds are also to be found in the (subtle) body' (Vasu 1975: 16). The subtle body is also called the seat/vehicle of the soul (*atma*) (Carter 1982: 122).

Among those who practise disciplines, physical and subtle bodies are not absolute categories. Exercise of one body is understood to naturally affect the other. They are fluid conceptual and practical counterparts. Specific parts of the subtle body are thought to correspond to specific places in the physical body. These are analogous/homologous correspondences and are never exact (Varenne 1976: 155). Yet the two are so fundamentally related that what affects one body is understood to affect the other. In classical texts and contemporary practice the physical and subtle bodies are so interrelated and the boundaries between them so fluid that descriptions of the subtle body refer to the physical body. *Yoga Darshana Upanishad* (4.7) records that 'the measure of the body is ninety-six finger breadths' (in Varenne 1976: 206). Many kalarippayattu texts, such as one Muslim master's text, *nadi sampradayam* ('traditional knowledge of the channels' see Appendix I), record similar details: 'The study of the human body is part of kalari practice. The height of a person is eight widths of the hand (*can*); four (*can*) is the width of the chest below the breast. There are 362 bones in the human body. 96 are hollow.'

Hatha-yoga-pradipika (II.21) takes careful note of the humoral condition of the practitioner: 'He who is of weak constitution and phlegmatic, subject to *kapha* disorders, should first practise *satkarma*. Those not suffering (constitutionally) from the (main) disorders due to *vata*, *pitta*, and *kapha* do not need it' (Reiker 1971: 80). Like preliminary kalarippayattu practice, it both warns of the dangers to healthy balance among the humours of incorrect practice, and touts the disease-freeing results of correct practice. Incorrect practice of special breathing exercises (*pranayama*) brings 'all kinds of ailments' including 'coughs, asthma, headaches, eye and ear pain, as well as other sicknesses' (ibid.: 79). Correct practice of internal cleansing or mastery of a particular configuration of meditation (*mudra*) allows one to 'remove' or 'destroy all diseases' (ibid.: 83; *Siva Samhita* III. 77, Vasu 1975: 36).

Although in texts and practice the physical and subtle bodies are integrally related, the concept and specific inner alchemy of the subtle body historically developed separately from Ayurveda as part of ascetic and yogic practice (Eliade 1958: 234; Filliozat 1964: 234) and appears fully developed after about the eighth century AD in the *Yoga Upanisad* and *Tantra*. The essential elements of the subtle body usually identified in these texts, as well as in kalarippayattu versions of the subtle body, include structural elements, *nadi* and wheels or centres (*cakra*), and vital energy or wind (prana, vayu, or prana-vayu) and the cosmic energy (kundalini or Sakti) sleeping coiled within the lowest centre.

The first structural elements are the nadi through which wind or vital energy flows.[99] Various classical texts provide different speculative numbers. *Hatha-yoga-pradipika* IV.8 and *Yoga Darsana Upanisad* IV.6 each propose 72,000 and *Siva Samhita* 350,000—both are symbolic figures 'signifying a vast and indefinite number' (Varenne 1976: 231). Most texts identify around ten to fourteen channels, three of which are most important. *Ida* and *pingala* reach from the lower end of the spinal column (*muladhara-cakra*) up to the left and right nostrils. Between and intertwined with them is the central *susumna-nadi*. It also originates at the 'root' of the spinal column and stretches upward to the top of the head. All nadi originate at the lower end of the spinal column, forming an intricate network of hollow channels through the body linking the *muladhara-cakra* with all the various limbs and sense organs.

The second structural elements are the six or eight centres, or wheels (*cakra*). They take the form of a stylized lotus arrayed vertically from the base of the spinal column (and the corresponding central *susumna nadi*) up to and through increasingly refined and more subtle centres. These centres are places within the subtle body where latent functions, often represented as half-opened buds, await the invigorating exercise of the internal energy.

Based on classical yoga and tantra texts, martial texts include descriptions of the subtle body's channels and centres. Sometimes only a passing reference is made; at other times there is a complete description. For example, in the Muslim master's text cited above, immediately following the enumeration of facts about the physical body, the channels are described:

> And there are seventy-two thousand nadi. Seventy of these are the most important. And then of these seventy, three are the most important. The King of the nadi is one called susumna. This is like a golden string. If anything happens to it, the person will die. The other important nadi are pingala, idapingala, and valapingala.

Martial texts vary in completeness. A Christian master's text records brief descriptions of six centres (*cakra*), a Hindu master only lists four, and others like the following, contain a complete description of seven centres comparable to what is found in classical texts:

> The *susumna-nadi* is located in the middle of the body. Its shape is like a bamboo which has been cut or sliced diagonally. Its position is two fingers above the anus and two fingers below the root of the penis. The end of the nadi which has been cut like this stands at this place.

Below this is the cakram called *muladharam*. The colour of the cakram of muladharam is of heated gold. In this cakram lies in eight folds, kundalini. In that kundalini sakti Siva is located in the shape of Agni.

From the muladharam, two fingers above and two fingers below the root of the penis is *svadisthanam*. This is square shaped and is the colour of a red diamond. In that Siva is situated as Brahma in the shape or form of Agni.

From svadisthanam ten fingers above, with ten petals with the brightness of the sun is situated in the susumna-nadi, *manipurakam*. Here also is Siva in the shape of the sun (Vaghnirupam).

Fourteen fingers above the manipurakam-cakram with twelve petals and the colour of lightning is the *cakram-anahatam*. This is a heart-shaped lotus. Here Siva is located as Vishnu in the shape of life (*jiva-rupam*).

From the place of the heart, six fingers above in the neck, is located the *visuddhicakram*. This is sixteen petals with the colour of purified glass. Here Siva is located in the shape of Chandra, the moon, which is the *amrtam* (nectar).

From the vissudhicakram nine fingers above between the brows is situated *ajnacakram* ('the commanding power').

All of the above six *adharas* are located in the susumna-nadi. At the top end of the susumna with thirty-two petals, placed over the hole of the susumna-nadi upside down enclosing the hold, is the *sahasrara-cakram*.

For the neophyte, the subtle body is at first hidden. To discover it, he must vigilantly practise basic psychophysiological exercises. Most traditional kalarippayattu masters who interpret practice through this paradigm agree that the subtle body is gradually revealed as the student (1) develops both external and one-point focus (*ekagrata*), (2) corrects external physical forms and corresponding internal circulation of the vayu or prana-vayu so that alignment and movement are correct and within the limits of a form, and (3) develops proper breath control, and thereby circulates energy 'correctly'.

DEVELOPING ONE-POINT FOCUS (EKAGRATA)

Developing ekagrata begins with the first kick when students are instructed to focus the external eye on a place at the opposite end of the kalari. It continues as students are instructed on where to focus their eyes while performing body exercises—on the opposite wall, or on a specific part of the body such as the hands or the big toe. *Vayttari* for *meippayattu* have at least one specific command for the student to literally 'look' (*nokki*). In the C.V.N. style this command occurs when students perform the 'lion' pose where the left leg is drawn up along the body and the big toe is fully extended. 'Nokki' commands the student to take his focus from a place on the opposite wall the tip of the big toe, and then follow the big toe as it travels down along the line of his body as it is put forward in the next step. Development of internal focus is especially important in the advanced *kaikuttyppayattu* sequences where nine different times the students are ordered by its verbal commands to 'look' (*nokki*) at specific points: the palm, the top of the knuckle when a fist is made, or between the two thumbs when the two fists are in an extended position. Constantly bringing the student to specific points of focus prevents mindless habitualization where they vacantly go through the motions of an exercise, and helps develop a heightened state of internal awareness and correct breathing.

Fixing the visual focus on the teacher's eyes during weapons training continues the development of one-point focus. Achuttan Gurukkal explained, 'We should never take our eyes from those of our opponent. By ekagrata here I mean *kannottam*, keeping the eyes on the opponent's. When doing practice you should not see anything else going on around you.'

Achuttan Gurukkal's observation mirrors Drona's test of skill administered to his pupils at the end of their course of training in the *Mahabharata*. He asked each prince in turn to take aim with their bow and arrow at an artificial bird attached to a treetop 'where it was hardly visible'. He asked each, when he had drawn the bow and taken aim, whether 'you see the bird in the treetop . . . the tree or me, or your brothers?' to which all but Arjuna replied, 'Yes' (van Buitenen Vol. I, 1973: 272–3). All but Arjuna failed. He was the only practitioner who answered 'no' to all but the first question. He did not 'see anything else going on around' him–he and the target were one.

Masters have numerous practical techniques to further develop one point. During spear practice, students practise thrusts and swings by knocking a tiny matchbox off an upright mace placed at the opposite end of the kalari. During practice of the long-staff, C. Mohammed Sherif explains that the verbal command '*cherna*' literally means 'join', and is intended to 'call the practitioner's attention back to a specific point of focus', i.e. to 'join' with the opponent.

Given the fact that weapons are taught repetitiously as set-form sequences, there is a natural tendency for students to simply 'go through the motions' and *not* 'join' or meet the master's focus and internal energy with their own. One of the most effective ways of getting the student into concentrated single-point focus is for the teacher to simply attack a different vital spot. This usually 'wakes' the student up, and is followed by a verbal admonition such as 'look here', i.e. *really* look into the teacher's eyes, and see precisely where and when to defend against an attack.

DEVELOPING CORRECT FORM AND BREATH CONTROL

In hatha yoga, the practitioner must first be able to assume the basic forms or postures (asana). For the kalarippayattu practitioner, comparable to asana are preliminary leg exercises and *vativu*. Assuming an asana or moving into and out of a vativu, the structural physical body of bones and muscles maintains alignment so that the breath is controlled or 'stopped'. The spinal column is the central axis of the physical body, which must be kept in correct alignment even in vigorous movement.[100]

When a practitioner learns to assume the 'correct position', moving into that position is understood to make the wind course through the body, controlling and harmonizing it. *Siva Samhita* (III.90) states, 'by performing and practising this posture (*padmasana*), undoubtedly the vital airs of the practitioner at once become completely equable, and flow harmoniously through the body' (Vasu 1975: 39). Certain poses are considered important in developing control of the breath and the wind humour. In the *Siva Samhita* (III.96) assuming *svatiskasana* is understood to bring 'regulation of the air . . . he obtains *vayu siddhi*' and thereby becomes accomplished in controlling the wind or breath (Vasu 1975: 40).

Each pose/form has its own limits which circumscribe and precisely define how it should be performed. K. Achuthan Gurukkal stresses that 'correct practice also means breathing naturally and therefore having the breath properly coordinated with performing the exercise or pose'. Correct breathing is understood to develop naturally over months of practice. Neelakanthan Namboodiripad told me that while doing all the preliminary exercises, breathing 'should be automatic and effortless, which comes from continuous practice. Inhalation and exhalation should be the maximum possible, but there is no retention'. Teachers tell their students to 'breathe through the nose; don't open your mouth'. Keeping the mouth closed, the hands raised, and the spinal column firm in its natural alignment during leg exercises forces the student to begin to develop deep diaphragmatic breathing from the navel region and is intended to prevent the tendency to take shallow breaths from the chest. As Kallada Balakrishnan explained,

'When the straight kick is done fully and correctly and the foot touches the hand above the head, there is correct breathing.'

In addition to the natural coordination of breath with exercise, some masters also practise special breath control techniques understood to help activate and circulate the practitioner's 'internal energy' or prana vayu, thus filling out each form or pose. There are two types of special exercises: (1) yogic pranayama which require repetition of the fourfold pattern of *puraka* (inhalation), *kumbhaka* (retention), and *rejaka* (exhalation), retention/pause, and (2) special kalarippayattu breathing exercises, often called *swasam*, which require continuous deep inhalation and exhalation without retention or pause.

One Christian master teaches a special form of pranayama called *bhramanapranayamam* in which the breath is coordinated with *cuvadu*. Strength is developed through repetition of the usual pattern prior to and after body exercises, and for bare-hand techniques. For him 'breath control exercises are superior to all other forms of exercise. The vital energy (prana-vayu), mind, intellect and *balam* are all closely related'. Neelakanthan Namboodiripad says that practising pranayama leads to 'control over the mind as well as the body's metabolic functions' and therefore to correct martial practice. Narayanan Nayar told me that practising pranayama brings 'concentration', and eventually 'air strength' (*vayubalam*), identical with the manifestation of sakti itself.

Simple *swasam* are practised 'to gain balam and power (sakti)'. Haji N.M. Kutty practises thirty-three different exercises, while Mohammedunni Gurukkal practises twelve. Both emphasize deep inhalation/exhalation to develop what Mohammedunni calls 'wind power' (*vayusakti*) 'so that I will have firm steps and for application (in combat)'. When performing these exercises, 'your mind is simply on what you are doing. There is a grip or power in the stomach at the full point of inhalation'. Haji N.M. Kutty explained the practical application to fighting: '. . . especially arm movements for specific offensive or defensive reasons, the breath may be held or retained for control. Exhalation accompanies an attack, with the sound of the breath coming out strongly.'

Mohammedunni Gurukkal explained how the strength of retention below the navel allows one 'not to be injured there . . . if an attack comes here'. Neelakanthan Namboodiripad has a similar interpretation: 'In pranayama there are two retentions, one after inhalation and one after exhalation. The one after exhalation is not strong. Therefore when you give a blow it comes with exhalation. But strong defence comes with inhalation.'

During vigorous practice deep breathing is coordinated with strenuous exercise. One of the most important signs of correct practice and internal coordination of breath is when there is a 'gripping' (*piduttam*) which comes naturally to specific places (*sthanam*) of the body, especially below the navel. This is where the *kacca* is wrapped in order to provide firm support in the abdominal region, and to 'hold in' the life force (Figure 2.1).

As both posture and breath are controlled, the physical and subtle bodies maintain the alignment necessary for quietening and balancing the three humours *and* for purification of the nadi. The channels are ordinarily thought to be clogged and impure, part of one's encasement in a state of illusion (maya). As *Hatha-yoga-pradipika* (II.21) states,

> When the *nadi* are impure, breath cannot penetrate into the *susumna*. Then the yogi achieves nothing, nor can he reach the state of deep concentration . . . Only when all the *nadi* which are still impure are purified can the yogi practise *pranayama* successfully (Reiker 1971: 73).

Simply mimicking an external form during practice is not enough to attain inner actualization or awakening. Gurukkal Govindankutty Nayar explained:

> Almost all practice you see is partial. It is not complete. Even with advanced students practising, their form may be good and correct in (external) form, but it is still lacking something. It is lacking that spark or life (*jivana*) that makes this a real and full practice. They do not yet have the soul of the form.

The external form remains empty, 'life-less', and a mere shell if the internal wind or energy, or the 'soul' of the form, is not manifest. The internal 'life', 'spark', or 'soul' of the form is the degree to which the practitioner activates and circulates the energy (prana-vayu) and awakens power (sakti).

THE INTERRELATIONSHIP OF THE GROSS AND SUBTLE BODIES IN PRACTICE: RAISING THE VITAL ENERGY (PRANA-VAYU) AND POWER (SAKTI)

The wind, breath or vital energy (vayu, prana or prana-vayu) is conceptually and practically the link between the physical and subtle bodies. Filliozat (1964: 185) traces both the organic sense of breath and the association between wind and breath from the period of the Vedas through the classical Ayurveda of Susruta and Caraka and the psycho-physiology of yoga. As early as the Vedas breath (prana) and wind (vayu or vata, from Indo-Iranian pre-history 'the principle of activity') were assimilated to each other (ibid.: 184). The technical vocabulary of the Vedic texts was later developed into a full 'system of pneumatic cosmo-physiology' in which the animating power of wind took the shape of breath (prana) or atman (ibid.: 65–6). The *Atharvaveda* affirmed the identity of breath and wind; 'it is the wind which is called the breath; it is on the breath that all that was and all this is, all is based' (ibid.: 64–5).

The natural form that the wind humour took in classical Ayurvedic texts was its form in nature as wind or breath. Filliozat notes that all three major classical texts of medicine are 'unanimous in making the wind as the soul of the world and of the body' (ibid.: 218). Wind spreads throughout the body and is responsible for all activity, just as atmospheric wind is thought to be responsible for all natural activity. Within the physical body, specific activities are identified with specific forms of wind or breath. The *Susruta Samhita* (*Nidanasthanan* I.7–12) recorded the winds as (1) prana, 'the breath of the front' located in the mouth and ensuring respiration; (2) *udana*, 'the breath on high, superior wind, goes upward' and producing sound; (3) *samana*, 'the concentrated breath' which circulates in the stomach and intestines for digestion; (4) *vyana*, 'the diffused breath' which circulates throughout the limbs of the body making possible perspiration, blood flow, etc.; and (5) *apana*, 'the breath below' which has a downward action or tendency and makes possible excretion and birth (Filliozat 1964: 210–11). Although prana is one of the five specific winds, the term is also used generically to refer to any type of wind activity within the body, whatever its specific form. In this more general sense, prana or the compound prana-vayu refers not just to breath, but to breath-as-life, or the essential vital energy of life itself. 'Who am I? My hands, legs, nose, etc.? Who am I? My hands, legs, breast? That, all of these, is prana. Just to close your eyes—that is one prana. Yawning is another prana. Therefore, life itself (*jivana*) is prana.'

This equation of wind as vital energy (prana) with life itself (jivana) was made by many masters. Another defined prana as 'the vayu which rules the body as a whole. Prana is the controlling power of all parts of the body. Vayu is not just air, but one sakti (power). That is what rules us completely. Prana means jivana, "life," individual soul.'

Although the classical Ayurvedic texts do not give a precise physical account of action of wind within the organism (Filliozat 1964: 204), the later Tantras and Yogas do describe the action of wind in the subtle body. At the same time they accept the Ayurvedic understanding of the wind humour, and the notion of specific organic winds. Just as wind is the source of cosmic, natural and organic activity, it is the source of activity within the subtle body. In the midst of its discussion of techniques of breath control, *Yoga Darsana Upanisad* (IV.23–IV.34) lists the ten organic prana and describes the five most important ones (Varenne 1976, passim).

Some masters' texts describe these five or ten winds. The same Muslim master's text quoted above also describes ten organic winds as 'controlling the working of the human body, the most important of which is prana-vayu'. Another master's text identifies five organic winds: 'The direction of apana is downward so that weight is increased. Prana and upana have an upward tendency. And samana and vyana help circulation throughout the body.'

Figure 5.1 diagrams the conceptual and practical role that wind, breath or vital energy plays in relating the physical and subtle bodies. By controlling the downward action of inspiration (apana) and the upward action of

Fig. 5.1: *The Mediating Action of Vital Energy.*

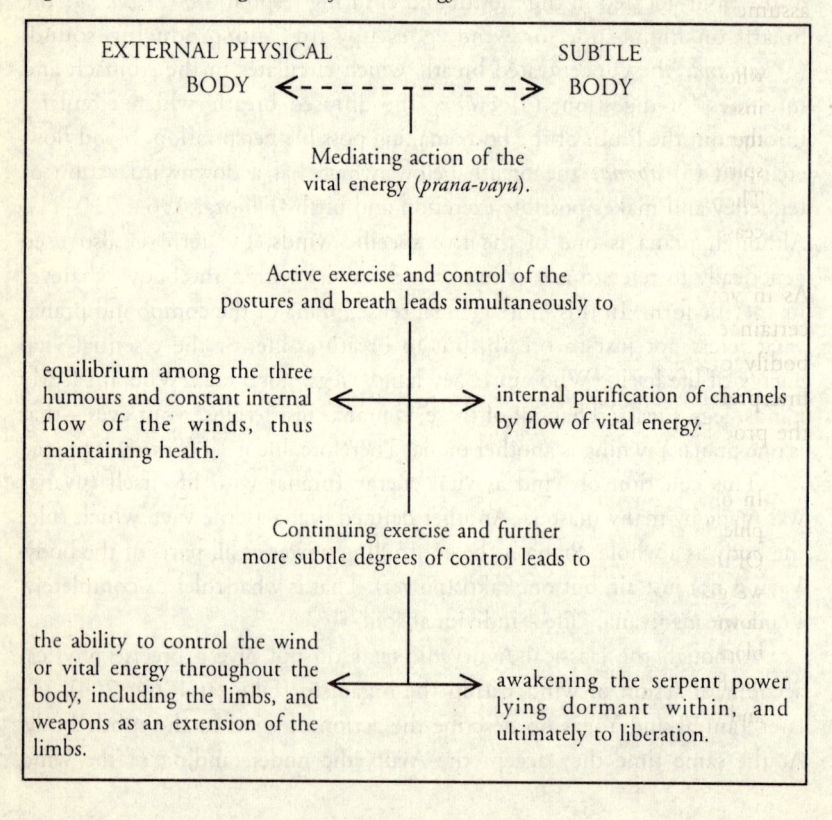

```
        EXTERNAL PHYSICAL                      SUBTLE
              BODY        <----------->        BODY
                                |
                   Mediating action of the
                   vital energy (prana-vayu).
                                |
              Active exercise and control of the
         postures and breath leads simultaneously to

  equilibrium among the three                 internal purification of channels
  humours and constant internal  <----->      by flow of vital energy.
  flow of the winds, thus
  maintaining health.
                                |
                  Continuing exercise and further
              more subtle degrees of control leads to

  the ability to control the wind
  or vital energy throughout the               awakening the serpent power
  body, including the limbs, and  <----->      lying dormant within, and
  weapons as an extension of the               ultimately to liberation.
  limbs.
```

expiration (prana) the practitioner simultaneously quiets and balances the three humours, purifies the channels of the subtle body, controls the movement of vital energy throughout the physical and subtle bodies, and develops control of his mind in single-point concentration (see Gupta *et. al.* 1979). As Gupta *et. al.* explain,

> *prana* in the generic sense is the cause of the particular breaths, and they in turn are the cause of the mind. Therefore control over the one leads to control over the other two. All are normally unruly, but by controlling the breaths the yogin calms down and controls the whole complex (1979: 168).

In kundalini yoga, control of wind eventually leads the practitioner to awaken the serpent power (kundalini) understood to lie sleeping and dormant. *Siva Samhita* explains that by controlling the downward wind the susumna-nadi is forced to open, thus awakening kundalini lying within. Once awakened she is raised through each succeeding centre until she breaks through to assume her place on top of the last centre:

> where the Cosmic Energy—the aggregate of all Kundalinis—resides in inseparable union with Parama Siva (Brahman, the Supreme Reality), and there merging her with the Cosmic Energy, the yogin is able to obtain spiritual release from bondage of this world and everything worldly ... The yogin's conscious identification of his self with his gross physical body ceases (ibid.: 171, 176).

As in yoga practice some martial masters assume that, when performing certain exercises like the 'cat' pose, the internal energy is controlled and bodily orifices are 'locked'.[101] This leads to manifestation of sakti, often interpreted as kundalini or serpent power. P.K. Balan Gurukkal described the process:

> In order to attain sakti for the body, you do the following: the wind, phlegm and fire are coordinated jointly and blocked (through exercise). Of these three the wind humour is most important. By controlling wind we get extra power. The body will become 'airtight'. If you block the downward trend of prana you will create an upward trend. We create this block by 'gripping' and through use of the *kacca*. The effect (of these methods) is the same as with pranayama developed through self-control and concentration.

When practising some techniques, the master momentarily stops or holds the wind in specific places (*sthanam* or *adharam*) of the body. Vasu Gurukkal practises a form of *brahmanaka pranayama* where he assumes kalarippayattu 'cat' pose, thereby 'locking' the anal and other orifices where his recitation of aum moves. In Gurukkal Govindankutty Nayar's practice, the wind is stopped in the navel region (corresponding to *svadisthanam cakram*) when performing the lion pose; in the throat (corresponding to *visuddhicakram*) when performing the horse pose; in the chest (corresponding to *anahatam cakram*) and navel when performing a jumping kick; between the anus and penis (corresponding to *muladharam cakram*) when performing the cat pose, etc.

A specific example of circulation and stoppage of the wind is the lion pose (*simhavadivu*) as interpreted by Gurukkal Govindankutty Nayar and Achuthan Gurukkal. For these masters there is a lower limit to the lion pose—if the student squats too low without keeping the spinal column aligned and without a firm grip in the navel region, the lower limit of the form will be 'broken' and it will lose its potential power. Figures 5.2–5.4 provide a record of what both these masters consider to be 'correct form'.

Figure 5.2 (a) With the hands/arms crossed over the chest and 'ready', the movement originates in the 'centre' at the navel—the leg is kicked up,

Figure 5.2: *The 'correct' way to perform the 'lion pose'* (simhavadivu).

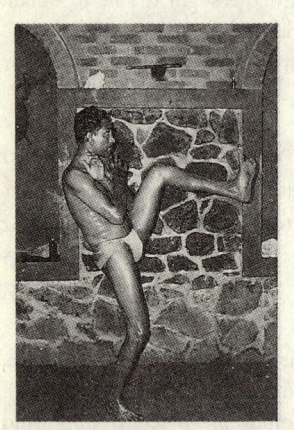

(a) With the hands/arms crossed over the chest and 'ready', the movement originates in the 'centre' at the nabhi mula: the leg is kicked up, energy flows from the centre out through the knee and up through the foot as it extends up...

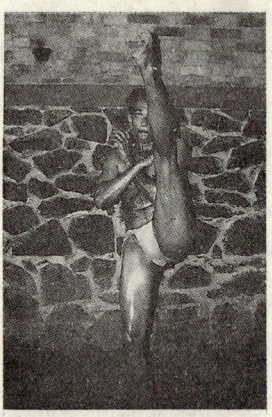

(b) to forehead level with the big toe extended.

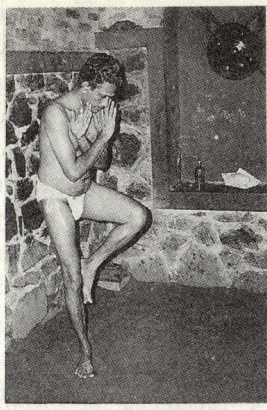

(c) The leg descends along the line of the body, the energy flow returning to the centre as the leg descends.

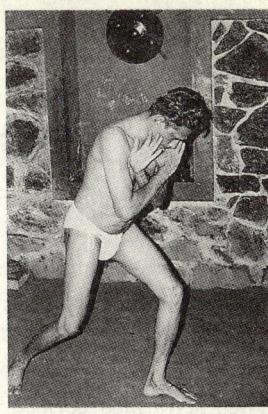

(d) The natural extension of the descent of the leg is a forward step in which the foot is firmly planted.

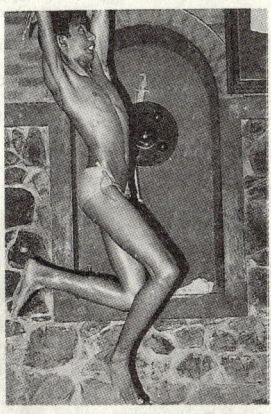

(e) The firmly planted foot provides the base for a jump, executed off the forward foot, as the hands extend behind the body, thus making the jump a total body movement, again originating from the centre.

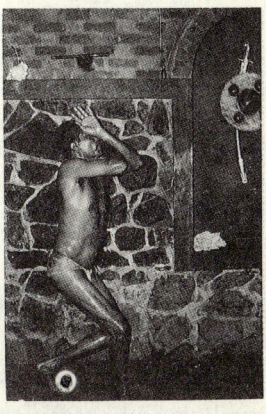

(f) Landing from the jump the energy is recycled and drawn into the centre as …

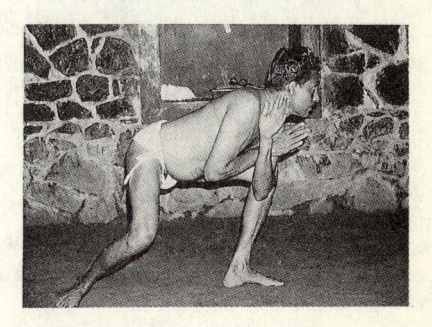

(g) the final position is assumed with the hands in front of the chest, in the 'lion' pose.

prana-vayu flowing up from the navel out through the knee and through the foot as it extends upward . . .(b) to the forehead level with the big toe extended. (c) The leg descends down the stationary leg along the line of the body, the energy flow returning to the navel region as the leg descends. (d) The natural extension of the descent of the leg is a forward step in which the foot is firmly planted on the earth. (e) The firmly planted foot provides the base for a jump, executed as the weight is taken on the forward foot, as the hands extend behind the body, and supported by the navel/hip region. (f) Landing from the jump the energy is recycled and drawn into the navel region as . . .(g) the final position is assumed with the hands in front of the chest, in the 'lion' pose.

When performed 'correctly' the spine has a firm and natural alignment. The spine must never collapse or the shoulders round, as often happens when beginning students try to assume the pose and 'push' the leg upward as they kick. Achuthan Gurukkal explained his understanding of how power is raised in the pose:

> When a student does the lion pose . . . if the left foot is simply placed forward into the step without bringing it correctly to here (indicating the navel) and then drawing it down along the body, there will be no power in the step. But if it is done with correct way (as described above), if it is done this 'scientific way', then there is sakti.[102]

Throughout the exercise there is a natural 'gripping' (*piduttam*) at the *nabhi mula*. One master's text records the following: 'When doing the action stay firmly in the *vadivu*, planting the foot in this position, holding the breath firmly in the *nabhi mula* (thus) raising to life (your) balam.'[103] The 'grip' is a physical, muscular sensation in the region just below the navel which is simultaneous with a 'stopping' of the wind/breath in that place as the pose concludes. While performing the entire pose, the air is not only 'in' that one place, it simultaneously spreads throughout the body and is manifest in the hands which are 'ready' to attack or defend from their place at the chest, and in the extension and return of the leg/foot/toe in the forceful kick which might be directed towards an opponent's vital spot.

Sakti as well as balam are manifest in the dynamic quality of oppositional energy in the pose, i.e. as the practitioner moves into the final position (Figures 5.3–5.4), the gripping in the navel region is experienced and manifest as an oppositional set of forces—outward and forward from the navel along the spinal column, continuing out through the arms/hands and

Figure 5.3: The flow of energy and movement in the lion pose: a summary of Figures 5.2 (a-g).

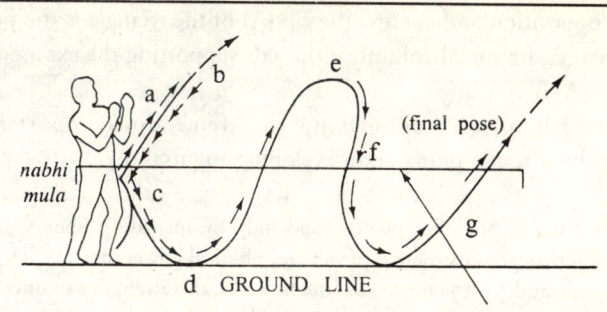

nabhi mula

(final pose)

d GROUND LINE

the constant centre to which and from which movement and energy returns and originates

Letters a-g indicate the photos in Figure 5.2.

The arrows indicate the direction in which the internal energy flows.

- - -> indicates the flow of energy beyond the body—the extended energy constitutes an offensive move (the kick with the big toe at the peak or a defensive posture of strength in the 'final' pose (g). Even the 'final' pose is a position poised for an ongoing offensive attack or defensive move.

—> indicates the flow of energy from and back to the 'centre' in the navel region.

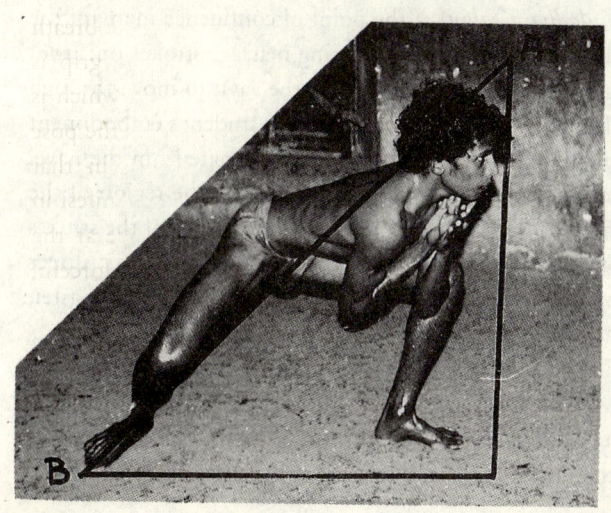

Figure 5.4: The oppositional flow of energy in the final position of the lion pose. This opposition creates the triangle which is the solid base and source of strength of the lion pose. Note also that the central axis of the spine follows the long line of the triangle.

eyes; backward along the same line to the earth. The body forms a solid triangle (Figure 5.4): the base of the triangle (B) is the ground point of downward opposition and energy; the tip (A) of the triangle is the point of outward energy; the spinal column is the axis supporting the exposed tip of the triangle (A–B).

A Christian master summed up the tremendous importance of controlling the internal prana and developing vayu-sakti:

> It is the basis of all other powers, and only by increasing one's wind-power will that person's mental power and physical power increase. These *cuvatu, nila,* and *prayogam* need *balam*; however, this strength can only be acquired when one has control of the vital energy. Only by taking the breath in and retaining it under the *nabhi* can the practitioner spread the 'special' power situated in the inner parts through the external organs.

As the master controls the vital energy, he is able to use that energy positively as he administers therapeutic massage. He channels the appropriate degree of power into each stroke, and his own vital energy and/or power are transmitted directly through the palm, foot or forearm into the student/patient's body, thereby stimulating the internal wind of the student, or quieting the enraged wind humour when giving a massage as a treatment.

The special kalarippayattu massage is also understood to not only affect the humoral balance and alignment of the body, but affect the subtle body as well. According to a number of masters, the full-body massage originates and terminates at the small of the back opposite the navel region (corresponding to *muladhara-cakra*) at the point of confluence many of the major channels of the subtle body. Administering massage strokes out from and back to this region stimulates and circulates the vayu to move through the nadi of the subtle body, and thereby enhances the student's embodiment of correct form through which strength and power emanate from the navel region. The massage process begins by slowly stimulating the region of the small of the back, and hips (Figure 4.1). Gradually the patterns of the strokes extend outward from the navel region through the limbs (the legs, upper torso, arms). The internal wind, stimulated and manipulated by the master, is circulated as it should be during exercise.

Gurukkal Govindankutty Nayar explained that the full body massage concludes at the small of the back with a strong slap delivered with the right palm in the depression between the hips in order to 'awaken the vital energy and all the channels which originate here'. Similarly, in the midst of the massage, to complete strokes to the face and head, a firm slap is delivered directly to the top of the head where *sahasrara-cakra* is located to 'awaken the senses' (Figure 5.5). The master transmits his own vital energy into the student, implanting correct form in physical and subtle bodies, and awakening and raising kundalini sakti.

THE GODDESS (SAKTI), JOINING SIVA-SAKTI, AND THE ACTUALIZATION OF 'POWER' IN PRACTICE

For kalarippayattu masters who still interpret this wind-power as kundalini sakti, its awakening *within the bodymind* is that state of actualization toward which the entire process of training leads. Certain body exercise sequences are practised to help achieve this inner awakening of sakti and the joining of Siva/Sakti. Both *puttara tolil* and *kalari vanakkam* are understood to help raise kundalini sakti and internally join Siva and Sakti. Both sequences are performed toward the *puttara* in the south-west corner and include the embodied connection of a series of poses/prostrations which psycho-physiologically increase circulation of the internal energy.

As discussed in Chapter 3, the south-west corner of the kalari is associated with the goddess as Sakti, and the diagonally opposite north-east corner is associated with Siva. Many masters interpret the seven steps of the *puttara* as the seven *mahanadi* (great internal circuits through which the vital energy or sakti travels), or the seven cakra or adhara important in meditation. Kallada Balakrishnan gave the following interpretation:

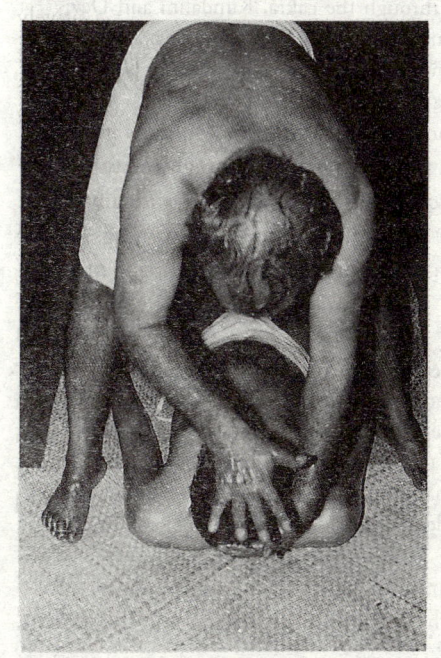

Figure 5.5: Sreejayan Gurukkal applies a firm slap with the palm to the top of the head where sahasrara cakra *is located to 'awaken the senses'.*

The first six tiers of the puttara are the six adharam or cakra, while the seven is Siva. The seventh cakra is at the top of the puttara. All siddhi is located at the top of the head. Correct breathing and correct practice of exercises alone will raise the kundalini from the muladharam up through all the cakra to the top.

Yogis pump this energy up by sitting and through meditation, but in kalarippayattu this comes by correct breathing and kalarippayattu exercises. The master never explains this to the student, but he will see in the student the raising of the kundalini through the cakra.

Nilakantha Namboodiripad explained his interpretation of performing the puttara tolil:

In doing the puttara tolil we are before Devi or Sakti, and in this action (when the hands come forward and outward from the region of the navel) we are moving the kundalini up through the cakra. Kundalini and Devi are the same. This action of the arms going out is called bodhaka mudra (the 'awakening' or 'arousing' movement). It is also in yoga and puja.

The hands are shaped like the hood of a cobra, and literally trace the movement of kundalini sakti from muladhara cakra through the top of the head. The difficult-to-attain physical positions of the body literally create an internal sensation of vibration through rotations and turnings of the torso as it moves from one position to another. Kallada Balakrishnan gave a similar explanation:

In the kalari the two corners represent Sakti and Devi (in the south-west) and Siva on the opposite side (north-east). In this action (when the body turns under 180 degrees while performing the serpent pose from south-west to north-east, or north-east to south-west), there is a joining of the two. We are all *ardanariswara*, 'half-man and half-woman'. This act is a joining of male and female, inside and outside.

Through this exercise in particular, sakti as kundalini is raised, Siva/Sakti are literally embodied, and ideally there is an inner awakening in the student. As one master explained to me:

The guru does not explain the centres or serpent power to the student, but he observes the changes in the student which come automatically through correct practice. He is observing the effect of the raising of the serpent power even though the student is not aware of it. He may all of a sudden see a noticeable change in the student. Everyone will not reach this stage, but if one does, whatever the student does will be in correct form.

Some of the traditional signs of the presence of sakti are the relative 'heaviness' with which a blow or cut is delivered to a vital spot, or the sensitivity of the hands and feet as the internal energy is used to apply the correct amount of pressure in massage. Once experienced and awakened, single-point focus and the power of kundalini can be further developed and refined through a variety of meditation and magico-religious techniques.

SUBTLER POWERS OF PRACTICE: MEDITATION AND MANTRAM

Kalarippayattu masters also practise a variety of meditation techniques to enhance their devotional life as well as develop subtler powers. Most important are stationary meditation and repetition of mantram. Practitioners learn these techniques from kalarippayattu teachers, yoga masters or wandering holy men. Some masters organize and conceptualize their experience around the conventional progression of classical yoga from ekagrata to more subtle, refined and stationary levels of meditation, i.e. to dharana and eventually dhyana where the 'object' of meditation (the deity, etc.) is transcended and a more complete state of non-duality is experienced. Whether this conventional identification is made or not, for the martial practitioner, achieving these higher/deeper states of internalization is both an end in itself—ideally leading to transcendence, enlightenment or union with Allah—*and* a means to an end, i.e. attaining the 'mental courage and power' through which the martial artist 'conquers' himself, i.e. his fears, anxieties, and doubts, and also gains access to specific and more subtle forms of sakti in martial applications.

Gurukkal Govindankutty Nayar performs simple meditation 'to increase my powers of concentration and the ability to consciously control my mind'. What differentiates a student from a teacher is that a master 'must follow a strict routine. One must have regular *nistha* (a standard set of ritual/ behavioural observances) that he follows each day of his life'. In this view, personal disciplines are a natural extension of daily practice of kalarippayattu, and the effects of both are closely linked.

Although the particular observances vary, one common form is *vratam*— simply sitting in an appropriately quiet part of one's house, and focusing one's mind on a deity through repetition of the deity's name. Performing vratam 'is always associated with sincere action where one's mental state itself is involved' (Moore 1983: 342). A similar form of a simple meditation is to simply 'sit in a relaxed position, with your back firmly supported in a natural position. In this position, listen to your breathing. You should do this five to ten minutes each day.' Once a student begins to manifest single-point focus in his practice, some masters teach specific forms of more advanced meditation, *dharana*, like the following:

> facing the puttara in the south-west corner, the student assumes the cat pose. Staying in that pose the student repeats all the verbal commands for the body exercise sequences one after another in his mind while maintaining long, deep, sustained breathing.

A similar but more advanced form is to mentally repeat the weapons forms, allowing the 'sounds of the weapons to fill your ears'. In these stationary forms, what is most important is that 'the mental eye visualize the self in exercise' so that all sounds are 'shut out except the sound of the self in exercise'. Repetition of these exercises is understood to lead to dharana, a state this master interpreted as continuous with, but 'higher' than one-point concentration.[104] It is 'higher' because it is both a more difficult, and more subtle form of exercise which leads to a heightened state of 'mental concentration'. This master went on to describe the effect:

> I can do these now, sitting here, in my mind, and I will begin to perspire. By doing *meiabhyasa* (body art) it is not just an external form, but internal as well, affecting the body's inner channels, and all parts physically. If you do these mental repetitions it will have the same effect as doing it physically. So at a certain point you can do these by mental repetitions all your life and it will produce energy or heightened awareness.

For this master, the highest level of practice is dhyana in which he fixes his mind on his personal deity:

> I sit in a relaxed position with a relaxed mind, and think about god according to my own belief. Slowly, with the help of my breathing, I concentrate on the deity in my mind. Gradually, an image of the deity forms in my mind. When I get the image of the deity in my mind, and am able to maintain it daily through practice, I gain mental courage and power.
>
> Then if I ever need this power, I take the image of the deity in my mind and from my repetitions of the meditation on that image, the power of the deity moves me automatically and allows me to be a conduit for this power in practice of the martial art.

Ubiquitous to Hinduism from as early as the Vedas and to all aspects of kalarippayattu, are repetition of mantram. Usually taking the form of a series of sacred words and/or syllables which may or may not be 'translatable', mantram are 'instruments of power' (Alper 1989: 6). As Andre Padoux explains in terms relevant to martial arts practice,

> Mantras rank among the courses of action men have devised to satisfy a deep urge within them to overstep their limits, to be all powerful and all knowing, a dream of omnipotence. There also is the wish to be free from fear, to fill the void men feel surrounds them. Hence, the magical words. Hence, mantras (1989: 315).

Harvey P. Alper describes a mantram as

> a tool designed for a particular task, which will achieve a particular end when, and only when, it is used in a particular manner. Mantras, according to this view, are as distinct from each other as are hammers from screwdrivers. More critically, they are taken to be as distinct from each other as are individuals (1989: 6).

In this sense, kalarippayattu practitioners traditionally possessed what might be called a 'tool box' of mantram—a collection of mantram each with a specific purpose including:

(1) worship/puja specific to a particular deity;
(2) personal mantram given by one's master according to the character of the student;
(3) vadivu mantram to gain superior power and actualization of a particular kalarippayattu techniques, especially its vativu;
(4) weapons/combat mantram to gain accomplishment in the use of a particular weapon or technique in the practice of a weapon;
(5) general all-purpose mantram to gain access to 'higher' powers generally, to be used to enhance the power of any technique of attack or defence;
(6) medical/healing mantram, i.e. a variety of specific mantram to be repeated prior to giving a particular treatment or preparing/cooking a recipe for medicine as part of achieving its efficacious healing effect.

Some of these are collections of sacred syllables, while others are a kind of prayer for a specific result or power.

Like most mantram, kalarippayattu mantram are traditionally given to a student by a master as *upadesham*. Mantram are secret, and like the vital spots, are revealed only to most trusted disciples. One master said, 'These higher studies are meant for a person who wants to become a master, and are only for the person who will take the great pains necessary to learn these techniques'. When taught, the student is told never to reveal the mantram since to reveal it would 'spoil the power of the *mantram*. Its *siddhi* (accomplishment through repetition) will be lost if it is ever revealed.' When concealed, it 'preserves the power of the mantram'. In fact, concealing a mantram over time is understood to increase the power of the mantram.

(For a mantram to be useful as a tool to achieve the desired result, it must be brought to accomplishment by repeating it by the required number of times.) The repetitions must never be performed perfunctorily, and therefore also serve to focus the practitioner's attention. Since each mantram 'has its own specific methods' followed in bringing it to accomplishment, they differ in precise number of repetitions, whether restraints must be followed, whether they are repeated aloud or silently, the number of syllables in the mantram and its degree of complexity, and whether special mudra are performed.

For example, before giving a personal mantram to 'guide that student's future', one master requires the student to bathe and abstain from sex, and while repeating the mantram to perform nyasa, i.e. touching various parts of his body in order to invest them with power or energy. Nyasa includes the use of mudra, recitation of the mantram through the various limbs of the body, repetition through the entire body beginning at the head and reaching the feet (*dyanamantram*), and imagining god from head to feet. Once received, this personal mantram must be recited daily the required number of times throughout one's life to maintain its power. According to this master, the result of attaining accomplishment in a personal mantram is that 'it increases the power of your mind; it strengthens the mind' through which 'one gains personal devotion, self-confidence and the complete eradication of fear'.

Vadivu Mantram

Vadivu mantram are specific to particular kalarippayattu poses—full power is attained when a practitioner is accomplished in the particular mantram associated with that pose. One master learned vadivu mantram particular to four of the eight poses he practises including (1) *Ganapadimantram* for bringing the elephant pose to accomplishment; (2) *Narasimhamantram* (the lion incarnation of Lord Visnu) for bringing the lion pose to accomplishment; (3) *asuarudammantram* (the 'good/right' goddess on horseback) for bringing the horse pose to accomplishment; and (4) *varahamurtimantram* (the wild boar incarnation of Lord Visnu) for bringing the wild boar pose to accomplishment. When taught, each of the four mula-mantram of the particular deity is given individually and brought to accomplishment in the pose. This master explained:

> Each root mantram must be repeated lakhs of times to gain accomplishment. For example, Rama has two syllables. If that were the root mantram for a pose, you would have to repeat Rama two lakh times. Narayana has four syllables. If that were the root mantram you would have to repeat it four lakh times. Root mantram are not long like some other kalarippayattu mantram. They are usually between one and ten syllables. If you are reciting Narayana ten thousand times each day, in ten days you can recite one lakh times, and within forty days four lakh times. After reciting it four lakh times you have brought accomplishment on that mantram.

When reciting a root mantram it is sometimes necessary to move the specific place of recitation within the body. For example, a mantram like Narayana moves through the fingers, then to the *nabhi*, heart (*hrydayam*), tongue and top of the head. Unlike personal *mantram* which must be repeated daily to continue to have their power, once a *vadivu mantram* is brought to accomplishment the practitioner only need 'take it in his mind' when he needs access to its power.

> When you stay or move into a particular pose, that particular mantram will come to your mind. This will give power (sakti) to the mind also, and put your feet firmly in that position, use your breath according to that and then recite the mantram and the pose will be one-hundred per cent successful.

The practical result is that 'you will be so firm (in that pose) that an elephant won't be able to move you'. Although the mantram is the final key to unlocking and giving the practitioner access to the full power of a specific pose and therefore must have been practised by nearly all masters in the past, very few of today's masters learn, use or teach these practical martial mantram.

Specific Weapons/Combat Mantram

These mantram allow the practitioner to gain access to the power of a specific weapon, or technique in manipulation of a weapon. Like vadivu mantram, in the past when the practitioner's life depended on gaining access to the full power of a technique or weapon, weapons mantram must have been commonplace. Since kalarippayattu weapons are seldom if ever used in life-or-death situations today, very few masters practise these mantram although some cite examples they learned or from their texts. One master's manuscript records that in 'leopard fight' (*puliankappayattu*) with sword and shield, after the two opponents salute one another, 'and after saluting the spirits of the old masters, take in your mind the goddess Kali. Taking the sword and shield, touch them, and after saluting them adopt an heroic attitude. Give salutations to Lord Siva.'

At particular points in the verbal commands, the manuscript records mantram to be recalled prior to a particular blow, thereby infusing that strike with 'full power'. Another master traditionally practised five different mantram to be used in fighting:

(1) *Sivakkaruttumantram,* when the encounter was mild.
(2) *Bhadrakalimulamantram,* when the encounter was angry or heated.
(3) *Hanumanmulamantram,* when jumping to attack or to defend.
(4) *Virabhadramulamantram,* only when it was necessary to vanquish and kill an opponent.
(5) *Pasupadam* (Siva's) *mantram,* to 'charm a weapon'.

General Mantram

More typical today are masters who practise general, all-purpose mantram understood to access 'higher powers' rather than powers specific to a technique or weapon. One master practises four mantram associated with each major deity propitiated in his kalari—Bhagavati, Hanuman, Ganapadi and past gurus. For this master guru mantram is most important:

> It is chanted in the mind before teaching any weapon. It is repeated before performing any item in class, or in a demonstration. Only by repetition of this mantram will the blows have their full force and power. It must be repeated if you want to do anything with combat application (ayudha prayogam) or to avoid injury.

Some kalarippayattu mantram are even more generic. Vasu Gurukkal practises brahymanaka pranayama—a form of breath control in which the breath moves to different places in the body. He coordinates repetition of the root mantram ('aum') with breathing and performance of special mudra (Figure 5.6).[105] For this the student undergoes bodily purifications and practises restraints, ritually enters the kalari, and participates as the master

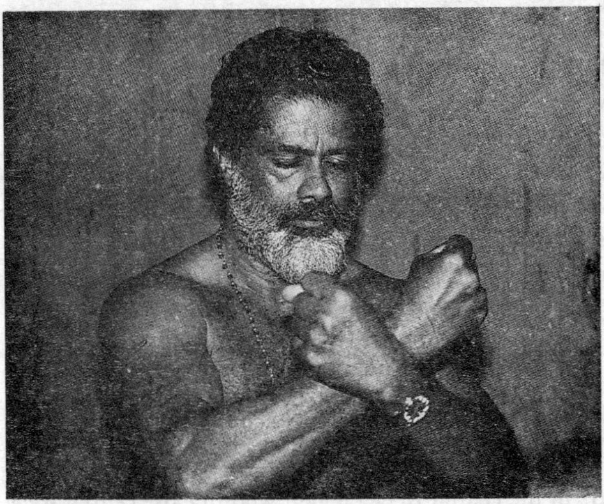

Figure 5.6: Vasu Gurukkal performs brahyamanaka pranayama *in which he moves the breath through various parts of the body while repeating the root mantram 'aum' and performing* vira *(the heroic) mudra with his hands.*

gives special offers to the kalari deities. The student assumes the cat pose (*panditamarman*), facing the south-west corner and the puttara where the guardian deity is located.

> In the cat pose with the right heel tucked under, touching the anus (thereby closing off this cavity), inhale with the back straight. This is *mulabandam* ('root' or 'source' posture—referring to the place between the genitals and anus). On inhalation the nabhi area tightens. As you exhale, make the sound, 'ahhhh'. (The continuous 'ahhh' sound keeps the navel tight through the entire exhalation.)
>
> Next, move through *uddiyanabandam* (the 'great flying bird' position) by breathing in slowly, and on exhalation sounding the second syllable, 'oooooo'—the sound resonating in the heart (hrdayam, i.e. chest) (as the diaphragm 'flies upward' pushing the breath up from the lower abdomen).
>
> Third, as you move through *jalandrabandam* (the 'net' or 'web' position) in which the chin rests on the chest (between the two collarbones), take the breath in slowly and on exhalation sound 'hummmmm' in the throat (*kandam*).
>
> On the next inhalation, take the breath in slowly, and now complete all three together on exhalation as a sounding of 'ahhh-oooo-mmmm'.

Simultaneously, the practitioner performs the vira mudra ('the heroic' or 'courageous' hand postures).

> The thumbs are joined slowly on the in breath. On exhalation the thumbs are unlocked and close across the chest into a double fist configuration.

In the cat pose (Figure 3.2) the anal cavity is closed, providing support for the breath. The three separate actions followed by the unison 'aum' are understood to move the vital breath up from the area of the navel through the chest cavity and finally to the throat.

Once the basic pattern has been learned, the student practises for forty-one consecutive days. On each day the length of time and number of repetitions increases. Vasu Gurukkal said that 'by doing this pranava pranayama for forty-one continuous days the practitioner acquires vira mudra', i.e. he can 'face any situation with no fear or danger and withstand any enemy's attack'.

THE ESOTERIC DIMENSIONS OF CENTRAL STYLE KALARIPPAYATTU

A number of masters in the central Kerala region who practise central style kalarippayattu techniques also practise mantra *vadyam*, healing through use of mantram. Hindu practitioners make use of Sanskrit mantram, while most Muslim masters of mantra *vadyam* have Arabic mantram written in Malayalam script.

The basic floor patterns described in Chapter 4 (Figure 4.19) are not only a pattern for steps, but are also understood as mystical yantra. By meditating on yantra secret application of steps, locks, etc. are revealed. In one kalam the two basic constituents of the design are the straight line and curved loop (Figure 5.7, a–c) combined to form a complex set of steps for attack and defence. For Hindus the straight line is interpreted as Siva (the lingam), and the loop as Sakti (the yoni) which, when combined, give the practitioner access to power. For Muslims the straight line is interpreted as *alif*, the first letter of the Arabic alphabet, and the loop as *lam*. Alif and lam are two of the most important syllables found in Muslim mantram.

There is also an internal style of central practice which is highly secretive and seldom taught. These yantra-like kalam are joined into more complex patterns, as seen in the combination of five basic squares (Figure 5.7, d). In this yantra, there are four gates to the four cardinal directions, each of which when discovered and accomplished reveals a set of offences or defences to the practitioner. Given this emphasis on esoteric practice, it is said that when applying these techniques to the vital spots, the attack directly affects the respiratory system.

Figure 5.7: Central style floor patterns at yantra.

Especially in central style bare-hand practice, basic floor patterns are not only a pattern for steps, but are also understood as mystical yantra (diagrams). By meditating on yantra secret application of steps, locks, etc. are revealed. In the first kalam the two basic constituents of the design are the straight line (a) and curved loop (b). For Hindus the straight line is interpreted as Siva (the lingam), and the loop as Sakti (the yoni) which, when combined give the practitioner access to power. For Muslims the straight line is interpreted as alif, the first letter of the Arabic alphabet, and the loop as lam. In (c) four of these patterns are joined representing a combination of basic footwork patterns.

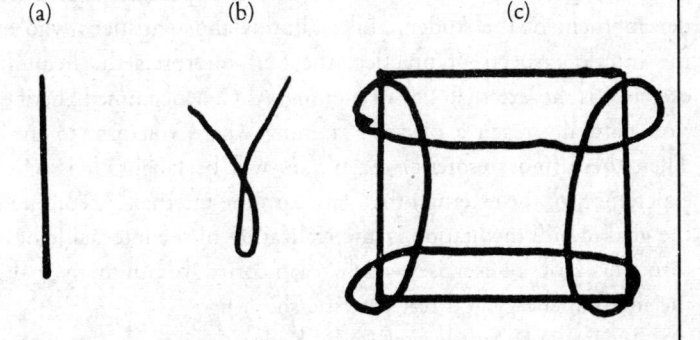

(a) (b) (c)

In (d) is depicted a pattern of five basic squares constituting a seldom taught and secretive internal style of central practice. In this yantra, there are four gates to the four cardinal directions, each of which when discovered and accomplished reveals a set of offences or defences to the practitioner.

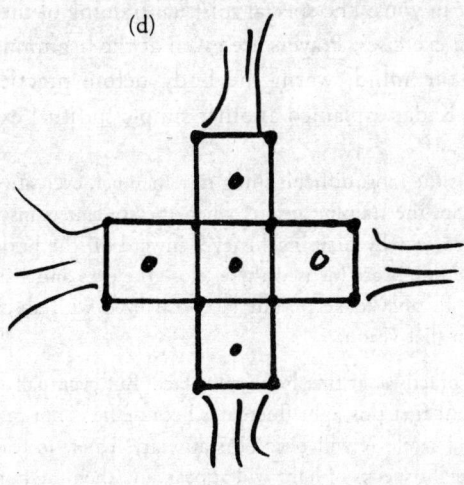

(d)

SPECIAL ESOTERIC SUFI MUSLIM PRACTICES

Just as Hindus practise *vratam* as part of their daily purificatory observances, among Sufi Muslims of the Kannur region of northern Kerala, some forms of Sufi meditation are part of Sufi kalarippayattu practice actualizing higher states of consciousness and power. In contrast to the legalism of some forms of Islam, in its formative period 'Sufism meant (...) mainly an interiorization of Islam, a personal experience of the central mystery of Islam, that of *tauhid*, "to declare that God is One"' (Schimmel 1975: 17–18; see also Eaton 1978; Miller 1976).

Among Sufi kalarippayattu practitioners, importance is given to spiritual development of the student. Like Hindus and Christians who emphasize the interior aspects of practice, the Sufi interprets the beginning body exercises as the 'external' side of training. As C. Mohammed Sherif explained, 'you naturally reach a place in training where you pass to the spiritual. Then these (more esoteric) techniques will be taught. It is only through experience (of the external) that you learn the internal.' According to Sherif, the goal of Sufi meditation is 'the realization of the internal light', achieved through a series of exercises which 'teach correct breathing (...) and awaken the internal energy and teach mystic shouting'.

According to Sufi master Abdul Kadar, the body is a microcosm of the natural world. The natural elements have their homologous elements in our experience—sneezing is like an earthquake, a shout like thunder, crying like rain and tears like salt water: 'First one must understand the body as part of the earth and the natural laws thereof. All the powers of the outside world are manifest in you.' The special spiritual training of the Sufi student begins with simple exercises. Prayers are given at the beginning and end of practice to calm the mind, warm the body before practice or cool it afterwards. Abdul Kadar explained another simple spiritual exercise:

> Your own face is the most difficult thing to remember, even after looking in the mirror. So, the training begins when the student is instructed to visualize his own face by focusing his eyes inward on the bridge of the nose. While the pupils are focused there, close the eyes and visualize the face. You must be able to keep your face visualized with absolutely no distraction from that vision.
>
> As the student practises, at first he sees his face. But eventually he sees a vision of light. At first this light fluctuates because he is not practised in this. But after a while it will become stationary. Later, instead of one light, seven or eight specks of light will appear, and then the number will

increase until they are all joined into one. At times the light will have six colours, but eventually it all vanishes and in its space it will be blank. When it becomes blank the student observes something. But what he sees depends on his individual constitution.

This practice continues for forty days, and results in the development of 'internal strength . . . the will power reaches a very high level'.

Sufis practise a series of *dhikr*—methods of remembrance or recollection of god performed silently or aloud (Schimmel 1975: 167ff; Arberry 1970: 89ff). A dhikr may be as simple as the repetition, 'O Allah! O Allah! O Allah!' first one a day, then two, and continuing until the practitioner is '"habituated to saying those words"' (Schimmel 1975: 169). The purpose of dhikr is to reach 'the stage in which the subject is lost in the object, in which recollection, recollecting subject, and recollected object become again one . . .' (ibid.: 172). Similar to mantram, when learning dhikr, the student obeys dietary and sexual restraints. Kalarippayattu dhikr are practised privately for a specific number of days, usually twenty-one or forty. Some dhikr must be repeated three thousand times in one day to gain their full effect.

Sufis also practise a collective form of spiritual awakening (*ratheeb*) to further develop spiritual power through group chanting. Master Abdul Kadar explained that both dhikr and ratheeb transport the participants into an 'altered state; your mind becomes completely absorbed in the sounds you are making'. Ratheeb serves as a form of purification through breath control (Figure 5.8):

> The breath is taken into the body and then the breath goes out through the body openings. It is purified. All impurities are expelled. Sound is coming outside while the breathing goes in.[106]

> '*Hi um kai um*' is chanted. It is another word for jivan. It must be done slowly at first, and then build to a very fast tempo. When doing this you are inhaling and exhaling inside the body.

The repetitions move through seven stages of chanting, each with its own unique variation. At the height of the seventh stage, all light is extinguished as the entire group joins in the unison chant—'Allah'—the unitary sound. A state of ecstatic union is achieved in which there is one sound, one light and one power—Allah. After the ritual chanting reaches its crescendo, and gradually subsides through a series of short culminating unison chants, the participants share a late night meal.

Both ratheeb and dhikr are essential to Sufi kalarippayattu practice. Ratheeb 'increases your mental and physical strength', leads to breath control, and therefore concentration. It 'gives strength' through absorption and union with Allah. Schimmel, translating Abu'l-Qasim al-Qushayri's *Ar-risala fi ilm at–tasawwuf*, notes that "*dhikr* is the sword by which he threatens his enemies, and God will protect him who remembers Him constantly in the moment of affliction and danger"' (1975: 167).

TOWARD RENUNCIATION

The yogic paradigm of subtle, internal practice, inevitably is understood to lead the practitioner inward and to produce specific results. 'If you do exercises which affect the six adharam (of the subtle body), then you naturally begin to develop a spiritual attitude.' For those students who begin to develop this 'spiritual' attitude, their relationship to exercise and practice changes—they may begin to 'enjoy' the feeling with which they are left at the conclusion of practice. According to this paradigm, the student gains better health by keeping the humours in balance, gains mental equanimity which is reflected in behaviour, and begins to manifest superior concentration, control and power in practice. As one master explained, when the student begins to discover the subtle body, 'he will develop wisdom and not go astray'.

Another master explained the logical conclusion of this paradigm of practice:

> The aim of kalarippayattu is to be able to fight, but when you learn the system very well you will find yourself moving away from an interest in fighting and toward more spiritual goals. I don't take as much interest now as I used to in kalarippayattu because of a growing sense of detachment in my life which has come from practice of the martial art. The physical exercises have contributed much to this, and also the kalari itself which is a place where god is present. When you enter the kalari, salute the deities, and perform the other rituals of the kalari, you slowly find yourself getting closer to god.
>
> Now I practise meditation every day. Meditation and kalarippayattu are closely related, and my own practice of meditation is a result of my martial practice.

Occasionally a master, to fulfil the cultural model of the spiritual renunciant, will leave his martial and medical practice for weeks, months or permanently to seek liberation.

Like any other mode of cultural practice, long-term kalarippayattu practice shapes the practitioner's state of mind and being *in* practice, as well as his behaviour as a person. Chapter 7 further explores the state of 'mental courage' or 'mental power' assumed by many traditional practitioners to be that ideal state of actualization in combat, and Chapter 8 discusses the process of cultural negotiation through which practitioners craft themselves as persons.

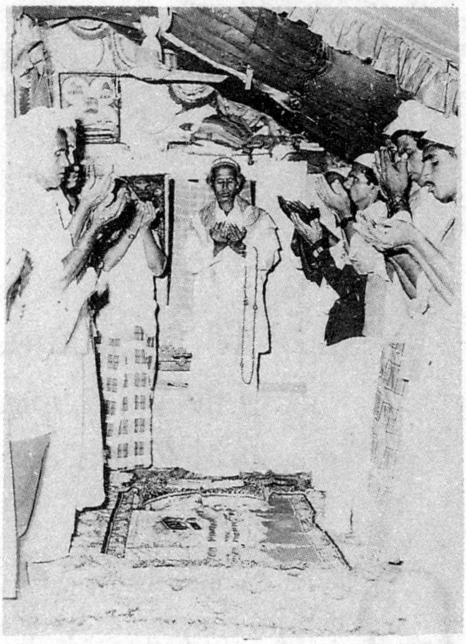

Figure 5.8: Sufi Master Abdul Kadar leads a late-night ratheeb *which through group chanting leads to at-onement with Allah and the concentration and focus of greater spiritual powers for the martial practitioner. (Photo courtesy of Kerala Kalarippayattu Academy.)*

Chapter 6

To Heal and/or To Harm:
The Vital Spots of the Body and Practice

One of the most important parts of the physical body of bones, muscles, ligaments and joints are its junctures or vital spots (Skt. marman; Mal. marmmam; Tam. varmam). This chapter focuses on the central role that the vital spots play in kalarippayattu, as well as in varma ati. Both martial arts share with antique Sanskrit medical sources a similar concept of the vital spots and their role in martial and medical practice. Knowledge of the vital spots was the most important part of a practitioner's training since his life and livelihood depended on the ability to attack the vital spots to kill, stun or disarm an opponent, to defend one's own vital spots and to heal injuries to the vital spots affecting the circulation of the wind humour. As a practical, hands-on art, applications (prayogam) to specific vital spots and treatments for penetration of them are usually taught together. Due to the life-threatening nature of knowledge of the vital spots, such knowledge has always been secretive, taught last in training, and given only to students in whom the master has complete trust. This chapter identifies both the common and unique ways in which these two martial systems interpret the vital spots and make use of their interpretations in practice. I briefly discuss the vital spots in Ayurvedic history. Following a description of the textual sources available for specific study of the vital spots, I provide a working definition of 'vital spot' based on these sources. This is followed by a detailed account of the vital spots in kalarippayattu and varma ati, including the esoteric, subtle concept of the vital spots of the subtle body. The chapter concludes with a discussion of the local nature of this knowledge which requires the practitioner to have a 'doubtless mentality'.

To Heal and/or To Harm • 155

THE VITAL SPOTS IN THE ETHNOGRAPHIC PRESENT

In the popular imagination, a martial master's powers of attack and revival can appear miraculous. Stories and lore abound. K.P.K. Menon's 1967 account of the life of Chattambi Swamigal, the great scholar-saint of southern Kerala (1853-1924) records how this great holy man was known as a master of many traditional arts—wrestling, healing, yoga and the 'art' of the vital spots. Menon records the following account of the swami's use of his knowledge to defeat and then revive some troublesome youth:

> One day he was on his way from Kollur to Alwaye with two disciples. When he had reached the spot in front of the church at Edappalli, his progress was interrupted by a band of young men who were drunk. Asking his companions to hold him by the back, he held his stick horizontally in front of him and with bated breath he bounced forward. Those who felt the touch of the stick fell to the ground. Thus he continued his journey without difficulty. It was only the next day on his way back, after he had administered the counter stroke that the ruffians were able to get up and move away.[107] (Menon 1967, p. 134)

Like other such stories, a mere tap with a finger, hand or stick to one of the vital spots can incapacitate an attacker. Some practitioners of varma ati like to demonstrate this spectacular effect by putting a rooster to sleep by pressing on a vital spot (Figure 6.1).

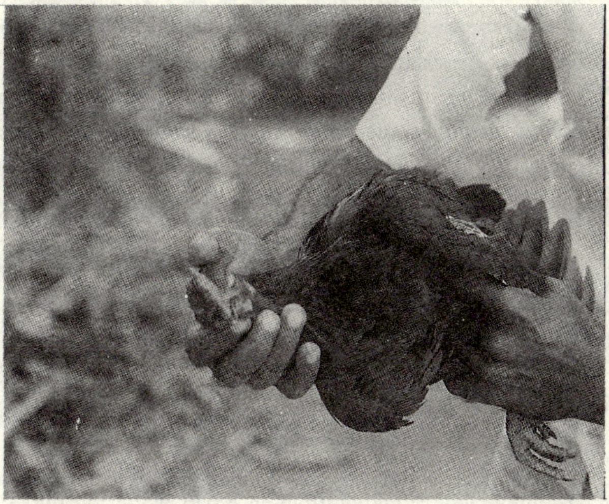

Figure 6.1: A master demonstrates the principle of attacking the vital spots by pressing one of the vital spots of a rooster, rendering the rooster limp in his hands. He then revives the rooster with a counter-application.

Masters like Kalathil Krishnan Vaidyar of Alavil recount stories like the following about their skills at revival:

> There was a young boy who wanted to buy tickets to go to the local cinema. So he went to someone's property to pluck cocoanuts. Unfortunately, when he climbed the tree, it fell over with him on it. He clung to it as it fell and landed against a wall. He was unconscious when he was taken down. A modern medical specialist was called. Several Ayurvedic doctors were also called. But no one could revive him.
>
> A taxi came to pick me up and took me to the place. (After learning what had happened), I asked for a sari and a bronze vessel. I covered his body with the sari (so that no one could see the revival technique), applied pressure to one nerve and the boy urinated into the bronze vessel. The boy immediately regained consciousness and I was given a gift of 101 rupees.
>
> The secret of this technique I will only give to one of my students on my death bed.

Like other miraculous healing narratives in which the healer's powers are sought as a source of final resort, Krishnan Vaidyar conceals his revival techniques, imbuing them with an aura of mystery.

For those who witness a Chattambi Swamigal or a master like Kalathil Krishnan Vaidyar render an attacker unconscious, suddenly revive someone who appears to be dead, or supposedly attack a vital spot by simply pointing or looking, a martial master's powers can seem as miraculous as those of the ancient yogis whose powers were said to tame and control people, animals or the elements. Helping create this impression are cheap popular editions of martial techniques and the vital spots which, along with other paperbacks on everything from astrology to dating and home remedies, are available at book vendors' stalls at railway stations or bus stands. In 1983 for Rs. 3.50 anyone could purchase C.K. Velayudhan's *Kalarippayattu and the Pointing Vital Spots* (*Kalarippayattu and Marmmacuntaniyum*) which advises its readers on how to attack the vital spots by pointing (an important part of the tradition to which I shall return later):

> The 64 'practical vital spots' (*abhyasamarmmangal*), their contents, and how to point at those vital spots with the forefinger while reciting a sacred formula (*mantram*) should be learned not only by reading this book but also by obtaining some practical training from an expert master on the vital spots . . . (This knowledge) can only be used at a time when his life

is in danger. At that time he can point at the enemy's vital spot with his forefinger and recite the 'pointing magic formula' (*cuntumantram*). If he uses the sacred formula known as 'Sri Bhadrakali Mantram' without any mistake, he can defeat his enemy. (1983: 14)

Popular stories have made such an indelible imprint on the Malayali imagination that the concept of the vital spots is a commonplace in vernacular folk culture. When someone wishes to refer to a person who knows a subject so well that he has a special knowledge of the particular knack necessary to do something, marmmam may be used to refer to such knowledge, whether in earnest or in jest. Connoisseurs of the well-known Kerala dance-drama, Kathakali, may refer to the acting of a great performer like Krishnan Nayar as 'knowing the marmmam of acting', i.e. he can act a role with brilliant attention to its specific details. In response to an article by freelance journalist K.K. Gopalakrishnan in which he was critical of a Kathakali performance of a new play ('People's Victory'), Arikkattu Setumadavan wrote to the editor, 'From his article, the writer very clearly knows the vital spots (*marmmam*) of *Kathakali*' (1987). Likewise, a politician might be referred to as one who 'knows the marmmam of politics'—a tongue-in-cheek reference to a politician's ability to win influence by applying pressure at the right points through influence peddling.

Just as common as vernacular uses of marmmam are other tales which make light of the difficulties of obtaining and using this knowledge. K.K. Gopalakrishnan shared the humorous story of a Kalari master who was faced with a dilemma when a cow strayed into his compound and started eating up all the vegetation. He could not decide which part of the cow's body was safe to strike, as every spot appeared to be a 'vital spot' and a blow there could be fatal!

TRADITIONAL TRANSMISSION AND CURRENT STATE OF KNOWLEDGE

Given the esoteric and highly secretive nature of this traditional branch of knowledge, it is virtually impossible to know precisely how much practical knowledge anyone possesses of the subject. A master's reluctance to impart information, whether to his own students or to a researcher asking questions may be due to either a genuine desire to follow a tradition of secrecy, or to hide the fact that he really doesn't have full knowledge of the vital spots.

As reflected in Monier-Williams' definition of the Sanskrit marman, 'the core of anything, the quick . . . anything which requires to be kept concealed, secret quality, hidden meaning, any secret or mystery' (1899: 791)—the tradition of secrecy is antique and reflects the secondary vernacular Malayalam meanings discussed above. In keeping with the potentially deadly nature of this knowledge, transmission is surrounded by protective rituals and a discourse of secrecy. Moolachal Asan's varma ati text, *Agastyar Cutiram*, records the following typical admonition about transmission:

> (Knowledge of the varmam) has been made for everyone in the world to know. You should know this perfectly. People may come and try to praise you, but don't give this out. Rather, watch (a student) for twelve years and only then give this knowledge. Do not give this to anyone who is cruel, but only to one who is a Siva yogi.[108]

A kalarippayattu master's text records the following conditions under which the vital spots are taught:

> If you have ten students, you have to take care of their hearts, you must maintain care over their development, and you must sustain their devotion. But among these there may be only one who emerges as part of your soul, like a son. To him you can give the knowledge (abhyasam).

Only the student who is pure of heart, devout, and has complete trust in the master (*gurutvam*) is to be taught.

> You take him to the kalari, close the door, offer prayers and puja to the various deities, and prostrate yourselves before the deities. Then perform special puja to all the deities. Only then do you begin to teach him.

Taught in secret, learning the vital spots may involve the repetition of mantram and other special rituals to protect the student from injury when learning. Once learned, this special knowledge should never be exhibited in public. As T.N. Ganapathy explains, any desire or attempt to attract

> popular notice through a display of siddhis (accomplished abilities) show immaturity. As Pambatticittar says: 'Those who have attained self-realization will not exhibit it and those who have not attained self-realization are those who exhibit it' (1993: 53).

Knowledge of the vital spots is taught fragmentarily and gradually. As one long-term practitioner commented, 'No one parts with this knowledge completely. A student today is very lucky if he is given 70 per cent of one master's knowledge. At least 30 per cent will always be left out'. Among students who follow tradition and study with masters for years, most are not taught full knowledge of the vital spots. Since students have no right to question a master, their only recourse is to learn what they can from different teachers.

As one informant told Ananda Wood during his research on traditional knowledge in Kerala, the consequence is that 'many people make exaggerated claims of their skill and knowledge in marma vidya' (1985: 115). My experience confirms this observation. One gurukkal who is a master of massage and treatment happily shared his knowledge of several of his texts on the vital spots with me; however, it had been so long since he had used this knowledge that he was unable to clearly explain the locations, symptoms of injury or methods of attack of a number of specific spots.

Another practitioner in his late 20s was born into a Nadar family where the grandfather was a traditional practitioner of varma ati. Although this young man's father had not learned varma ati, he was consumed with a passion to learn the martial and medical system and began training at his grandfather's feet from a young age. But as so often happens, masters only gradually reveal the secrets of practice to their students, even within their families, and often vow, like Kalathil Krishnan Vaidyar, to withhold revelation of their most secret techniques until 'on my death-bed'.

Unfortunately, his grandfather died in 1982 before he was able to share knowledge of the location, methods of attack and treatment of all the vital spots, leaving him unable to decipher and use as much as three-fifths of the original palm-leaf manuscript he inherited which recorded all of the traditional techniques. Frustrated, he sought out other masters to teach him how to use and interpret his family's text. So much variation existed between his own family's text/practice and that of other masters he consulted that numerous contradictions and inconsistencies appeared; therefore, he is unable to interpret and use much of his family's text. So contradictory can versions of the vital spots be that, as Balachandran Master laughingly told me, 'you will either become a renunciant or a mental case. If you just go to one master, fine. You learn what he knows (even if that is incomplete) and there will be no confusion; but if you go to more than one master!'

The confusion reflected in these stories is not recent. As early as 1957 in his preface to Sreedharan Nayar's comparative study of Sanskrit, Tamil and Malayalam sources on the vital spots, Narayanan wrote soberly about the condition of this knowledge:

> We have all heard a lot about the vital spots. But usually what we hear is unclear or full of fantastic information. To achieve a systematic life, a clear and perfect knowledge is needed. But in naming, locating, and explaining the vital spots, even what teachers say is uncertain (C T.S. Nayar 1957: 1).

The gradual breakdown in the process of transmission as well as lack of practice in use of some techniques has resulted in confusion and uncertainty among some of today's masters. Like others who try to preserve systems of traditional knowledge from the past, Narayanan problematically assumes an idealized past:

> At one time there were well-developed laws of martial, massage, and vital spot practice. When we look to Kerala's past, we can believe that at one time there was both a scientific and full knowledge of these vital spots (Ibid.).

This picture of an idyllic past in which knowledge was perfect assumes that in this 'Kali Yuga' all knowledge, morality, and the quality of life has 'degenerated'.[109] In contrast to this idyllic picture of a past in which knowledge was perfect, I would suggest that, like other esoteric and secretive systems of practice/knowledge, contentiousness, confusion and lack of clarity has always surrounded this specialized and potentially very dangerous system of attacking/defending the vital spots of the body, and that the multiple interpretations of the vital spots we find today are because the martial traditions have by necessity always been relatively closed and secretive.

From the perspective of some varma ati practitioners, 'knowing' the vital spots is not a 'knowledge' that can be taught, but only intuited experientially, as a mode of 'revealed' knowledge. As R. Perumal Raju explained in a lengthy personal correspondence:

> Mere knowledge (of the vital spots) is not experience. A marker can only give knowledge to a certain extent, and that knowledge can't be experience. Even thousands of volumes and talks of the masters cannot explain or give knowledge about the sweetness of sugar. One can experience the sweetness of sugar only when some sugar is put on his tongue.
>
> Then how that experience was given by the great masters in ancient days is a matter of wonder!
>
> This varmam art is like meditation in the yogas. It is just like an uphill task. Suppose one climbs up a hill fully covered by thick forest. He will

struggle day in and day out not knowing when he would reach the top and see the other side of it! That moment comes suddenly to him—he finds himself at the top—sees the other side and will be thrilled by the experience.

So also the master will give knowledge of the subject through some exercises, practice of certain movements according to their tradition. All these exercises and movements become a sort of meditation. Even without their knowledge they will start moving inwardly. *By the grace of the Master all of a sudden they will have the darsan* or visually see the whole mechanism and the movements inside the body! The entire body—the skeleton, the bones, flesh, nerves, blood, glands, *vayus* and all with their movements will become crystal clear to him. This is some sort of Enlightenment—such as that of Buddha. The inward eye experience will be wonderful. Then he need not grope for a centre or a spot in the body. He can touch it in a given moment.

To summarize thus far, knowledge of the vital spots is not a 'seamless' non-contradictory body of 'scientific' information practised in exactly the same way or with exacting precision by all those who claim to be masters of the martial tradition, but rather a cultural commonplace in South India which has found many forms of popular expression, been open to many interpretations, and which in some ways has fallen into misuse. I will situate the concept and practice of the vital spots within three interpretive communities in which they developed (antique Ayurvedic physicians, kalarippayattu and varma ati), accepting the fact that numerous 'contradictions' exist both between their interpretations as well as within each tradition.

THE VITAL SPOTS AND AYURVEDIC HISTORY AND PRINCIPLES

The earliest textual evidence of the concept of the vital spots dates from as early as the *RgVeda* (*c.* 1200 BC) where the god Indra is recorded as defeating the demon Vrtra by attacking his marman with his vajra (Fedorova 1989: 1). From this and numerous other scattered references to the vital spots in Vedic and epic sources, it is certain that India's early martial practitioners attacked and defended the vital spots; however, we possess no martial texts from antiquity comparable to the Sanskrit medical texts in which a systematic knowledge of the vital spots is recorded.[110]

By the time Susruta's classic Sanskrit medical text had been revised in the second century AD, (Kutumbiah 1974: xxx)107 vital spots of *sthulasarira* had been identified as an aid to surgical intervention:

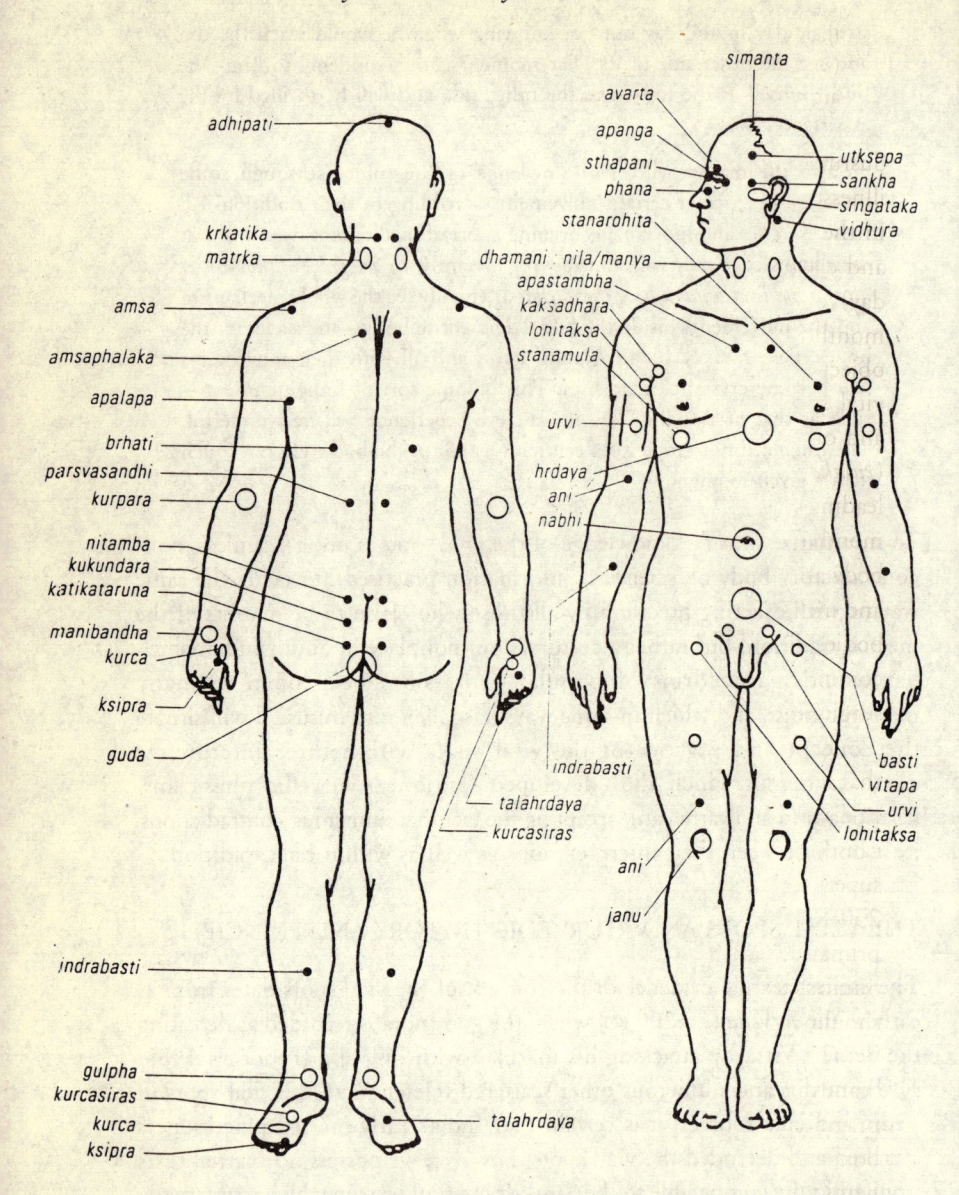

Figure 6.2 : Location of the marmans *of*
Susruta Samhita *as interpreted by Fedorova (1989).*

the areas where muscles, vessels, ligaments, bones, and joints meet together (...) which by virtue of their nature are specially the seats of life (Singhal and Guru 1973: 132) (Figure 6.2).

Susruta knew the importance of avoiding vital spots in surgery, identified illnesses caused by direct and indirect injury to them, and diseases situated in them. He asserted that direct penetration of many vital spots was fatal, and classified these trauma as *sadyah-pranahara* (causing death within one day) or *kalantara-pranahara* (causing death within fourteen days to one month). He also observed that death could be caused by extracting a foreign object from a wound to a vital spot (*visalyaghna*), that some wounds to the vital spots might result in maiming or deforming injuries (*vaikalyakara*), and other times penetration of vital spots only resulted in painful injuries (*rujakar*). Of the 107 vital spots he identified, Susruta listed fifty-one as leading either to immediate death, death within twenty-four hours, or one month. Limited emergency measures included surgical removal of the foreign body and amputation. Susruta established a close connection between combat and medical intervention. Surgery was called *salya*, which referred to 'foreign bodies of every kind ... but ... specifically ... the arrow, which was the commonest and most dangerous foreign body causing wounds and requiring surgical treatment' (Kutumbiah 1974: 144).[111]

Knowledge of the vital spots shares the general Ayurvedic principles that health is a state of humoral equilibrium. Susruta identified seven kinds of diseases, one of which was *samghata-bala-pravrtta*, 'the traumatic type ... caused by an external blow or ... due to wrestling with an antagonist of superior strength' (Susruta, Suthrasthana XXIV, 6; Bhishagratna trans., 1963: 230). All combat injuries fall into this class. Susruta related them to the primary humoral body by explaining that traumatic injuries enrage the wind humour in the area of injury. The first action of the attending physician should thus aim to calm the 'enraged wind humour (*vayu*).'[112]

This principle guides the kalari master's medical practice which, as a 'hands-on' therapy learned through apprenticeship, is always practical and pragmatic. The therapeutic action of all *marmma cikitsa* treatments such as bone-setting (Figure 6.3), massage and administration of bags of medical herbs dipped in heated oil (*kili*, Figure 6.4), is produced by fomentation from massage which affects the wind humour, and works its healing power 'in due time' (Govindankutty Nayar, Interview).

The legacy of identification, classification and treatment of the vital spots established by Susruta, and in south India by Vagbhata, was a rational system based on humoral theory and therapeutic intervention applied to observations of wounds received in combat. It was never a closed, secret tradition since its purpose was to save lives. The tradition eventually passed to martial specialists for whom the combat *prayogam* of their specialized knowledge was just as important as medical intervention.[113]

TEXTUAL SOURCES FOR THE STUDY OF THE VITAL SPOTS

Kalarippayattu masters possess one or more of three types of texts on the vital spots: (1) those like the *Marmmanidanam* ('Diagnosis of the Vital Spots') which are ultimately derived from Susruta's *Samhita* and enumerate for each vital spot its Sanskrit name, number, location, size, classification, symptoms of direct and full penetration, length of time a person may live after penetration and occasionally symptoms of lesser injury; (2) those like *Granthavarimarmma cikitsa* which also identify the 107 vital spots of the Sanskrit texts and record recipes and therapeutic procedures to be followed in healing injuries to the vital spots; and (3) much less Sanskritized texts like *Marmmayogam* which are the kalarippayattu practitioner's handbook of empty-hand practical fighting applications and emergency revivals for the 64 'most vital' of the spots (*kulabhysamarmmam*).[114] As detailed below, these kalarippayattu texts could be characterized as rather straightforward descriptive reference manuals cataloguing practical information.

In contrast to the straightforward descriptive nature of these texts are the varma ati master's highly poetic Tamil texts which were traditionally

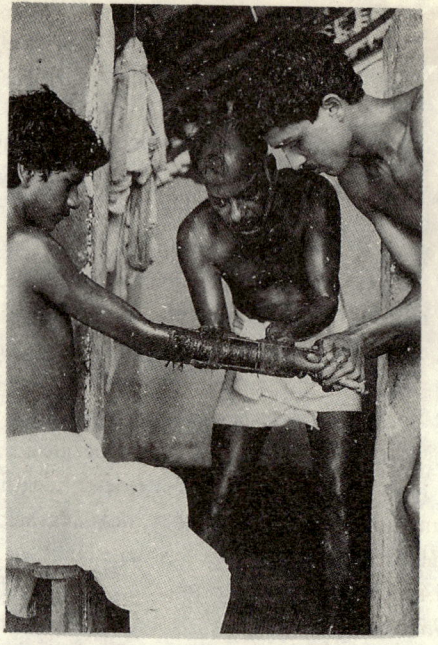

Figure 6.3: Assisted by his son, C. Sankaranarayanan Gurukkal places a new cast on a broken arm. Once a broken bone is set in a temporary plaster, the patient returns every three days to have the limb massaged with medical oils, and a new cast applied. The cotton bandages have been soaked in medicinal oils and are being wrapped around splints.

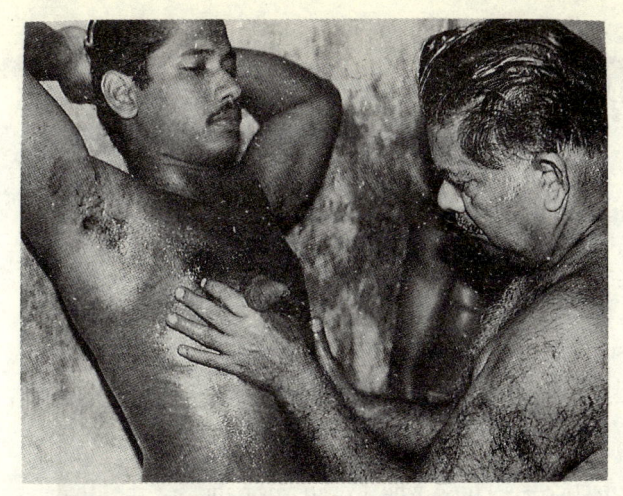

Figure 6.4: One important massage therapy in the repertory of many practitioners is application of cloth bags (kili) of specially prepared medicine herbs for injuries, such as this 'catch' in the student's chest. Here Gurukkal K. Narayanan Nayar treats one of his students.

sung and taught verse by verse. Some texts like *Varma Cuttiram* located at the University of Madras manuscript library (#2429) are relatively short (146 sloka) and focus on one aspect of practice. Longer texts like *Varma Oti Murivu Cara Cuttiram* ('Songs [concerning] the Breaking and Wounding of the Vital Spots') include more than one thousand verses and provide names and locations of the vital spots, whether it is a single or a double spot, symptoms of injury, methods of emergency revival, techniques and recipes for treatment of injuries not only to the vital spots but also to bones, muscles, etc. As a comprehensive medical text its purpose is clearly sung:

10.1 Oh leader of the world, since human beings (receive) cuts, fall down, (receive) blows,
10.2 lose their grip and fall down from high places—for all these reasons parts of the body are broken,
10.3 and for these same reasons for so long now people have suffered or died, and the vital spots of their bodies may have been wounded.
10.4 Because of all the suffering caused by these injuries, I am going to recount the various oils, internal medicines, and tablets (to give).

The text admonishes the student as he learns these verses to

12.1 Proceed by giving massage with the hands, legs, and bundles of medicinal herbs,
12.2 with confidence set fractures. I am explaining all this carefully, so listen and follow what I say.

12.3 With piety take your guru and god in mind, and treat other lives as your own.
12.4 With thinking and doing together as one, search out the vital spots, fractures, and wounds.

These texts reveal that the varma ati system was traditionally a highly esoteric and mystical one since *only* someone who had attained accomplishment as a Siddha yogi could be considered a master of the vital spots. In keeping with the commonplace Tamil expression, 'without knowing myself first, I cannot know about others', the poet who authored *Varma Oti Murivu Cara Cuttiram* explicitly states, 'Only by practising the five stages (of yoga *kantam*) in the six *ataram* (locations within the subtle body for meditation and generation of internal vital energy) will you get (a clear understanding) of the 108 vital spots (*varmam*)' (17.1). Tirumular's classic definition of a Siddha is implicit in this practice—'"Those who live in yoga and see the divine light (*oli*) and power (*cakti*) through yoga are the *cittar*"' (Zvelebil 1973: 225; *Tirumantiram* 1490).[115]

As anthropologist Margaret Trawick Egnor notes, 'the language of Siddha poetry is notoriously esoteric; modern students of it say it was deliberately made so, so that the Siddha knowledge would not become public' (1983: 989). The difficulty of interpreting the obscurities of these texts on the vital spots is in keeping with the nature of all Siddha poetry:

> Whenever the Siddhas use ambiguous language, it is on purpose; they are obscure because they want to be obscure . . . In fact, according to the living *cittar* tradition, the texts are a closed mystic treasure-box bound by the Lock of ignorance, and only a practising Siddha yogi is able to unlock the poems and reveal their true meaning (Zvelebil 1973: 229).

As reflected in R. Perumal Raju's traditional assertion that knowledge of the vital spots is revealed 'like a meditation', only a practising Siddha yogi can intuitively unlock the secrets of a text and apply them in locating, attacking and/or healing the vital spots.

DEFINITION OF THE VITAL SPOTS

Given its relationship to the antique Sanskrit medical sources, kalarippayattu's medical texts define the vital spots in terms whose source is certainly Susruta. For example, the anonymous undated, *Marmmanidanam*, in the possession of a north Kerala master records the following:

> If a person is hit anywhere in his body with a punch, and the strength of

the pain (where he has been hit) constantly fluctuates, increasing and then decreasing, this is known as a marmmam. Flesh, bones, tendons, veins, arteries, and joints, all these six are places of marmmam. These are the seats of life (jivan).

This definition combines Susruta's anatomical understanding of the vital spots with the martial practitioner's rational observations of the throbbing pain produced when a vital spot is hit or penetrated. Other definitions, like the following from *Marmmarahasyangal* ('The Secrets of the Vital Spots'), are less explicit: 'If at any place there is injury from weapons or hits due to which death occurs, this is known as a vital spot.'

The varma ati texts I have examined do not give a precise anatomical definition. In keeping with the more esoteric and poetic nature of Tamil cittar literature, the vital spots are explained suggestively, as in this passage from *Varma Oti Murivu Cara Cuttiram*:

14.1. Only by searching have you discovered the secret of the secrets of all these details (of the varmam).

14.2. If you understand and locate the wonderful places where (the varmam are situated) which are hidden (inside the body), (you will experience these as) being cooling places (if injured).

What is common to Sanskrit, Malayalam and Tamil sources is that the vital spots are places where the life force in the form of the internal breath or wind (prana-vayu) is situated, and therefore vulnerable to attack. As discussed earlier, wind is understood to be spread throughout the body and responsible for all activity, and the terms prana/prana-vayu refer not just to breath, but to breath-as-life, or the essential vital energy itself. Varma ati master Sadasivan Asan of Thiruvananthapuram defined the vital spots as 'where the vital force passes when there is an injury'. In keeping with the importance of the breath as it has been defined by the classical Siddha therapeutists like Roma Rsi (Zvelebil 1973: 224ff.), Moolachal Asan explained in more detail the relationship between the breath and the vital spots:

If a person has no breath, there is no varmam. Vayu (breath) is varmam. Varmam are those places where the breath collects while doing meditation. Varmam means breath comes through the ida and pingala nadi. A healthy man takes 21,600 breaths per day. The channels through which the breath passes are called varma nila where if you strike, the vayu will be stopped, and then symptoms will be shown. Then the blood will clot. When the breath is blocked, various diseases will result.

Some masters say a full understanding of the vital spots is possible only with knowledge of astrology. One informant asserted, 'The heart of the vital spots is time (kalam), and time is ultimately controlled by the stars'. One's internal life force (jivan; prana-vayu) is constantly circulating throughout the body in conjunction with the periodic fifteen-day cycles of the waxing and waning of the moon. Raju Asan of Vizhinjam explained how

> an expert in varmam must know and be able to spot specifically where the jivan is located at any given time. The life force is only in one specific vital spot at any specific time. And only if you attack this specific spot where the life force is located at that time will it have its full effect.

Therefore, a master must know that on the first day of the new moon the life force is located in the vital spot at the tip of the nail of the big toe, in the *nakannmarmmam*. For masters who follow this esoteric logic, the vital spots listed in medical texts are simply *sthanam* on the physical body. Only when the vital energy is located in a particular place at a particular time is it actually a marmmam in the original sense of the word—a spot on the body which, if hit or penetrated, will result in death, i.e. the stoppage of the vital energy. Following this logic, only a master fully accomplished in Siddha yoga, astrology, as well as the practical techniques of fighting applications has the requisite skills to be able to successfully locate and attack the particular vital spot vulnerable at the specific moment of attack.

DETAILS OF THE VITAL SPOTS IN THE KALARIPPAYATTU TRADITION

As illustrated in Figure 6.5, among kalarippayattu practitioners following the Susruta tradition, the majority identify 107 as the total number of vital spots. The master-as-physician ideally knows all 107 in order to treat injuries to the spots themselves and to give massage therapies without applying pressure directly to the spots and thereby causing injury. Two typical kalarippayattu texts, *Marmmanidanam* and *Marmmarahasyangal*, follow Susruta's *Samhita* in using 43 names to identify a total of 107 vital spots.

Examining the *Marmmanidanam* more closely (Figure 6.6), of the forty-three names given, nine located on the limbs identify four vital spots each, twenty-six identify two spots each, six are single spots located along the centre line of the torso, one name identifies a total of eight spots in the neck, and one name identifies five spots on the skull. In contrast to simpler

Comparative Chart of Vital Spot Distribution in the Body

Key
- # 1 = Susruta Samhitā
- # 2 = Marmmanidānam ('Diagnosis of the Vital Spots')
- # 3 = Marmmarahasyangal ('Vital Spot Secrets')
- # 4 = Chandran Gurukkal, Azhicode
- # 5 = Kalattil Krishnan Vaidyar, Alavil
- # 6 = Sadasivan Asan, Thiruvananthapuram
- # 7 = Moolachal Asan, Mekkamandapam
- # 8 = Varma Oti Murivu Cara Cuttiram ('A Set of Songs [Concerning] the Breaking and Wounding of the Vital Spots')

	SUSRUTA			KALARIPPAYATTU			VARMA ATI	
Name	#1 / 43	#2 / 43	#3 / 43	#4 / 54	#5 / 55	#6 / 108	#7 / 108	#8 / 108
Arms	22	22	22	24	16	14	10	10 [24]
Legs	22	22	22	22	14	14	11	11 [26]
Stomach	3	3	3	3	9	9	TORSO 34	34 [60]
Chest	9	9	9	7	21	45		
Back	14	14	14	17	38	*	16	16 [28]
Neck/Head	37	37	37	35	9	25	37	37 [57]
Total	107	107	107	108	107	108+	108^	108 [195]

- * = Sadasivan Asan includes those on the back in his count of the torso.
- \+ = Sadasivan Asan also includes 'one special secret spot' to give a total of 108.
- ^ = Moolachal Asan also recognizes two special vital spots not counted as part of the *sastric* 108.

Figure 6.5: *Comparative chart of vital spot distribution in the body.*

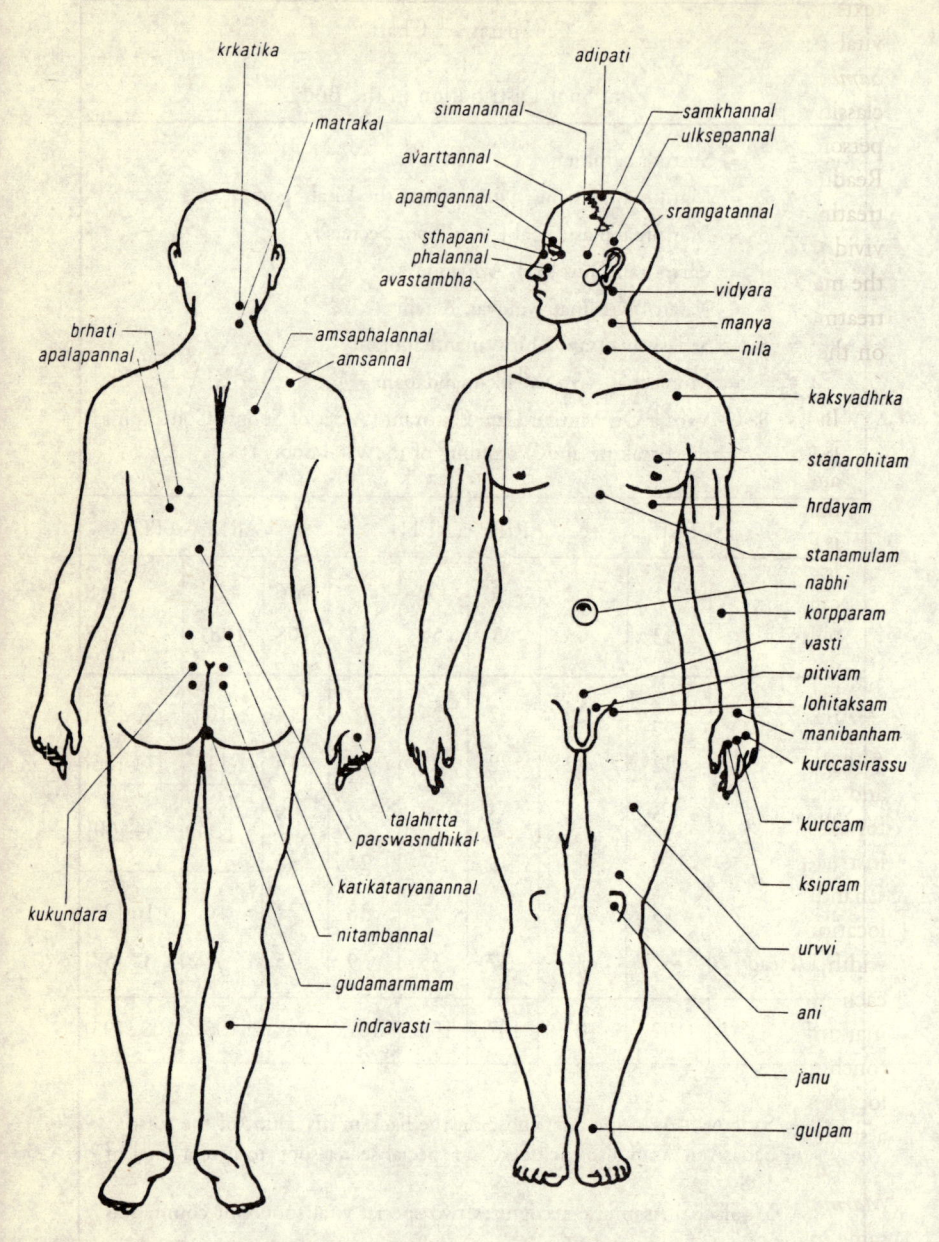

Figure 6.6: The locations of the vital spots on the body according to one kalarippayattu text, the Marmmanidanam.

texts like the *Marmmarahasyangal* which only records the locations of the vital spots, the medically-based *Marmmanidanam* is similar to Susruta's *Samhita* in enumerating for each vital spot its name, number, location, size, classification,[116] symptoms of direct and full penetration, length of time a person may live after penetration and occasionally symptoms of lesser injury. Reading like a manual for a battlefield surgeon faced with recognizing and treating blade wounds to the vital spots, the *Marmmanidanam* contains vivid descriptions of these injuries, but no information of practical use to the martial artist on attack, defence, or counter-applications for emergency treatment to the vital spots. Typical of the majority of the text is the entry on the first vital spot with the Sanskrit name, *talahrttu*:

> In the sole of the foot and the hand, straight in front of the middle finger is the *marmmam talahrttu*. There are four which are 1/2 finger in width and which are *mamsa marmmam*. (If injured) at first the pain is not strong, but it slowly increases with continuous bleeding. The colour of the blood is like the colour of blood when you are washing meat. The flow of blood is gradual. (As a result), the body becomes pale. The five senses lose their capacity (to feel). The injured person will live for a maximum of one to one and a half months. If the pain is only slight, it can be assumed that only the edge of the vital spot has been injured and it was not directly hit.[117]

Although these texts give a general idea of the location of the vital spots and may indicate that a spot is located a specific number of *angulam* away—for example, two finger widths below the nipple—only through hands-on instruction does a student discover the precise location of each marmmam. Chandran Gurukkal maintains that the only precise way of measuring the location of the vital spots is by taking the measure of a person's own finger width, and then using this specific measure (marked on a string) to locate each of the vital spots (Figure 6.7). Locations are usually taught either by marking each with rice paste or a special grass (Figure 6.8), or by carefully touching/probing each spot on the student's body so that he feels the precise location. The text serves as a manual to which the master refers while showing a student the location of each of the vital spots.

Other than the specific information on the location of each spot, the *Marmmanidanam* is as formulaic as the *Samhita*, providing virtually the same information for all the vital spots in each class, as the following entries for the seventeenth and eighteenth-named vital spots illustrate for two-vein (sira) marmmam.

In the centre of the body between the large and small intestine, nabhi marmmam is located. It is the centre of all the nadi. It is the measure of the palm. It is a sira marmmam. If it is injured, (the result is) immediate death. Symptoms include thick blood continuously flowing in large quantity resulting in anaemia, thirst, head spinning, breathing difficulty, hiccups. He will live a maximum of seven days.

In between the breasts where the abdomen and chest join, at the hole of the abdomen the hrdayam marmmam is located. It is the measure of the palm and is connected with the sira (veins). When injured, (the result is) immediate death. Symptoms include thick blood continuously flowing in large quantity resulting in anaemia, thirst, head spinning, breathing difficulty, hiccups.

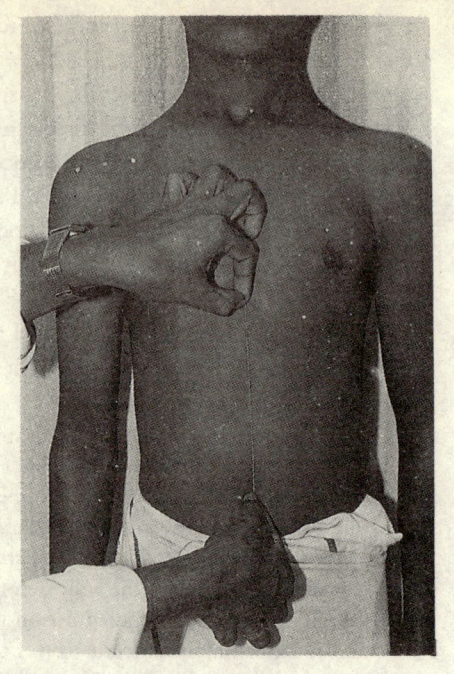

Figure 6.7: Chandran Gurukkal demonstrates how he precisely locates nabhimarmmam (at the navel) by measuring the correct distance from hrttamarmmam.

Again like the *Samhita*, *Marmmanidanam* clearly differentiates between penetration of the vital spots and other battlefield-type injuries, and provides additional practical information on amputation.

> When an injury occurs at the vital spots before the vayu travels upwards, the upper portion should be immediately amputated at the point (of injury). When amputation is done the veins and joints shrink and bleeding stops, and therefore the person lives.
>
> If injury occurs where there is no vital spot, even though bleeding results the person will not die; however, if it is a vital spot which brings immediate death, then even if penetrated with the tip of the stem of a grass, the person will not live. By some chance due either to the skill of the physician or if the injury is not deep, even if the person lives he will be handicapped . . .

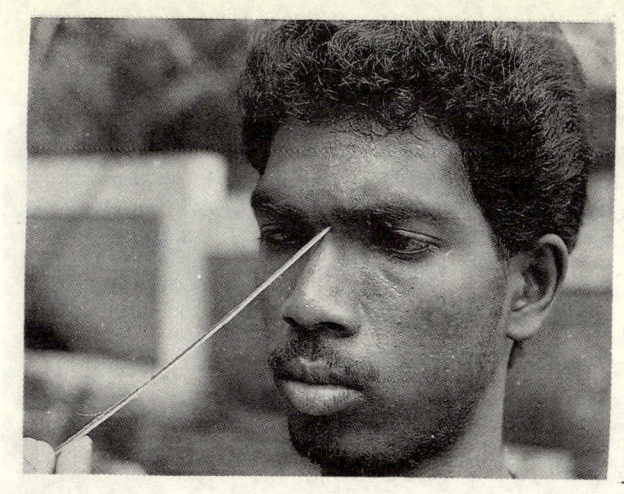

Figure 6.8: Using a stiff piece of straw, Balachandran Master demonstrates one method of teaching students the locations of the vital spots—in this case, tilartakalam, *one of the twelve death spots in the* varma ati *system.*

If even a small cut or injury occurs to a vital spot, it brings great pain. Just like this, even if treated well many diseases affecting the vital spots create great difficulty.

Apart from the symptoms mentioned above, you may also see: contortion of the body, faintness, trembling of the body, a feeling that the heart is burning, disorientation and eventual death.

When an injury occurs where there is no vital spot, even if there is great bleeding, the person will not die; therefore, even if 100 arrows penetrate (where there are no vital spots), the person will not die. A person who is pure and whose fate is to live a long life on this earth will not die in any manner.

If the *Marmmanidanam* and other similar texts traditionally served the martial artist-as-physician as a diagnostic field manual helping him identify the characteristic features of battlefield-type cuts or penetrations of the vital spots, his practical training taught him specific weapons techniques used to penetrate, cut or defend some, if not all, of these 107 vital spots. Although most of today's kalarippayattu masters learned practical methods of attacking and defending the vital spots while learning either *verumkai* techniques or the special wooden practice weapon (the *otta*), many practitioners of the past probably learned the vital spots during training with weapons. C.C. Velayudan Asan, then 87, told me in 1983:

> In my family tradition the vital spots were learned while doing spear. The tip of the spear is very sharp and small, and the vital spots are very small,

specific points. The student first learned thrusts to various body parts and specific spots, as well as how to defend against those thrusts. Once he began to learn these techniques, standing at a distance he was taught to throw the spear at a human target aiming at specific vital points. Only when he was able to hit all those specific places by throwing the spear was he taught the specific names of the vital spots. In our tradition we identified thirty-six death marmmam. There are thirty-six methods of attacking. Everything is contained in those thirty-six methods of attacking the thirty-six death spots.

Masters like Velayudan who still practise traditional combat weapons, especially sword/shield and spear, still attack and defend the vital spots in their daily practice.

For treatment of penetrating injuries to the 107 vital spots identified by Susruta, some masters also possess a second type of text, like either the *Granthavarimarmma cikitsa* or *Marmmani cikitsa*, which record recipes for medicinal preparations and therapeutic procedures for treatment. Regarding penetration of *talahrttu* described above, the *Granthavarimarmma cikitsa* records the following course of treatment:

> If talahrttu is injured you give dhara (continuous pouring of any type of liquid on any part of the body) with gingili oil and ghee for three hours. After dhara is complete, grind gingili oil with butter and rub it on the place. To the top of the head apply a mixture of jasmine flower and butter. After three hours it should be wiped off. Then all over the body apply a mixture of water, oil, ghee, and Aloe Vera(*kattavala*); if not, ghee, oil and tender coconut water.

Masters still use these recipes and therapeutic procedures to treat injuries to the vital spots.

Although attacks and defences of specific vital spots are taught as part of all weapons practice, kalarippayattu masters possess a third type of text which specifically enumerates the names, locations, symptoms of injury (*laksanam*), empty-hand techniques of attack or defence, and emergency counter-applications (*marukai*, literally, 'opposite hand') for blows to the sixty-four (or seventy-two) *kulabhyasamarmmam*—the 'great practical vital spots'. These empty-hand techniques must have been important when a practitioner lost or broke his weapon in combat, or when attacked while unarmed. Although some masters maintain that the sixty-four practical spots are 'the most important vital spots of the 107', and therefore are sixty-four of the same 107 vital spots identified by Susruta, others insist that perhaps only one-half of them are included in the 107 identified for medical purposes.

Some masters classify the sixty-four practical spots, according to the results produced by their penetration as either the 'most vital' spots (kula-marmmam) whose direct penetration could bring death or very serious injury if a counter-application is not applied; 'catch' spots (*kolu-marmmam*) whose direct penetration produces a freezing pain which incapacitates an individual temporarily and may lead to death; or 'practice' spots (*abhyasa-marmmam*) whose penetration causes less serious injury. In theory, only when a master intends to kill an opponent would he attack the most vital spots. When wishing to disarm or incapacitate an opponent, he would attack a catch spot. In the least dangerous situation he should overcome an opponent by attacking a practice spot.

These differences reflect the fact that, as Sreedharan Nayar noted in 1957, there is no uniformity about either the titles or locations of these sixty-four practical vital spots (Figure 6.9). Whether part of Susruta's 107

Figure 6.9: Comparative locations of kalarippayattu's 'practical vital spots' (kulabhyasamarmmam).

Comparative Locations of Kalarippayattu's 'Practical Vital Spots' *(Kulabhyasamarmmam)*		
Key # 1 = Marmmadarppanam (Chirakkal Sreedharan Nayar, 1957) # 2 = Marmayōgam (Kunnhikannan Gurukkal)		
Name	# 1 37	# 2 34
Arms	12	10
Legs	10	10
Stomach	3	3
Chest	12	15
Sides/Back	7	7
Neck	7	6
Head	13	13
Total	64	64

or not, these sixty-four spots are learned in advanced training in unarmed combat.

The following two examples from Kunnhikannan Gurukkal's *Marmmayogam* text, counterparts of the Susruta-based nabhi and hrdaya marmmam recorded above, illustrate the type of information in these manuals:

> *Jalapantam* is one-half finger width below the navel.
> Block with the left, take a right step and chop with the right hand. He will lose consciousness and urinate. (To revive your attacker) six finger widths above where the legs join, at the centre of the backbone, (apply the counter-application) punch. Sometimes blood may ooze out (of the penis). Then apply pressure at the base of the vertebral column (with the base of the palm).
>
> *Trisankupuspam* ('three conch flower') (Between the nipples) below the chest and above the abdomen, this spot is liquid in nature and shaped like the bud of the lotus, a bit tilted to the right, and you must locate it with your heart. Defend the hit with your left and attack this spot with the right elbow. (To revive) just on the opposite side of the back, punch.

As noted earlier, *verumkai* techniques are an integral part of training and, as Velayudan Asan explains, 'taught last because the teacher must have an understanding of the mind of the student' from observing him. Only he who has mastered the correct forms, developed consummate *ekagrata* and is able to channel his inner vital energy (prana-vayu) has the ability to make these techniques effective fighting techniques.

A few examples of specific empty-hand applications illustrate how kalarippayattu's empty-hand methods of attack and defence were directed to penetrating or protecting the vital spots. In Figures 6.10–6.11 Gurukkal Madhavan Panikkar demonstrates how he defends an attack to his forehead with his left hand, and returns an attack to his opponent's *sankapuspam-marmmam* located between the breasts with a right step forward and a thrust of the elbow. An alternative move is to counterattack to *mukkatappan marmmam* (located on the bridge of the nose) with a downward right cut with the outer edge of the hand (Figure 6.12). This same master defends against a right overhead blow to the forehead with a double-hand block (Figure 6.13) by stepping forward with his left leg and thrusting downward with his left elbow to *tarippan marmmam* (Figure 6.14). Higgins Master of the P.B. Kalari, Trissur, who specializes in empty-hand techniques and applications, illustrates how he defends against a knife attack, and counter-attacks by grabbing the attacker's hair with the left hand to expose *manya marmmam* on the neck for attack with his right elbow (Figure 6.15). Likewise, *otta* techniques attack and defend the 64 *kulabhyasamarmmam* (Figures 4.30–31).

Figures: 6.10–6.11: Gurukkal Madhavan Panikkar of Pallikkar in Malappuram district demonstrates how he defends an attack to his forehead with his left hand and returns an attack to his opponent's sankapuspam marmmam *located between the breasts with an elbow thrust.*

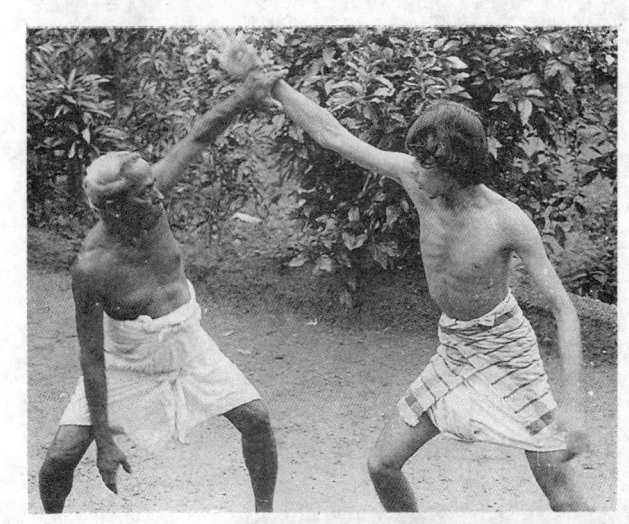

Figure.: 6.10

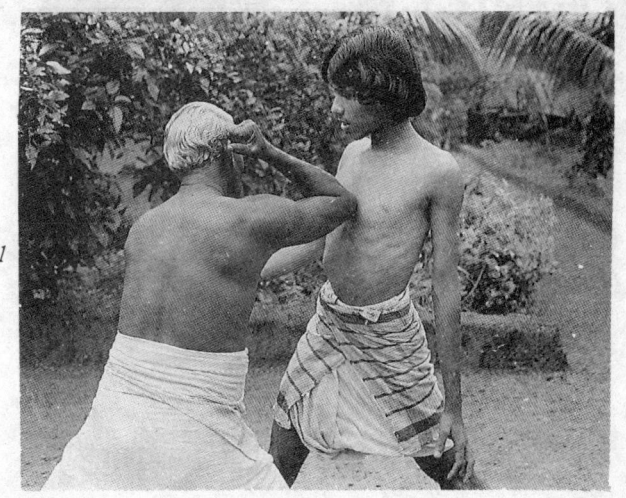

Figure.: 6.11

178 • When the Body Becomes All Eyes

Figure 6.12: An alternative counterattack is made to mukkatappan marmmam *located between the eyes on the bridge of the nose. After blocking with the left hand, Madhavan Panikkar attacks with the right hand, hitting downward with the outer edge of the bone.*

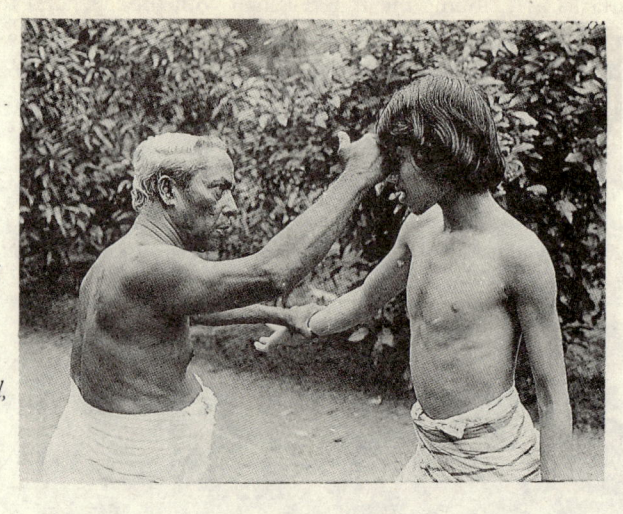

Figures 6.13–6.14: After defending an overhead blow with crossed fists, Madhavan Panikkar counter-attacks with a left forward step behind the attacker's right leg and an elbow thrust to tarippan marmmam *('jellyfish vital spot') located in the middle of the thigh.*

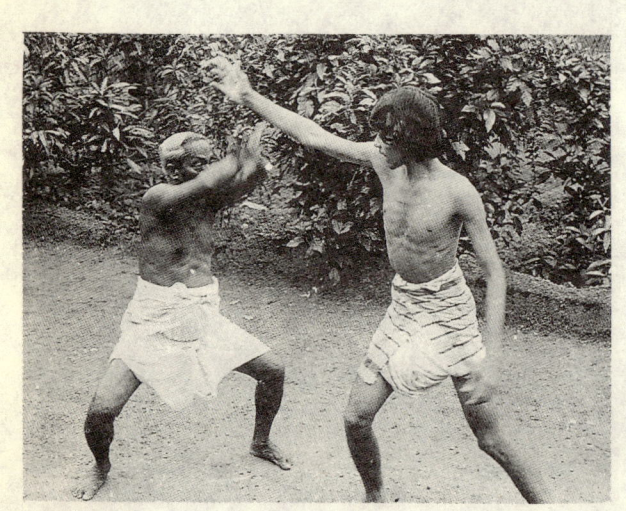

Figure.: 6.13

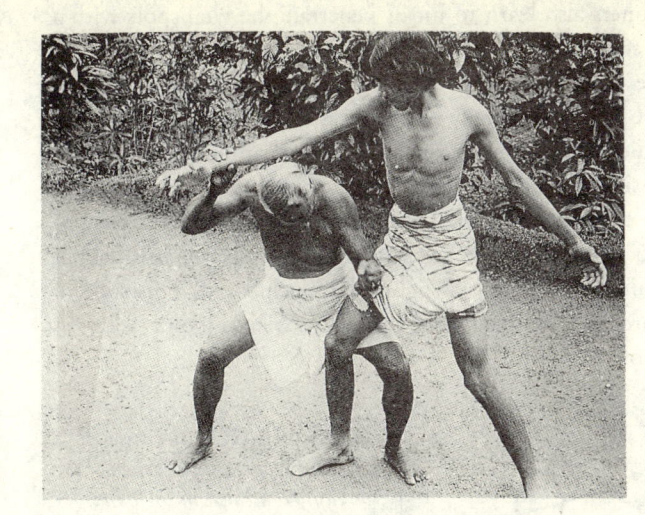

Figure: 6.14

Figure 6.15: Higgins Master of the P.B. Kalari, Trissur who specializes in empty-hand techniques and applications, illustrates how he defends against a knife attack, and counter-attacks by grabbing the attacker's hair with the left hand to expose manya marmmam *on the neck for attack with his right elbow.*

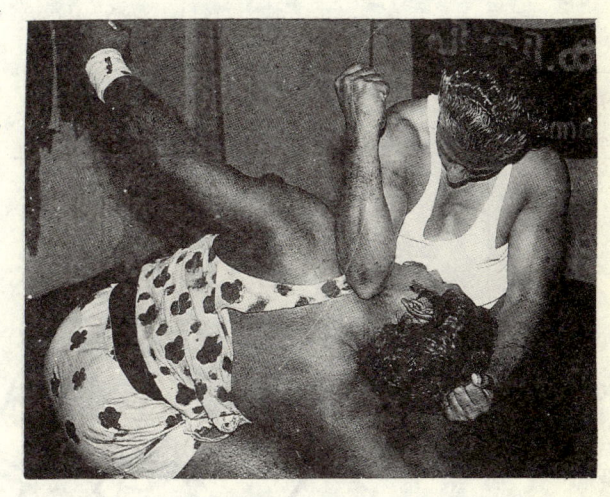

Some practitioners also learn to hit or penetrate the vital spots with a *cottaccan*, a small stick designed to be easily concealed in the hand. The stick measures one *can*.[118] One type of cottaccan is the stick rounded at both ends (Figure 6.16), occasionally tipped with brass, and always held by the palm in the middle of the stick so that an equal amount of the stick extends from each side of the palm. This style of cottachan is used to thrust with the forehand or strike with the back of the hand. A second style of cottaccan (Figure 6.17) is more like a very small billy-club which is held at the narrower gripping-end and has a slightly larger club-end. This style of stick is used for forehand and backhand thrusts, as well as blows delivered with a quick flick of the wrist.

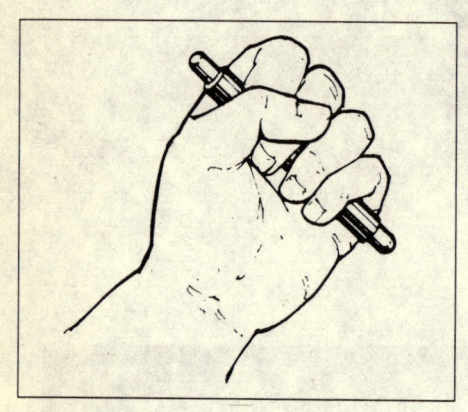

Figure 6.16

Figures 6.16–6.17: Two styles of cottaccan: *small sticks designed to be easily concealed in the hand. The first style is rounded at both ends, occasionally tipped with brass, and held in the palm of the hand for either forward or backward thrusts to the vital spots. The second is more like a small billy club held at the gripping end. The vital spots are attacked either with thrusts or with a quick flick of the wrist.*

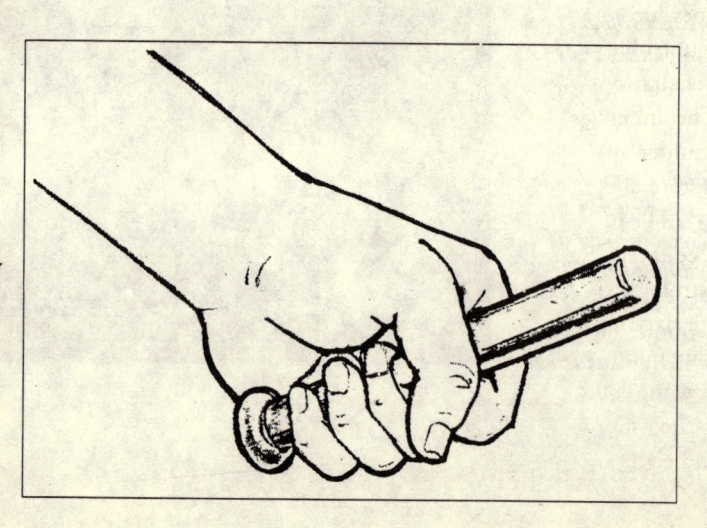

Figure 6.17

According to some masters, even if a practitioner knows the specific locations of the vital spots, if someone hits or even penetrates a spot it may have little result, or at the most produce a numbing, freezing pain. It certainly will not lead to death. The only way to actually kill an opponent when attacking a vital spot is to have learned a special knack for 'opening' the vital spot being attacked. This interpretation of the vital spots assumes that the vital spots are normally hidden or 'closed', and only when the spot has been 'opened' can a penetrating attack result in death. Among the various ways masters understand what it means to 'open' the vital spots are the following:

(1) The position of the body/limb and/or direction of attack must 'open' the vital spot to allow a deadly attack.
(2) Another secret method of 'opening' a vital spot is by disrupting the breathing pattern or rhythm either by attacking a specific secondary part of the body, or by recognizing the predominance of left or right nostril breathing.
(3) A third explanation is that a vital spot may also be 'opened' by stretching the opponent in a certain manner, for example, in a grappling situation, then attacking the exposed vital spot.

Techniques of Revival Through Counter-Application

As important as attacking and defending the vital spots is the practitioner's ability to revive an individual whose vital spots have been penetrated. When a vital spot is penetrated by a sharp weapon, death results when vital energy goes 'up' or 'out' through the wound. When there is penetration with a blunt object, the vital energy or internal wind is stopped at the point of penetration, and the entire structure may collapse and death may result. The inner system of *nadi* reverberates from the shock, and emergency counter-application must be given within a prescribed period of time to restore circulation of the wind humour as well as structural balance.

The fundamental measurement used to determine the time within which a counter-application must be given is the nalika—the basic time unit in astrology. One nalika is the period during which one star stands, and there are sixty nalika in a twenty-four hour period, i.e. one nalika equals twenty-four minutes. For example, Sreejayan Gurukkal's *Kulamarmmangal* records how the counter-application for penetration of *karnnapilikakanna marmmam*, located four finger widths above the ear, must be given 'within eight nalika and eight *vinalika*' on the 'opposite side four fingers above the ear'.

Kalarippayattu masters administer *marukai* applications to 'straighten out' a channel after it has collapsed and contracted when struck, and to thereby unblock the stopped and enraged internal wind. The antique Indian counterpart of modern emergency revival techniques, these are usually a strong slap with the palm of the empty hand and/or fist to precisely the same spot on the opposite side of the body. The counter-application restores structural balance, stops the blockage of the flow of the internal wind humour, and thereby brings the patient out of immediate danger. The master's ability to produce an effective counter-blow and bring the person out of danger is dependent upon his embodied ability to transmit the appropriate degree of energy/power (sakti) when channelling his own vital energy through the palm in the form of the slap.

In addition to counter-applications, kalarippayattu masters also use general revival techniques when the precise marmmam penetrated is unknown. When an unconscious patient is brought to Gurukkal Govindankutty Nayar and all he knows is that the injury was above the waist, he gives the following set of counter-applications intended to get the patient out of immediate danger: a firm slap with the palm to the top of the head, followed by the application of pressure with both palms to the patient's ears, followed by a twisting and jerking of the legs while applying pressure to certain vital spots. The head is slapped because this is understood to be the central 'channel of the vital energy'. Pressure is immediately applied to the ears to compress the effect of the slap on the vital wind. The legs are jerked and twisted to stimulate the vital energy/wind to begin recirculating.

Once the superstructure is out of immediate danger of collapse, the patient's humoral imbalance (also resulting from penetration of a vital spot) is treated through massage therapy and prescribing internal medicines. The counter-application and ensuing quieting massages are complementary emergency and longer-term therapies.

When the practical texts are examined closely and compared to the Susruta-based medical texts, five further observations may be made, each of which will be elaborated below: (1) although the names of the practical vital spots are occasionally the same Sanskrit names as in the medical texts, more often the names are colloquial and descriptive Malayalam; (2) all of the attacks and defences recorded are executed with bare hands; (3) likewise, the symptoms of injury never indicate that the vital spot has been cut with a sharp weapon like a sword, arrow or spear, but rather are the result of either a blow or penetration of a spot with a blunt instrument—either a part of the body or perhaps a stick; (4) the bare-hand attacks are intended to temporarily incapacitate an opponent with the most typical results being paralysis, numbness, loss of consciousness, wasting of the limbs, mental agitation and/or internal injury causing vomiting of blood; and (5) as long as a counter-application is given within the stipulated time period, only rarely does a text indicate that an attack to one of these sixty-four spots with a blunt object or part of the body will result in death.

More common than Sanskrit names are colloquial, descriptive ones like the vital spot located four finger widths below the ears known as 'lip twister' (*cirikotan*), or 'lightning flash' (*itiminni*), referring to the flash of light one sees when hit between the eyebrows. A few names are descriptive of the shape of the bare hand used to attack the spot such as 'like the serpent's hood' (*ittirapatti*) where the attacking hand takes the shape of a serpent's hood.

Even in those versions of the practical vital spots that use the same Sanskrit names as Susruta's *Samhita*, the information provided is quite different. For example, the *Samhita* records the vital spot *ksipram* as located 'at the junction of the thumb and index fingers' (Bhishagratna 1963: 275). It is classified as *kalantara-pranahara* (death within fourteen days to one month) and is said to lead to 'death from convulsions' (Bhishagratna 1963: 275). As noted above, texts derived from the *Samhita* like the *Marmmanidanam*, record details similar to those in the original text, in this case the following:

> In between the thumb and the forefinger is *ksipram* . . . Due to (the injury) of the two winds (*ayamam* and *aksepakam*), paralysis and strong pain (result). He will be unable to move the limbs of the body. Gradual death will come within one to one and a half month.

In contrast is *ksipram* as recorded in one master's text which identifies the symptoms of injury: 'the hand goes limp; thirst, belching, and burning sensation; nerves become taught; possible unconsciousness'. More typical than Sanskrit *ksipram*, this spot is called 'finger vital spot' (*angulamarmmam*) by one master, while in Kunnhikannan Gurukkal's *Marmmayogam* this same spot is named 'the sneezing hand finger press' (*tumbikaiviraluni*). 'Sneezing hand finger' clearly describes the result of the practical application recorded in the text: 'Block and catch hold of the palm and apply pressure. (The opponent's) hand will be immobilized.'

Some descriptions, like that for *kaikulappan marmmam* in Kunnhikannan Gurukkal's *Marmmayogam*, clearly indicate that these bare hand techniques were to be used to disarm, immobilize and then revive an attacker:

> Inside the elbow, below the bend (in the arm) is kaikulappan. Block and apply pressure with the right hand. (The attacker's) hand will be weakened and the weapon will fall from his hand. (Apply the counter) above that in the middle of the bend (of the elbow) and the shaking of the hand will be stopped.

In keeping with the emphasis on self-defence, in the texts I have been able to study in detail, only one vital spot, *vayuccini* ('spreading out the air') located 'in the depression on top of the head where the hair circles' indicates that death might result from a blow or penetration: 'If injured, difficulty in breathing, burping, etc. will occur. The head shivers. If the pupils of the eyes turn up, death occurs' (C.T.S. Nayar 1957: 42).

To summarize, it is clear that the Susruta-based 107 vital spots and the sixty-four practical vital spots were complementary systems equally important to the traditional kalarippayattu practitioner. It was to the Susruta-based system of 107 vital spots that the martial practitioner learned to aim the thrusts and cuts of his weapons on the battlefield, and it was also this system which guided the practitioner in locating the vital spots, identifying symptoms of battlefield-type injuries, avoiding these spots while giving massage therapies, and in treating penetrating wounds. Complementing this weapons-based system were the sixty-four vital spots of the bare hand practical repertoire with its techniques for defence, disarming an opponent, and temporarily stunning/disabling an opponent.[119]

DETAILS OF THE VITAL SPOTS IN THE VARMA ATI TRADITION

As illustrated in Figure 6.5, varma ati practitioners usually agree that 108 is the sastric number of vital spots identified by the Sage Agastya.[120] Unlike Susruta's 107 which is the total number of vital spots identified by forty-three names, 108 is the number of names. Since some names identify single spots, and others are double, the number of vital spots can total more than two hundred. *Varma Oti Murivu Cara Cuttiram* records forty-six of the 108 as single and 62 as double—a total of 170 (44.2).

Of these 108 vital spots, ninety-six are classified as minor spots (*thodu varmam*) and twelve as the major deadly vital spots (*padu varmam*).[121] The most vulnerable/dangerous *padu varmam* are those which, when penetrated deeply enough, cause instant death. The more numerous minor spots are not as dangerous when penetrated but cause great pain to an attacker while incapacitating him.[122] Tamil scholar M. Manickavasagam of the University of Madras explained that the difference between the two types of vital spots is due to how close the vital wind passes to the surface of the skin, i.e. when the vital wind is near the surface and therefore more exposed to stoppage through penetration it is a *padu varmam,* and when the vital wind 'goes around the side and/or circles the spot' it is a minor spot.

Like kalarippayattu, the information in varma ati texts provides colloquial names, specific locations, symptoms of injury/penetration with a blunt instrument or part of the body, and methods of emergency revival. *Varma Oti Murivu Cara Cuttiram* records the following for one of the twelve deadly spots:

45.1 *Kontakkoli* is correctly located at the top of the head. Listen to the symptoms if it is seriously injured.

45.2 My dear student, his head collapses completely and there is spontaneous ejaculation.

45.3 Life-endangering convulsions and chilling of the body occurs. If directly affected, death occurs.

45.4 You must know that even though an expert physician treats this injury the patient will die.

Varma Cuttiram, one manuscript in the possession of Moses Thilak in Madras, records the following name, location, symptoms and counter-application for another of the twelve deadly vital spots:

In between the eyebrows just one rice grain (nil) below, the name of the centre is *tilada kalam.*[123] As you strike, if it breaks, he will die. The deadly centre is tiladakalam. If the spot is struck (without it naturally breaking), he will open his mouth and look at the sky. He will be there for 3 and 3/4 nalikai (90 minutes). I will teach you the quieting techniques. Grasp the hair (tied in a knot on top of the head) and make him sit up, and slap at the centre of the crown of the head. (Massage) the *pinkalai* (the two nadi running up the back of the neck to the ears). Chew dried ginger and blow it (into the nose and ears). When you give boiled rice water, noble soul, it is certain that he will be all right.[124]

Sreedharan Nayar's 1957 Malayalam translation of Agastyamuni's student Bhogar's Tamil *Varmasastram* records the following account of one of the less dangerous ninety-six minor spots, *mukkuvarmam* ('nose vital spot'):

If a punch or hit comes to the centre of the nose, there is loss of the senses, the lights dim, blood flows from the nose, and faintness occurs. For this give a suitable blow to the top of the head. (1957: 53)

There are two results of penetration of a vital spot—those impossible to revive and resulting in death, and those it is possible to revive. According to Moolachal Asan, penetration one *matram* (or *angulam*) deep of one of the twelve deadly vital spots with a part of the body or blunt instrument is impossible to revive. But when a death spot is penetrated only one-half a matram, revival is possible.

Although texts *per se* do not record techniques of attack or defence, each master's practice is his repertoire (Figures 6.18–6.20). Since basic defensive and offensive moves are taught in four directions to guard against attack from all sides, varma ati techniques always open within an evasive move and/or block since philosophically one is never supposed to attack first. When a counter-attack is launched to one of the vital spots, some are to be attacked straight ahead, some from a forty-five-degree angle, and others must be caught inside and pulled in order to achieve the full result.

Like kalarippayattu, varma ati techniques include a variety of methods of attack with the hands, fingers, elbows, etc. and some masters provide esoteric explanations of the potentially deadly significance of each part of the hand:

> The thumb is the mother finger of the hand. The right index finger is the guru. The second (middle) finger is Saturn, god of death. The third finger is directly connected to the heart, and the fourth is for tantric practice . . . When you want to kill an opponent use the second finger of death (to penetrate a vital spot). If you only want to incapacitate your opponent use Saturn supported by the guru finger so that you only penetrate half-way (and therefore do not cause death).

Fig. 6.18: Having defended against an attack with the right fist, Sadasivan Asan demonstrates a counter-attack to the vital spot located on the bridge of his opponent's nose (paalmarmmam or mukkuvarmam).

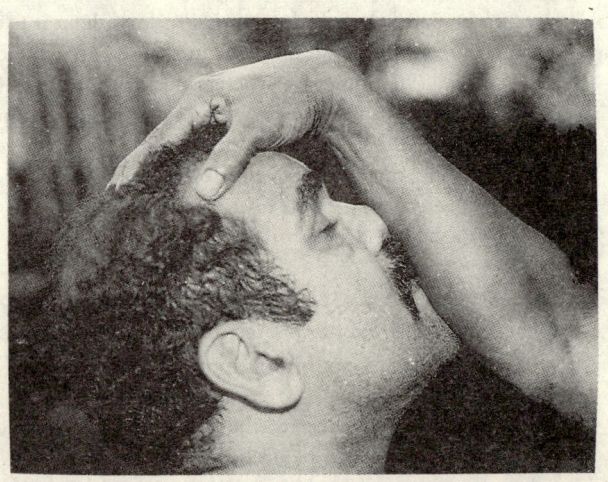

A unique method of bare hand training for attacking the vital spots was explained to me by Raju Asan. Chelayan Asan taught him the appropriate amount of pressure to apply and depth of penetration for each type of attack by having him apply each technique with the fingers, hands or fist to the trunk of a banana log—a surface which approximates remarkably well in its texture and resistance to penetration of skin and muscles.

Figures 6.19–6.20: Balachandran Master demonstrates a threefold counter-attack beginning with a right elbow attack to nermarmmam *located between the breasts (6.19), followed by a blow to* tilartakalam *between the eyes with the right knuckle, and concluding with a fist attack to the two* vittiumarmmam *located on the scrotum (6.20).*

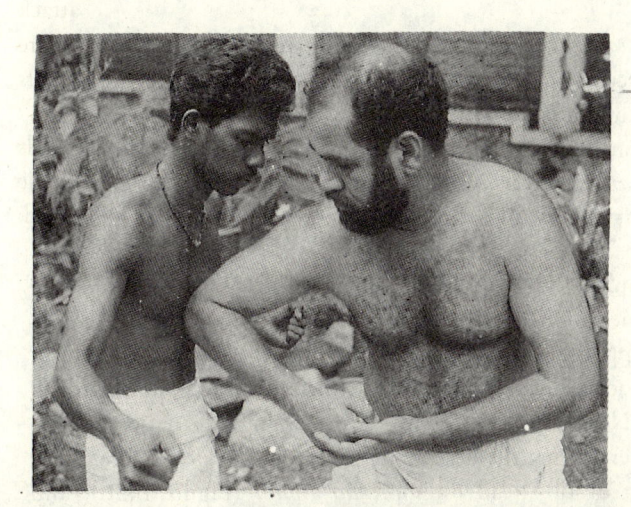

Figure 6.19

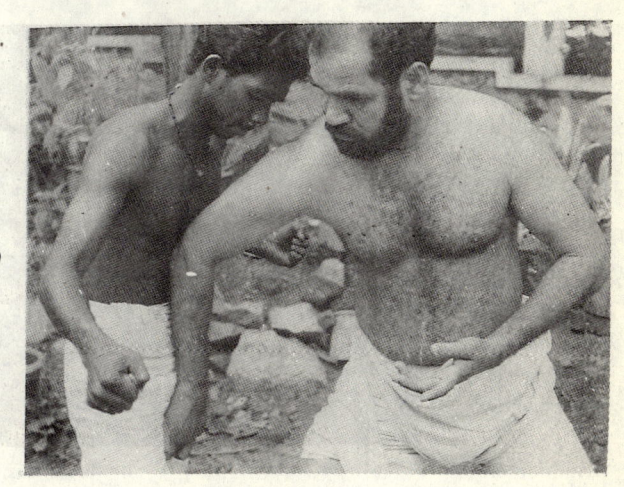

Figure 6.20

188 • When the Body Becomes All Eyes

As in the kalarippayattu system, according to varma ati practitioners when a vital spot is penetrated the internal wind or vital energy is understood to be stopped. While they too recognize the concept of *marutattu* for each vital spot, the main revival technique is to make use of one of twelve to sixteen *adangal*—methods of massaging and stimulating the revival spots among the 108. Since all the vital spots are understood to be connected through the internal *nadi* to these twelve (or sixteen) revival spots, stimulating the appropriate vital spot through an *adangal* application 'straightens the (contracted/collapsed) channel' so the internal wind moves freely again, and, as *Varma Oti Murivu Cara Cuttiram* explains, 'brings (the injured) back to consciousness'.

One simple *adangal* Chelayan Asan uses to revive '70 per cent of all injuries' is to directly stimulate *kavalikalam* with his thumb (Figure 6.21). When spasms occur and/or the face begins to contort from penetration of a vital spot, Chelayan Asan simultaneously stimulates *amakaalam* in the calf and *koncanimarmmam* in the ankle (Figure 6.22). Were *koncani* to be stimulated without also pressing *amakalam*, there would be an adverse affect on the patient.

A more complex revival technique is Chelayan Asan's techniques of counteracting penetration of *nerumarmmam* located between the breasts. Pressure is first applied with the knee against *vayukalam* (Figure 6.23) in the small of the back while the patient is supported on the opposite side at *nerumarmmam*. Next, the master rubs down along the patient's sides (Figure 6.24). Then, lifting the head under the chin upward (Figure 6.25), he slaps the top of the head on *unnimarmmam* (Figure 6.26), and

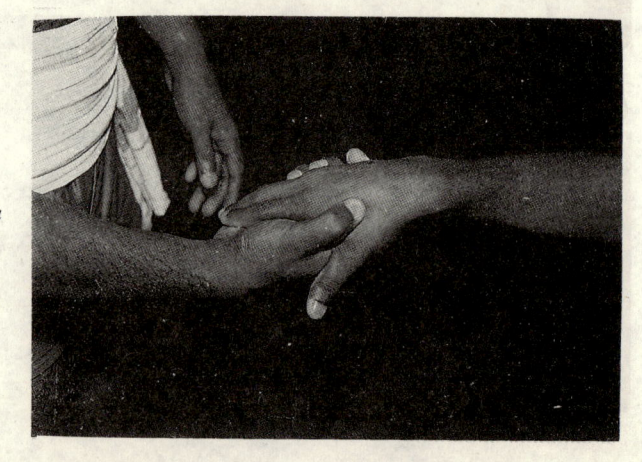

Figure 6.21: Raju Asan, student of Chelayan Asan, demonstrates how he stimulates kavalikalam *by applying pressure with his thumb.*

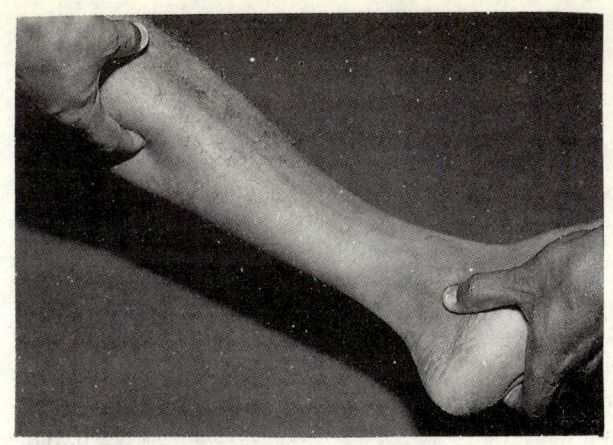

Figure 6.22: When spasms occur and/or the face begins to contort, Raju Asan demonstrates how Chelayan Asan simultaneously stimulates amakalam *in the calf and* koncanimarmmam *in the ankle.*

Figure 6.23–6.27: This set of photographs illustrates one of Chelayan Asan's complex sets of counter-applications for penetration of nermarmmam *located between the breasts. Pressure is first applied with the knee against* vayukalam *in the small of the back (6.23) while the patient is supported on the opposite side at* nerumarmmam. *The master rubs down along the patient's sides (6.24). Lifting up the head under the chin (6.25), he slaps the top of the head on* unnimarmmam *(6.26), and concludes by reaching under the patient's shoulders from behind, gripping, lifting sharply (6.27), and shaking.*

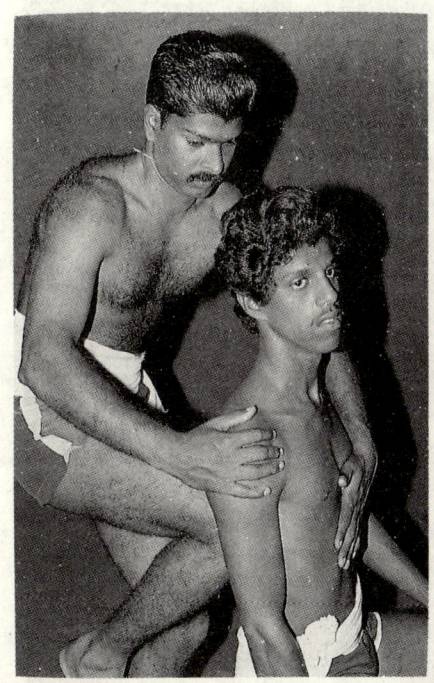

Figure 6.23

finally reaches under the patient's shoulders from behind, lifting sharply (Figure 6.27) and shaking the patient.

Before performing any of these techniques, varma ati practitioners are admonished to take in mind their guru, momentarily focus their mind through dhyana, and only then apply the revival techniques. When applying any *adangal*, the practitioner must be careful to 'not apply more pressure than needed' since that could lead to further injury. When giving an *adangal*, *Varma Oti Murivu Cara Cuttiram* instructs the practitioner to

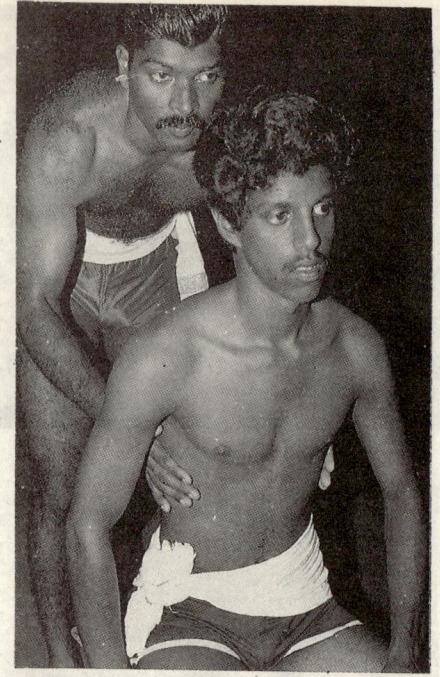

Figure 6.24

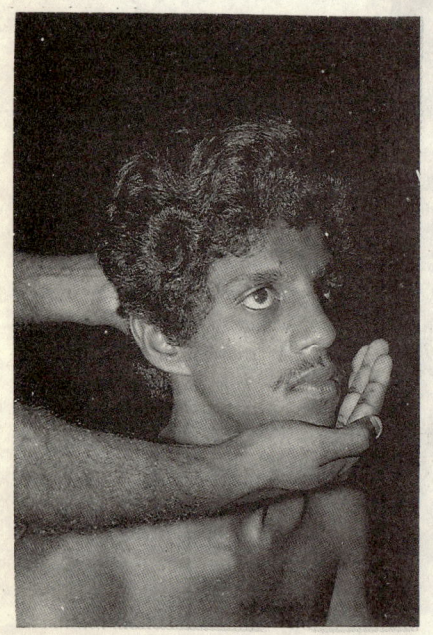

Figure 6.25

84.3 . . . inhale the adequate amount of air needed, and hold it firm

84.4 Keeping the breath inside, and knowing the correct period (of application), without hesitation do this and you will have success and bring him back to consciousness.

Like kalarippayattu emergency revivals, once a patient has been revived and is out of immediate danger, a variety of external therapies and internal medicines are prescribed.

Before giving an emergency revival, varma ati practitioners are warned to differentiate between what is treatable or untreatable. *Varma Oti Murivu Cara Cuttiram* says,

> 11.2 ... If, after determining that the condition (of a patient) is very serious and he is going to die, leave that place.
>
> 11.3 (If the symptoms do not indicate that the patient is going to die, stay) correctly read the symptoms of a wound,
>
> 11.4 and through treatment preserve each life, except for that of the cruel person (*kacataru*) whom you should never treat ...

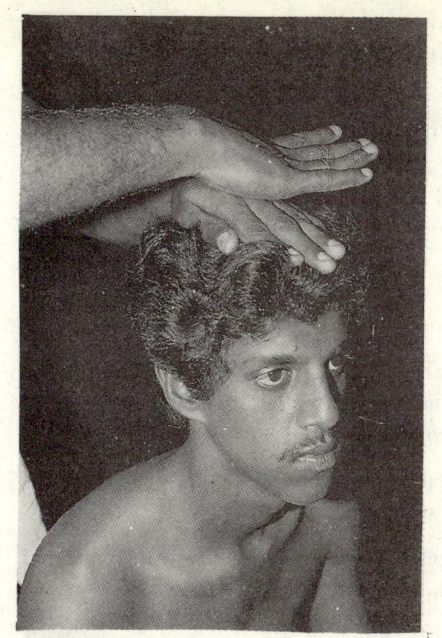

Figure 6.26

Some entries, like the following for *katirvarmam* located 'below the neck where you wear jewels', explicitly tell the master not to treat someone injured in this vital spot if the appropriate period for attempting counter-application has passed:

> 86.1 Hear me for I am telling you the different symptoms when *katirvaramam* is affected.
>
> 86.2 Others will become frightened because his eyes will protrude, his head will collapse, and the neck will bend forward.

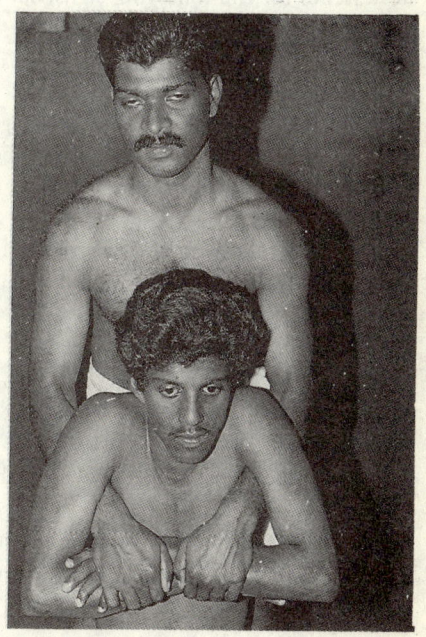

Figure 6.27

86.3 Following this he will have troublesome vomiting and hiccups. I tell you the period (for counter-application) is thirty-four *katikai*.

86.4 I tell you, do not do the impossible. Do not give him medicine, but leave him (to die).

Masters are advised to read a wide variety of signs before determining whether to treat a patient:

13.1 When you see bad symptoms from which you know death may arise, leave.

13.2 Good man, if the symptoms you see are positive, surely you can apply your touch (*adankal*) and cure the patient.

13.3 If you see symptoms indicating life will pass away, able man, never go there (to give a revival or treatment).

13.4 If you stand as firm as a pillar, you will see very clearly the drama (of the symptoms) and find the correct (diagnosis).

When someone approaches Moolachal Asan to give an emergency revival, he watches for the following signs, 'all of which indicate sure death';

If the messenger scratches his head while asking.
If he argues with you.
If he arrives leaning on a walking stick.
If he indicates the place where the injury has occurred.
If he reports the leg is broken at the mid-foreleg.

If any of the following cuts/injuries resulting in the vital energy 'going out', i.e. death, are reported to him, Moolachal Asan will not go to attempt a revival:

If the small of the back or back of neck is broken.
If the big toe is cut off just below the nail line.
If the centre foreleg is broken in two.
If the points of the hipbone are broken.

Moolachal Asan explained that if any master attempts to treat a case whose signs are hopeless, 'it will bring misfortune to him'.

THE ESOTERIC/SUBTLE POWERS OF ATTACK AND THE MARMMAM OF THE SUBTLE BODY

This description of the vital spots has focused on the places of the gross *sthula-sarira* which, when penetrated or cut, may cause death. Clearly the symptoms of injury from either a weapon or a blunt object are based on rational observation of the physiological results of penetration. As discussed in Chapter 5, just as the practitioner's entire training process begins with the external, gross body and is understood to eventually move inward toward the discovery of the *suksma-sarira*, likewise there exists a more esoteric, subtle means of attacking the vital spots by looking (*nokku-marmmam*) or pointing (*cundu-marmmam*). Such attacks are made on either the 107–8 vital spots of the gross, physical body, or a separate set of thirty-two vital spots of the *suksma-sarira*. No actual physical blow, cut or thrust with a weapon or bare hand is said to be needed by a master who develops the higher mental powers (*manasakti*) necessary to make such attacks.

Belief in these subtle powers is a logical extension of the yogic paradigm of practice and accomplishment through which the individual is able to concentrate his powers through meditation in order to control everything in his environment. As Lee Siegel describes it,

> Through ascetic practices, wandering sannyasis were (and are) believed to attain supernatural powers, the powers of Shiva, *siddhis*, which, like every other aspect of life and death in India, have been systematically catalogued and normatively categorized: *animan* (the power to become minute or, for the magician, disappearance) and *mahiman* (the power to become large); *laghiman* (the ability to become light, to levitate) and *gariman* (the power to become heavy); *prapti* (the skill of obtaining things, effecting materializations, or, as explained by the traditional commentators on the *Yogasutras* of Patanjali (3.45), having the ability to touch the moon with one's fingertip); *prakamya* (the power to will things so—telekinesis); *isitva* (a power over the will of others—hypnosis) and *vasitva* (a power to subdue one's own will—self-hypnosis). Demonstrations of any of these skills are proof of holy perfection and perfect holiness (1991: 150).

As Krishnan Vaidyar succinctly stated, 'In order to practise advanced techniques of the marmmam a person must be spiritually pure, have concentrated patience, and not become easily upset'. To have attained the ability to attack the vital spots by pointing or looking is, like other yogic powers, a demonstration of a master's 'holy perfection and perfect holiness'. For Tamil siddhas, gaining accomplishment in such powers which can be demonstrated and practised in the material world is the rightful phenomenon of a successful *yoga* practice. Tirumular calls them as the 'seal of *yoga*' . . . the *siddhis* are integral elements of *yoga* practice and they are the modes of the *yogin's* being; they are the products of the natural unfoldment of consciousness in its evolution towards perfection (Ganapathy 1993: 53–4).

Stories about masters who possess such esoteric, subtle powers still circulate. Cheap paperbacks like *Kalarippayattu* and *Marmmamcuntaniyum* provide tantalizing bits of information on these seemingly miraculous powers of attack by looking:

> There is a bone in the neck known as *kalayellu*. If anyone points his finger at this spot which is nearly one inch from the *kalayellu*; the victim will fall unconscious and his urine and excrement will come out. This can be cured by lifting the chin (Velayudhan, n.d.: 28).

Magical, short-hand formulas are recorded for some attacks, such as '*a, a, kai ta ma va. Olinnumuttuinnakam*'. The author explains what the shorthand, apparently copied from an old manuscript, means:

> . . . if we point at the elbow with the thumb, the breath will be stopped, a kind of mucus will be discharged through the mouth, and the victim will also start bleeding. If not cured, the victim will die within forty-one days. But, after doing this vital spot, if remedial measures are quickly taken, the victim will be saved, i.e. by pointing at a spot one inch on the right side of the forearm from the elbow (ibid.).

These popular accounts elide superstition, magic and yogic powers of concentration, and continue to be very much a part of attempts to actualize this esoteric/yogic paradigm of practice.

In 1989, while a student of Chandran Gurukkal of Azhicode in both yoga and while learning a special form of yoga massage (*nadi sambradayam*), I asked Chandran if he had ever heard of these claims to yogic powers through which one might attack the vital spots by looking or pointing. An unassuming youth, in his early thirties at the time, and trained in both kalarippayattu and yoga, Chandran surprised me when he casually gave an account of this paradigm of subtle practice and its specific techniques based on his own experience. In a matter-of-fact manner, he recounted the story of how he had been initiated into, but never completed, the higher meditation techniques intended to allow him to gain the power to attack the marmmam as part of advanced yoga training. Chandran described the first time he witnessed his own teacher demonstrating these powers:

To Heal and/or To Harm • 195

One day my master came to my house. We were relaxing in my house chatting, when my master pointed to a cock and asked, 'Why is it standing still?' I said, 'I don't know.' So the master told me to throw some stones at the cock. I obliged him. But still the cock stood there. I went to catch it. It would run a few feet, and then stand still. My master teased me, 'Why can't you catch it?' In this way, I saw that my master could control everything.

Figure 6.28: The thirty-two yoga marmmam

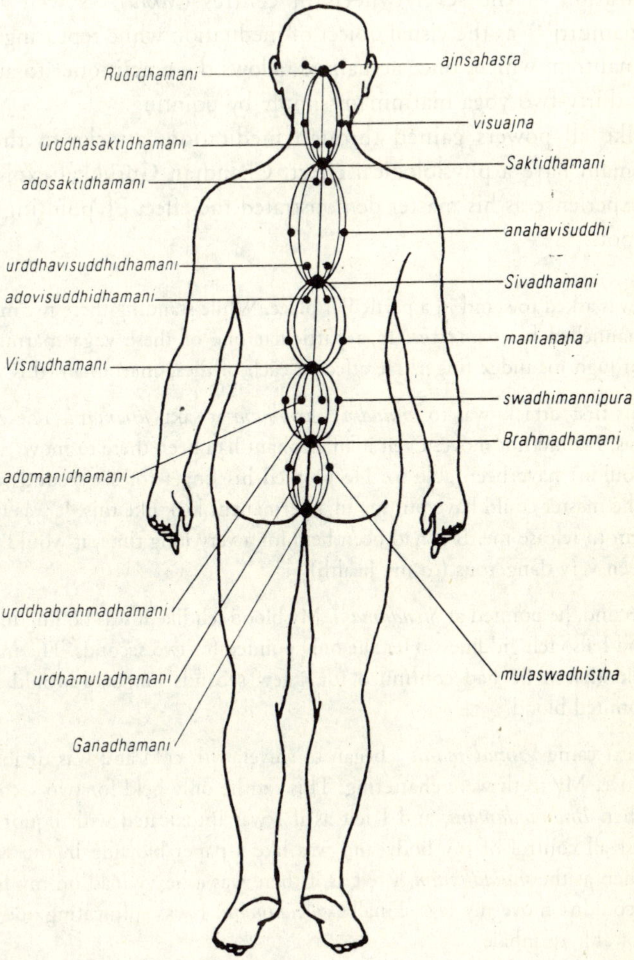

Rudrahamani
urddhasaktidhamani
adosaktidhamani
urddhavisuddhidhamani
adovisuddhidhamani
Visnudhamani
adomanidhamani
urddhabrahmadhamani
urdhamuladhamani
Ganadhamani

ajnsahasra
visuajna
Saktidhamani
anahavisuddhi
Sivadhamani
manianaha
swadhimannipura
Brahmadhamani
mulaswadhistha

| Fourteen marmmam at the ends of the interior subtle nadi | Six adharam marmmam | Twelve marmmam at the meeting of the nadi between the adharam |

Chandran Gurukkal explained that the vital spots attacked through accomplishment in higher meditational techniques are the 'yoga marmmam'—a set of thirty-two vital spots associated with the subtle body (Figure 6.28) and separate from the sixty-four or 107–8 vital spots of the gross, physical body. According to Chandran Gurukkal the power to attack these subtle yoga marmmam can *only* be generated through a forty-eight day period of initiation during which the practitioner fasts, practises restraint (brahmacharya), and special meditation techniques including time-specific visualization of the seven wheels or centres (*cakra*), as well as taking Dhyanamurti[125] as the visual object of meditation while repeating a special yoga mantram which, once actualized, allows the practitioner to attack any of the thirty-two yoga marmmam simply by pointing.

Like all powers gained through meditation, attacks to these yoga marmmam have a physiological effect. Chandran Gurukkal explained his own experience as his master demonstrated the effect of 'pointing' at these vital spots:

> I was asked to stand in a particular place. While standing there my master channelled his *manasakti* to a particular one of these yoga marmmam through his index finger. He affected each of these marmmam this way.
>
> His first 'attack' was to *visuddhi marmmam* at sakti *dhamani*. The effect was, I could not move. Even if an elephant had been there to move me, it wouldn't have been able to. He pointed his finger for six seconds only. The master could have put me in a permanent lock like this. It was up to him to release me. If it had been held for a very long time, it would have been very dangerous (to my health).
>
> Second, he pointed at *Sivadamani*. My blood felt like it was boiling inside, and I also felt giddiness. Here he only pointed for two seconds. The master said that if he had continued for a few seconds longer, I would have vomited blood.
>
> Next came *Visnudamani*. I began to shiver with cold and was unable to move. My teeth were chattering. This too he only held for two seconds. Then *Brahmadamani*, and I felt as if I was intoxicated with liquor as I lost all control of my body and was like a paper blowing in the wind. Then at the *muladharam*, I felt as if there was a heavy load on my head. I couldn't move my legs. Finally *gurudamani*. I was suffocating and was not able to inhale.

The subtle, esoteric ability to be able to attack the vital spots of either the gross or subtle bodies by pointing or looking is understood, like meditational practice itself, to extend the capabilities developed through psycho-physiological exercise of the gross body to an ever subtler level of accomplishment and actualization of 'powers' which produce physiological, rationally observable effects. However, accomplishment in such 'powers' is *always* relative and contingent. After noting how it was 'something great' that Chandran and his gurukkal actualized these thirty-two yoga marmmam since 'their perception was more subtle than normal people, so they perceived such delicate subtle centres', R. Perumal Raju went on to observe that 'if there is somebody whose perception is still more subtle, they will perceive still more centres! In fact, counting such centres is nothing less than counting the stars in the sky.'

Local Knowledge and Having a 'Doubtless Mentality'

I wish to return to some of the vernacular meanings and folk stories surrounding the concept of the vital spots with which I began this chapter. As a researcher who has gathered fifteen different versions of the vital spots among today's South Indian martial practitioners, I feel somewhat like the master who saw so many vital spots on the cow in his compound that he froze in inaction, unable to hit the cow anywhere. Were I to systematically collate *all* of these versions into a master chart of the human body, we too would see vital spots materializing everywhere we looked on the body, and as countless as the stars in the sky! What are we to make of this variability?

As we have seen the basic concept of vital spots, first identified in the *RgVeda* as those places where the vital energy is located, and which when penetrated have the potential to cause death or serious injury, has remained relatively constant. But it has also been a fluid concept, available to many modes of interpretation and popular, vernacular expression. Reflecting the skill which a martial/medical practitioner had to have in order to precisely penetrate a vital spot or revive someone, marmmam/marman/varman also refer to the 'core of anything, the quick'. Reflecting the secrecy which necessarily surrounded this dangerous knowledge as well as the fact that these spots are 'hidden' unless one knows where they are or how to see them, marmmam also refers to anything which is kept secret or hidden inside.

The concept of the vital spots has been subject to a variety of interpretations within particular interpretive communities—Ayurvedic physicians whose understanding of the vital spots was based on observations of battlefield injuries, martial practitioners whose lifetime of training was devoted to developing practical expertise in attacking and defending the vital spots, and martial/meditational practitioners who developed an esoteric interpretation and set of techniques for attacking/defending the vital spots based on their experience of the subtle body, and an accomplished ability to accumulate and concentrate 'power' through meditation. More specifically, kalarippayattu and varma ati practitioners developed their own context-specific versions of names, locations and practical techniques of attacking, defending and/or treating the vital spots.

From the perspective of a kalarippayattu or varma ati master who has been given full knowledge by a master within a particular lineage of transmission, his own particular, local practice possesses its own internal logic, coherence, efficacy and therefore appears normative. As Gurukkal Govindankutty Nayar explained:

> What we do is just follow (our particular) tradition. Other kalari have their own explanations and theories. In either case, if they simply believe it, it will have its own power. You must follow your own (local) tradition. If you change the forms (you) have received, it will not have its power (sakti).

Following Govindankutty Nayar's logic, one's powers of practice are derived from attaining accomplishment in those particular techniques given as a gift to the student by his master. And as R. Perumal Raju asserts, 'even within the followers of the same tradition, individual differences are bound to be there because each individual is a separate entity and their perceptions also vary'.

Balachandran Master's observation that as long as a practitioner learns from only one master the vital spots make complete sense, reflects the fact that a martial practitioner's knowledge of the vital spots must be 'doubtless'. Unlike the modern researcher or 'David' whose understanding of the vital spots is a blurred mass of confusion which results from attempts to cobble together coherence from several different traditions of interpretation, the practitioner is supposed to develop full confidence in the efficacy of his own techniques. Gurukkal Govindankutty Nayar explained:

> Being doubtless is the utmost target of the student. Therefore, whatever you do should be made perfect. You should never have doubts. Just do it! . . . You must have a doubtless mentality. Others may not have full confidence in themselves yet, and so they may have some lingering doubts. To have confidence you must have a pure heart and be true to yourself. You must not be proud or vain. One of the first steps toward doubtlessness is to have no pride; but you must have great belief in what you are doing. Then only will you know what to do at the proper time.

When one is doubtless his practice is instinctual. There is no premeditation, only action. He embodies the common folk expression of the ideal state of the martial practitioner—'the body becomes an eye' (*meyyu kannakuka*). What is done is done with the power and force appropriate to the moment—whether in giving a counter-application to a vital spot for revival, a healing stroke passing over a vital spot in a massage therapy or a potentially deadly blow or cut to a vital spot to disarm or kill an attacker.

Between the Fakir/Charlatan and the 'Master'

As a closing interpretive caveat to this chapter and especially to the esoteric/yogic 'power' to attack by pointing and/or looking, it is important to remember with Lee Siegal that in India the fakir/charlatan and the 'master' are part of a dialectical continuum which, given the metaphysical assumptions which inform 'magic' (and therefore notions of agency and action), allow the 'true master' *and* the 'charlatan' to cohabit not only the popular imagination but the reality of one's everyday life (1991: passim). This is illustrated in the spectacularization of the paradigm of accomplishment that took place in 1993 when, contrary to the traditions of initiation in esoteric knowledge by a master in techniques that must remain secret, kalarippayattu master A.K. Prakasan decided to 'go public' with his claim to have discovered the '109th vital spot' and to have attained the ability to fend off an attacker by simply pointing to a vital spot. He offered interviews to journalists as well as demonstrations for photographers. Accompanying two French journalists to visit Prakasan at his home, he claimed that he knew 'no one who has these powers. People say there was such a technique in ancient times, but no one knows it today'. Admitting that he had no teacher to initiate him into this esoteric knowledge, he claimed to have gained accomplishment in this power by first having a vision/dream in which this type of knowledge was revealed to him, and then developing a practical knowledge of these techniques through reading 'the *Puranas*' and an eclectic variety of 'other books'.[126] After practising *dhyana* on his own to gain control of his own 'life force, I created pointing at the vital spots as my own technique'. At the ensuing demonstration of his 'powers' staged for the two French journalists, he performed his ability to render five of his attacking students senseless by 'redirecting the heavy force of the enemy to make consequences come to him'. The demonstration was well staged, as apparently it had been for Saslin Salim of the English language weekly, *The Week*, who wrote in his 28 March 1993 colour photograph-illustrated story entitled, 'Finger Fighter: Prakasan can knock out opponents from a distance of 10 feet':

His index finger is his warhead. Prakasan Gurukkal makes challengers bite the dust by pointing it at them with all his might. The effect is devastating: opponents lose their senses and sink to the ground. Only Prakasan can bring the dazed men back on their feet. When charged up, he can knock out half a dozen men from a distance of ten feet (Salim1993: 20).[127]

Prakasan's public claim to such powers created protests from a number of kalarippayattu masters reported in the Malayalam dailies. A staff reporter for the 10 June 1993 *Malayala Manorama* quoted Muralidharan Gurukkal's public challege to Prakasan:

> Can you defeat me by pointing your finger? It is known that he defeated his own disciples this way. But this techique has to be tested with others who are in no way related to him . . . Agasthyar Muni's texts only refer to 108 vital spots. In *Susruta Samhita, Astanga Hrydaya,* and *Charaka Samhita* only 107 vital spots are mentioned. Nowhere is there reference to 'pointing *marmmam*' . . . The meaning of 'pointing' in northern style kalarippayattu is 'piercing.' (ibid.: 8)

The 11 June 1993 *Malayala Manorama* reported Prakasan's response—he was unwilling to engage Muralidharan Gurukkal in an *ankam* since that 'age is over'. Following the yoga paradigm of the concentration of mental powers to its logical extreme, Prakasan concluded,

> it is a method of controlling the mind. A real practitioner is the enlightened one who can control his hands, body, mind and eyes. Such an enlightened person cannot accept challenges. (ibid.: 5)

Chapter 7

When the 'Body is all Eyes': Attaining a State of Transformative 'Fury', 'Doubtlessness' and 'Mental Power'

As John and Jean Camaroff assert, 'no ethnography can ever hope to penetrate beyond the surface planes of everyday life, to plumb its invisible forms, unless it is informed by the historical imagination—the imagination, that is, of both those who make history and those who write it' (1992: xi). Part of the 'archive' of the 'annals of a cultural imagination' through which an historical ethnography of the practice of martial power in Kerala can be constructed are the representations and enactments of power, sacrifice, and kingship in Kathakali—a form of dance-drama enacting stories from the epics and *puranas* dating from the late sixteenth century and directly derived from kalarippayattu (Jones, 1983: 15; Zarrilli 1984). As discussed briefly in Chapter 2, Kathakali dance-dramas of Kerala enact the trials and tribulations of epic heroes like Arjuna, Yudhisthira, Bhima, Rugmamgada, Nala, Rama and/or anti-heroes such as Ravana, etc. as they are called upon to exercise their powers in particular circumstances. Kalarippayattu practitioners were those local martial 'heroes' trained to actualize similar powers. In this chapter I read between representations and enactments of 'heroic' power, sacrifice and kingship in one Kathakali dance-drama, *Rugmamgada Caritam ('King Rugmaamgada's Law')*,[128] and some of the commonplace ethno-semantic representations of heroic power in the ethnographic present, in order to better understand 'power' as a complex, nuanced, contextually and historically specific set of discourses, practices and behaviours. I focus in particular on the state of mind/being of the martial practitioner at the moment he wields his sword to kill—that existential moment when he should ideally be 'doubtless', have 'mental courage', possess 'mental power', i.e. that moment when his 'body is all eyes' and he attains a state of transformative 'fury'. These commonplace expressions represent that idealized state or condition of selfhood to which martial artists aspire as they practise their bodily-based techniques to 'transform themselves in order to attain a certain state' (Foucault 1988: 18).

BETWEEN KATHAKALI TEXTS AND THE ETHNOGRAPHIC PRESENT

Like other texts, Kathakali dance-dramas are 'anchored in the processes of their production, in the orbits of connection and influence that give them life and force' (Camaroff and Camaroff 1992: 34). Patronized by Kerala's highest land-holding castes, Namboodiri brahmans and royal princely families (either ksatriyas or high-ranking Nayars—Zarrilli 1992a), and first enacted by their Nayar martial retainers pledged to their service, the values and behaviour reflected in these dramas and their enactment are

> neither documentary records of the ruler-warrior (ksatriya) caste (Nayars) nor the fantasies of poets writing in isolation. They are texts of imagination that weave together traditional epic, mythology, and normative classical learning. Although like most Sanskrit texts they habitually eradicate their situatedness in time and place, being rooted in patronage (of high caste landholding families) they are at the same time expressive, often in indirect ways, of the anxieties and concerns of specific royal political milieux. Out of these varied sources, the poets create the dream of an order, an ideal, playful world. It is the pleasure of the connoisseur to enter this world, the work of the scholar to understand its intersection with . . . the past (Gitomer 1996: 43),

and the present. Reading between a Kathakali performance text written by Mandavapalli Ittiraricha Menon (1747–94) and current ethno-semantic representations of power, my intention is not to eradicate the situatedness of either, but to examine a few of the continuities and discontinuities between the discursive constructs and modes of enactment of power prompted by the 'anxieties and concerns' of both.

Given the vagaries and bellicosity of the exercise of power in medieval Kerala, not surprisingly one of the central anxieties and concerns for Kathakali's ruling, landholding patron-connoisseurs was exploring the nature of 'the heroic'. Based on the epics and *puranas*, Kathakali plays were authored to elaborate upon one or more of nine basic states of being (*stayi* bhava), and thirty-four secondary or complementary states (*vyabhicari* bhava) of their primary characters in order for the audience to 'taste' or have an aesthetic experience (rasa) of that state.[129] Within the traditional Kathakali repertory, the 'heroic' (utsaha bhava; vira rasa) and the 'erotic' (rati bhava; srngara rasa) are the two states around which many plays are primarily organized, and which other states complement and/or elaborate upon.

The heroic state is embodied by Kathakali's 'green' (*paccha*) make-up type—a class of characters which includes divine figures like Krishna, kings such as Nala and Rugmamgada, the five Pandava princes (most importantly Yudhisthira, Arjuna and Bhima) of the *Mahabharata*, as well as Rama. The predominant 'green' colour of the make-up reflects this character's basic moral uprightness, inner refinement and calm inner poise—the 'royal sage' of Sanskrit drama whose task as ksatriyas is to uphold dharma. Visnu's stylized mark is painted on the forehead with a yellow base and markings of red and black, and the white rice-paste base and frame sets off the predominant green in the make-up, reflecting the noble task of the type in life, and basic inner refinement. Within the basic type, characters range from Arjuna, Nala and Rugmamgada who most 'fit' the ideal, to Bhima who is something of a 'misfit'. Bhima belongs within the pacca type because he is a ksatriya, but whenever he is on stage he behaviourally and temperamentally tests the limits of the moral uprightness of the type. He must constantly be constrained by his brothers.

As represented in most Kathakali plays, the 'heroic' is a state dramatically marked by the hero's sacrificial act of bloodletting, usually accomplished through warfare when one or another demon or demon-king is dispatched by the end of the performance as in *Kichaka Vadham* ('The Killing of Kichaka'), *Duryodhana Vadham, Bali Vadham, Baka Vadham*, etc.[130] Fuller's assertion, noted earlier, that 'warfare itself is a reiteration of the idea that an ordered cosmos is created by sacrificial destruction' (1992: 124–5), is played out time and again on the Kathakali stage, traditionally toward the end of the play at dawn when the killing takes place. The predominance of the ritual of battle with its numerous killings in the Kathakali repertory is further evidence in support of Freeman's assertion that in medieval Kerala battle was a 'dominant metaphor for conceptualizing relations of spiritual and socio-political power' (1991: 588). Especially during Kathakali performances when stage blood is used for the disembowelment of Dussassana by Bhima or Hiranyakasipu by Narasimha, Kathakali can be seen as reflecting Kerala's 'harvest of war' where 'blood becomes the central metaphor for the essential fertilizing fluid of life' through 'the cutting of heads' or disembowelment, thereby promoting 'the health and fertility of the kingdom' (Freeman 1991: 289). My interest in the remainder of this chapter is in precisely *how* this act of sacrifice is enacted, i.e. in the state of mind/being of the martial/princely sacrificer in the act of bloody sacrifice.

THE 'FAILURE' AND EXERCISE OF POWER IN RUGMAMGADA'S LAW

Authored by Mantavappalli Ittiraricha Menon (1747–94), *King Rugmamgada's Law* enacts a version of the Abraham/Isaac story in which god tests his most avid devotee:

> King Rugmamgada, renowned devotee of Visnu, is so virtuous that the gods are jealous of him. They send Mohini, the celestial enchantress, to test his devotion to Visnu by leading him astray. Rugmamgada falls in love with the enchantress. She agrees to live with him as his consort on condition that he will never deny her anything she desires. He agrees on oath.
>
> On *ekadasi* day—the day most sacred to Visnu—after undergoing the necessary purificatory rites, King Rugmamgada begins meditating on Visnu when Mohini approaches him in an amorous mood. He tries to dissuade her, explaining that as a devotee of Visnu he must remain pure the entire day and can only fast and meditate. Mohini reminds him of his vow. She challenges him—she will only allow him to continue his fasting and meditation if he beheads his only son, Dharmamgada,[131] in his mother's (Sandhyavali) lap. Rugmamgada begs her to relent from her demand. She refuses.
>
> Dharmamgada himself comes forward and reminds his father that for members of their clan (ksatriyas), a vow must always be honoured. Rugmamgada undergoes the emotional torment of the contradictory demands of his situation, but finally knows he must sacrifice his son. Just as he raises his sword to strike, Visnu appears, and after blessing Rugmamgada, takes him to Vaikuntha, the heavenly abode.

My interpretation focuses on the section of the performance text in which Rugmamgada's state of mind is dramatically elaborated in performance. The great king has been reduced to pleading with Mohini, '. . . do not deceive (us)!'[132] Mohini responds by reminding him of his oath, and of the weight of its obligation:

> MOHINI: If you observe this rite today and do not kill your son, (your) vow will be broken—O King! Understand (this)!

In the sloka which follows, the result of Mohini's unexpected demand on Rugmamgada's state of mind is enacted:

sloka:
> When all of a sudden Mohini's unkind words fell on his ears, the king became greatly delirious because of the weight of (his) grief, and (he) fell, fainting, to the ground . . .

Even in the face of the extreme and unexpected demand Mohini makes of him, as a celebrated king and 'royal sage' Rugmamgada ideally should have been able to 'control his senses', maintain an inner equilibrium, and fulfil his duty by sacrificing his son. Recovering from his faint, but still in a state of distress and imbalance, Rugmamgada prays to the reclining form of Visnu, Sri Padmanabha, to protect him, 'the tormented one'.[133] Visnu does not come to his aid.

Then Rugmamgada's son, Dharmamgada—the literal embodiment of sacred law or duty (dharma) and continuation of divine rule within his kingdom—and his wife, Sandhyavali, enter. Dharmamgada bows respectfully at his father's feet and dutifully recites the reasons a son is born into this world. Standing before his father as the literal voice and embodiment of heroic duty and behaviour expected of the ksatriya clan, Dharmamgada reminds his father that 'grief does not become you'. With Rugmamgada's honour *and* sword on trial, Dharmamgada picks up the sword—indexical icon and vehicle of divine, royal and martial power—and tells his father,

> This is the sword. Please hold it. O protector of the people! Please preserve your vow! . . .

With the sword now in his father's right hand, he requests him to perform this 'graceful rite (vratam) (of sacrifice) with delight'.

In the performative interpolation (*ilakiyattam*) which follows between Rugmamgada, Mohini and Dharmamgada.[134] The focus is on the complex set of competing demands which Rugmamgada faces: the demand that he exercise the power of his sword as a ksatriya to uphold the truth of his vow and maintain the sanctity and legitimacy of their rule, and that he do so by engaging in an act of transgression by killing/sacrificing his son. Dharmamgada tells his father to 'protect the truth (*satyam*) to increase the fame of our own dynasty'. Rugmamgada responds by reflecting on his mental state:

> RUGMAMGADA: Alas! Such a fate (lit. 'head writing') has happened to me. This entire time I have not knowingly committed any sin. Yet this has happened to me. Why? O seat of affection, your father, this sinner

doesn't know what to do. I am immersed in an ocean of sorrow. Because my mind is not firm and brave, I acted like this . . .

Had Rugmamgada kept his mind 'firm and brave', he would not have fainted or experienced disequilibrium, but maintained the optimal state of 'doubtlessness' (*vita sankam*) reflected in the *Bhagavad Gita*, and been able to bring himself to sacrifice his son. In the *Gita* the ideal

> is that one should not be perturbed by feelings and emotions and lose one's balance . . . the mature person is one in whom desires enter without upsetting him. The analogy of the sea is given. Though rivers discharge their water continuously into the sea, the sea is ever motionless. In the same way the mature person experiences continually feelings and emotions, but he does not allow himself to be overpowered by them or to be swayed by them (Kuppuswamy 1993: 26; II.70).

Rugmamgada is suffering the somatic effects of mental distress which affects his ability to maintain utsaha bhava, and carry out his duty. When even a single 'doubt' or 'emotion' creates a ripple in one's consciousness, it is understood to potentially lead to that individual's ruin. In the *Bhagavad Gita*, when Arjuna's mind is 'distressed with sorrow', he too displays somatic effects like those of Rugmamgada:

> My limbs quail, my mouth goes dry, my body shakes and my hairs stand on end. The Gandiva bow slips from my hand and my skin too is burning all over, I am not able to stand steady and my mind is reeling (I, 23–30) (Rao 1978: 120).

Since 'the natural state of the mind/body is regarded in Hindu philosophy as basically flawed', one practises exercise, dietary and meditational techniques to compensate for 'natural irregularities' (Alter 1992: 95). Only when one achieves self-realization is perfect health and balance achieved—a state in which 'a person is not plagued by emotions of any sort' (ibid.). But even for epic and puranic heroes like Arjuna and Rugmamgada, the road to becoming a self-actualized royal sage is not easy, and one falters along the way. *Rugmamgada Caritam* dramatizes Rugmamgada's 'flawed' moment of weakness, emotional imbalance, and all too human 'doubt' along the road to actualization and release.

The dramatic and performative focus throughout this interpolation remains on Rugmamgada's mental state, allowing the senior actor playing the role to further elaborate the excruciating emotional roller-coaster ride that Rugmamgada takes as he attempts over and again to eradicate his 'fears', overcome the overwhelming pathos caused by the demand that he kill his son, make his mind 'firm' or controlled, and therefore regain his optimal state of 'bravery' and heroic demeanour so that he can fulfil his duty.

> ... (*Dharmamgada takes the sword and gives it to his father. Looking at the sword, and talking to it as a personified being.*) This sword has drunk the blood of many of my enemies. Will you cut this boy's neck and lick his blood? No, I have no fear.

By erasing his personal 'fear' and anguish in this situation, he attempts to regain mental equilibrium, and thereby the 'mental power', necessary to sacrifice his son.

> I will cut the boy's neck and maintain the good fame of our dynasty. (*He raises the sword and is about to bring it down, but as soon as he focuses his eyes on his son, he begins to lose his inner resolve, drops the sword to the ground, and falls to the ground in a faint. Rising from the ground, he embraces his son, and then turns to Mohini*) ...

Desperate, Rugmamgada turns once again to Lord Visnu, and after performatively embodying and enacting Visnu's ten major avatars, demands of him,

> ... And you protected Prahlada! Now why can't you protect this boy? (*Taking the sword.*) O Visnu! Please give me courage to sacrifice my son, thus protecting the truth, in order to maintain the good fame of our dynasty. Please be kind. I sacrifice the boy to protect the truth! (*Again he raises his sword, is about to sacrifice his son, but still is unable to do so.*)

Even calling on Visnu and taking him in mind has not completed Rugmamgada's transformation into a state which allows him to transcend the limitations of his feelings.

> (*Rugmamgada looks at the sword. Then immediately he looks at Mohini, then at his son. This is repeated as he enacts three complex and conflicting emotional states: his anger (krodha bhava) at Mohini for the demand she has placed on him, the heroic (utsaha bhava) resolve required of him by his duty as a ksatriya (represented by his sword), and the pathos (soka bhava) of the loss of his dear son whom he must sacrifice to keep his vow.*)

For Kathakali connoisseurs, this particular moment in the performance is the highlight when the actor sequentially enacts the three conflicting states which have produced Rugmamgada's mental confusion and inability to act.

> *In a moment of internal realization of what is demanded of him, Rugmamgada leans forward, and loosens his hair, drawing its long strands to either side of his head. As he raises himself up, his eyes are wide open, revealing his transformation into a state of 'fury' (raudra)* (Figure 7.1). O Lord of the world, please protect me. I have no fear. What you see with your naked eye is perishable. The truth is the only thing that is imperishable. Therefore, now what should I do? Cut the boy's neck and protect the truth itself. (*To Mohini.*) Watch what I do! (*Witnessing this transformation, Mohini herself is now unsettled emotionally and frightened.*)
>
> (*To Sandhyavali.*) You should not cry! Let all auspicious things come to you. (*He raises his hand to bless Dharmamgada.*)
>
> (*Rugmamgada now performs a choreography, raises his sword, and is about to cut his son's neck when Visnu appears from behind the raised curtain to grasp his raised arm and stop him. The auspicious conch shell is blown, and fresh flower petals rain down on Rugmamgada, marking Visnu's divine intervention.*)

What this Kathakali performance dramatically enacts is Rugmamgada's progression from the very familiar human condition of mental disequilibrium, lack of focus and loss of mental power 'caused' by our normative human frailties, to a transformative state of raudra ('fury') beyond all such potential distractions, and in which he is finally able to fulfil the 'heroic' demands of dharma by completing the ultimate act of transgressive blood sacrifice of his son. It is a state of concentrated awareness characterized by ekagrata in which all doubts, emotional upset and consciousness itself are transcended. It is an activated state (*rajasa*) of single-minded doing. At least temporarily entering into this transcendent state of raudra is necessary for the hero to ultimately be able to fulfil his duty by killing.[135]

Rugmamgada's entry into this state is clearly marked performatively when, unable to fulfil his vow after calling on Lord Visnu, he leans forward to loosen his hair. In other Kathakali performances, transformations into this state of 'fury' are marked by the loosening of the hair, as when beautiful women-in-disguise (*lalithas*) are transformed into demonesses (*Puthana Moksha* or *Kirmmira Vadham*), or when Bhima appears in his raudra form when is about to kill Dussassana by tearing out his entrails in *Duryodhana Vadham*.[136] The furious state is 'normative' for demonic characters whose fundamental nature (*gunam*) is to be (*tamasa*) shape changers who engage in transgressive acts. It is also the normative state of the goddess Bhagavati (Bhadrakali, Kali) in her 'terrifying' form (Caldwell 1995: passim) when she appears with her fierce, 'energized eyes', and whose total visual effect is to assume an expression that equally evokes vira rasa and raudra or fury— her inexorably conquering/victorious form as she defeats the demon Daruka (Jones 1981: 73). Iconographically with his wide-open eyes, Rugmamgada's state combining vira and raudra clearly articulates with that of the violent/ conquering Bhagavati.

But for pacca characters like Bhima and Rugmamgada who are required to engage in sacrificially transgressive acts of slaughter/sacrifice to fulfil their dharma, and for whom bloodletting is not 'natural', they can only do so when this state is appropriately marked as 'altered'. For Raudra Bhima this special role is played by an actor different from the one playing Bhima who appears in a special form of 'furious' make-up.[137]

In this state of single-mindedness, the royal sage Rugmamgada has overcome his emotional imbalance, doubts and sorrows, and stands without 'fear'. This state is marked by the signs of raudra in Kathakali performance and is distinct from the state of anger common to 'ordinary' experience. If it were not, it would be a state in which the practitioner was so absorbed in reacting *with* anger that he would not be in 'control', focused, or have 'mental power'. Rather, like Rugmamgada at first, he would be overcome by one or more emotion, and therefore be unable to fight with 'detachment'. The raudra state is a state of actualization quite different from a 'normative' state of consciousness. It is similar to that described in the 'Dhanur Veda' chapters of *Agni Purana* in which the martial practitioner 'conquers even Yama (the god of death)' (Dasgupta 1993a), i.e. conquers his 'fears' and 'emotions' and therefore is ready to die in battle. As represented in Kathakali, it is a state of heightened acuity in which the 'heroic' becomes realizable through one's actions in battle. For Rugmamgada, or Bhima, or the traditional kalarippayattu practitioner, everything is erased except the act of the 'sword'.

This is a state to which Mohini, hitherto in command and control, now responds with fear and distress. Seeing Rugmamgada before her in his transformed state, she is 'terrified'. She sees that he *will* complete this bloody sacrifice before her eyes. In this sense, when a hero embodies a state of 'raudra', it refers not to Rugmamgada's state of mind, but to the witness' experience of what happens when one *enters* this transformative state. In this state of sacrificial activation, the hero is as 'terrifying' as a demon, or

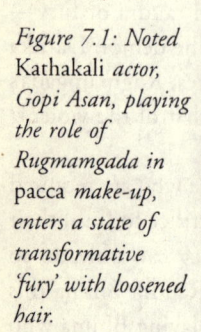

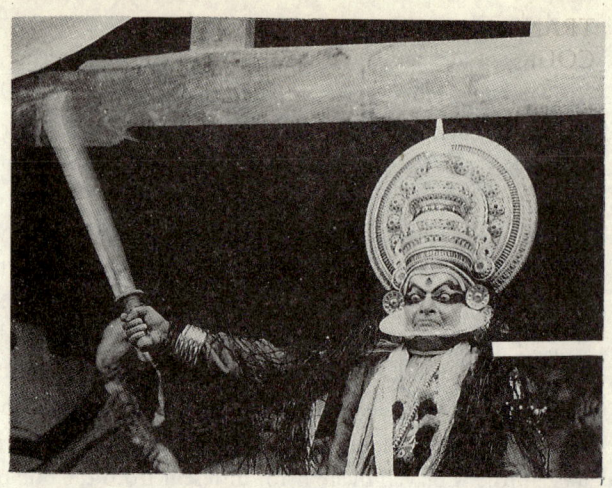

Figure 7.1: Noted Kathakali actor, Gopi Asan, playing the role of Rugmamgada in pacca *make-up, enters a state of transformative 'fury' with loosened hair.*

the goddess when she appears in her terrifying forms as Kali or Bhadrakali. Just as the Kathakali actor 'becomes' the character, so the martial artist 'becomes' a vehicle of the goddess' fury. The terror is in the eye of the beholder because of the 'terrible' things that happen when the divinely instantiated sakti concentrated in this state is unleashed. Mohini (and the audience) are 'terrified' of what Rugmamgada will do, just as villagers are 'terrified' of what the goddess might do.[138] And the most appropriate iconic index of this terrifying power is the sword where divine, royal and martial are manifest.

Sarah Caldwell asserts that in Kerala sexuality and war are both understood to 'release potentially uncontrollable passions leading to both life and death of sorts. Only heroic beings of great power can properly control these forces once they are unleashed' (1995: 308). When heroes engage in battle, a fight or an act of sacrifice like Rugmamgada, their predominant heroic state (utsaha bhava) must be complemented by moments of entering a furious state (raudra) when they must kill. It is the ability to enter this transformative state that allows the hero to 'properly control' the divine power and forces 'unleashed' by his practice which raise and actualize his 'powers'. When Kathakali's princes and kings enter this state of 'transformative fury' which allows them to 'act', they can become the 'heroes' they ideally aspire to be.

TRANSFORMATIVE 'FURY', 'DOUBTLESSNESS', AND 'MENTAL COURAGE' IN THE ETHNOGRAPHIC PRESENT

It may seem a long way from the late eighteenth-century Kathakali stage to the late twentieth-century kalari, but I think it no coincidence that the commonplace vocabulary masters use to discuss the optimal state of actualization of the kalarippayattu practitioner are terms describing the state that Kathakali's heroic characters like Rugmamgada had to achieve—a state where the practitioner is single-minded, 'doubtless', has 'mental courage', or attains 'mental power'. In the remainder of this chapter I explore these traditional discourses of practice, and the effect of practice on behaviour and lives in the ethnographic present.

In addition to congruence of the three humours discussed in Chapter 4, through practice one should 'naturally' begin to develop a calm and stable mental state. Gurukkal Govindankutty Nayar explained that 'kalarippayattu is 80 per cent mental and only the remainder is physical'. The 80 per cent mental is developed not only through the psycho-physiological martial exercises where single-point focus is first raised, but also, as discussed in Chapter 5, by following a strict routine of observances like Rugmamgada's observance of ekadasi.

> If you perform the exercises correctly and have the proper grip, then you begin to 'enjoy' practice. By doing this the whole body finds enjoyment. The mind won't be wandering here and there. You can do it with full confidence and courage. Your mind won't be in a flurry (*sambhramam*). Sometimes, in combat, one might become flustered. If an opponent is powerful, one might become nervous; so, slowly you must develop this ability to be calm, to have mental peace.

> What is most gratifying for an individual is when the mind is in a calm and stable state. What is ungratifying is when the mind is unstable and easily distracted . . .

This state is said to give the practitioner 'mental courage' (*manodhiryam*), i.e. the 'power to face anything that is dangerous to my health or mind. If I am confident of my art and health, then only can I have manasakti'.

Mental equilibrium is said to be 'read' on a person's face. 'If one faces an attack, relaxation of the face reflects mental equilibrium.' Ideally, this increased mental calm is not something esoteric, but of great practical use. Like the ideal epic hero, the ideal practitioner gains control of his emotions, achieves mental calm and courage, and becomes 'concentrated with a strong will'—a state of decidedness and singular focus on one's duty similar to the 'heroic' demeanour of the Kathakali hero.

The common Malayalam folk expression, *meyyu kannakuka* encapsulates the martial practitioner's idealized state of actualization where the bodymind is in such a concentrated state of acuity and awareness that, like Brahma, the 'thousand-eyed', the practitioner can 'see' everything around him, intuitively sensing and responding with his accomplished 'powers' to any/everything in the immediate environment. For the traditional martial practitioner, this state of superior actualization is developed in tandem with a notion of power (sakti) which, as we have seen, is not absolute, but highly ambiguous, contingent and context-specific. Having awakened and raised kundalini sakti within from the psycho-physiological practice of exercises, this 'power' was traditionally understood to take on the furious, raudra or destructive aspect of the goddess either alone or in combination with Siva as the fearful Kala-Bhairava. Through practice itself and/or realizing special *mantram* one might, as P.K. Balan described it, attain 'this special power of fury', i.e. reach an embodied state where 'fury' is concentrated and actualized.

I want to argue that this 'special power of fury' is comparable to the state of single-minded 'transformative fury' actualized by Rugmamgada—a state similar to that described by J. Richardson Freeman regarding Kerala's teyyam ritual performers. Freeman has observed that their bodymind state in performance 'entails no loss of consciousness, or "dissociation" in psychological terms, but rather a *heightened* sense of consciousness . . .' in which 'one's consciousness has not travelled somewhere else, shaman-like, but that instead, one's own body and mind are taken over and animated by a higher and more powerful (and I would add more concentrated) form of consciousness' (1993: 131). Some masters point out that the combination of self-confidence, doubtless heroism and internal fury manifest in the raising of kundalini sakti does not lead to emotional upset or anger, but rather to a state of intense concentration of energy (*aveshakaram*), 'the power generated from concentration'. In teyyam this heightened sense of consciousness takes the shape of 'performative acuity with regard to the rituals' (ibid.). For the martial practitioner, like Rugmamgada, it is a single-minded performative acuity with regard to wielding the weapon.

This ideal state of 'transformative fury' where the 'body is all eyes' and one possesses 'mental power' is, as discussed in Chapter 1, a discursive field of the possibilities for the exercise of power. But that power can only be manifest when exercised on a particular body in a context since 'power' only comes into being as it is practised. Kalarippayattu practitioners no longer pledge themselves to death on behalf of a ruler, nor do they form 'suicide squads' which would sacrifice themselves in the 'glorious' harvest of war on the battlefield of death, nor need they contend in a life-or-death situation with opponents who may have gained access to esoteric, seemingly magical powers and abilities. Since the kalarippayattu practitioner no longer necessarily uses his martial skills to kill or be killed, there is no longer an immediate need to be able to enter this state of 'transformative fury'; therefore, it is not surprising that just as the practice of the more esoteric aspects of kalarippayattu are becoming the exception rather than the rule, this state of actualization is only vestigially evident in the ethnographic present. But there are those rare occasions in the kalari when one witnesses a glimpse of this state of actualization. Although anecdotal, in Chapter 1 I described one such occasion, and my reaction to it:

> The master's eyes opened wide (see Figure 0.1), sparks literally flew from the student's shield from the tremendous force of the torrent of blows to the head, ribs and ankles he delivered as he backed the student into the corner of the kalari.
>
> The exchange momentarily took my breath away. At the time I could not explain why. I did not have an appropriate language with which to express what I had witnessed. In retrospect, my breath was taken away, not out of a sense of danger for either myself or the student practising, but for the fluidity and virtuosity of the exchange, the single-point focus, as well as the manifest power and 'danger' in the master's attack. But it was a 'danger' different from that I had experienced in Badagara where I had been afraid *for* students, not *of* the manifest (but controlled) power that was being unleashed, and that *could* and *would* do harm *if* unleashed.

What I witnessed then, and perhaps a handful of other times in a few other kalari I have visited over the past twenty years, is the concentration of the powers of practice in this optimal state of actualization. I experienced a practice so 'concentrated' with 'mental power', and so 'single-minded' that I felt the 'terror' of a state of (transformative) 'fury' that could do terrible harm.

In an era when the necessity of actualizing one's powers in combat have been narrowed from a panoply of forces and powers locally immanent on the field of battle and/or the duel platform, to the usually hypothetical arena of application on the streets, the demonstration stage, the training space, and/or the treatment room, the powers that might be visited upon one are becoming more tame and mundane, if no less important, than in the past. With rare exception, the practice of kalarippayattu is becoming more about actualizing and harnessing one's bodymind and powers for use in daily life than on the battlefield. But practice itself, and these traditional ethno-semantic understandings of practice exist as an elaborate set of metaphors useful to the practitioner for crafting his self *in* life. Chapter 8 explores some of the ways the practitioner's self is being crafted and negotiated today.

Chapter

8 | Repositioning the Body, Practice Power and Self in the Ethnographic Present

As suggested in Chapter 1, kalarippayattu is being practised, performed and its images produced in increasingly heteronomous contexts, and has therefore taken on new and highly divergent meanings within the transnational, global flows of 'public culture' (Appadurai and Breckenridge 1988: passim). Along with its complex political history and periods of rule by communists and/or left front state governments (see Nossiter 1982, 1988), Kerala has rapidly become a consumer capitalist economy. Carving out a niche for themselves in these new economies, kalarippayattu practitioners must run their kalari as small businesses—either as martial arts schools and/ or as clinics, and compete with other karate/self-defence schools, kalaris, or clinics for students and patients. The economic and social pressures to alter long-term kalarippayattu training to fit new images of 'martial arts' are compelling. When the Malayalam movie featuring traditional kalarippayattu, *Vadakan Veera Gadha*, was released in 1989, it created an immediate impact at some kalari in the number of students beginning training. But as Raghavan Nambiar explains, the initial enthusiasm was short-lived—'because of the rigorous and difficult training methods, those who joined the kalari left after one or two months' (Ajay 1993: 1). Like most other traditional arts, only a few masters are making a good living through their traditional practices. Especially those in small villages see little future in making a living by teaching the art. Puthuppanam Madhu, one of a number of younger teachers whose fathers are well known kalarippayattu practitioners and who are increasingly well educated (Madhu earned a graduate degree in economics), explained, 'Sometimes I think about stopping kalarippayattu, going into some other line of work. If I go to the Gulf, I can earn enough money to live . . . I worship kalari, but we can't eat it if we are hungry' (ibid.: 3).

How kalarippayattu practitioners think and talk about their art, and represent it to an increasingly diverse public is shaping the clientele attracted to study. In each context of its practice, presentation or representation the kalarippayattu practitioner's body, practice, power and self are constantly being repositioned for the practitioner himself, teacher and/or cultural consumers, thereby making available quite different images, discourses of power and agency, experiences, knowledge and meanings for them all. In addition to the 'traditional' paradigms, discourses and practices of power discussed above, I explore here several other examples of the dynamic and shifting set of relationships in the ethnographic present.

NEGOTIATING AND INTERPRETING KALARIPPAYATTU PRACTICE, SELF AND PERSON TODAY

The 'body is all eyes', as a special, virtuosic body of practice explored above, is not separate from the daily body inhabited by the practitioner. Rather, it is one mode of incorporation which is constitutive of the practitioner's horizon of experience. Along with other modes of incorporation and cultural practice, kalarippayattu is, as anthropologist Michelle Rosaldo explains, 'the very stuff of which our subjectivities are created' (1984: 150). It helps shape one's perceptions, experience and behaviour.

Today, practice is often understood to affect not just the gross, physical body of the humours and saps, but 'behaviour' as well. 'Good' health is viewed as equally dependent on maintaining equanimity among *all* aspects of one's life including body, mind and behaviour. As Sudhir Kakar points out, traditional Ayurvedic treatises 'are as much dissertations on correct behaviour as they are descriptions of pharmacological potencies and physiological equilibria' (1982: 220). One student at the C.V.N. Kalari, Palakkad explained how, in addition to better health, practice

> also increases stamina and concentration. Since I joined the kalari I have been able to obtain a high degree of concentration in my daily routines. Above all it has helped me to be calm in the midst of the people with whom I associate. In my experience kalarippayattu practice leads both to natural resistance in the body and to better behaviour.

As students advance they are expected to be able to control their feelings and emotions, respond calmly in an emergency, and possess the capability of resisting the 'temptations of modern life'. A student of Gurukkal Govindan Kutty Nayar explained how

There is a stability of mind that comes from practice. Just two days ago my son got milk caught in his nostrils while feeding, and began coughing and crying. Everyone got upset, but I remained completely calm and figured out what to do.

A group of students in Palakkad explained that if you practise kalarippayattu, 'you won't go for corruption'. The student should 'naturally develop wisdom and not go astray', i.e. he will avoid alcohol and drugs and be of 'good character'.

One master, well trained in both kalarippayattu and yoga, asserted that if one learns kalarippayattu properly, then 'he *should* gain release from unhappiness'; however, he also noted soberly, 'many practitioners have turned out to be wasters, drunks and of bad morals'. He cited the example of Chandu from the northern ballads, the infamous anti-hero who, bought off by money and a promise to win the affection of a beautiful young woman, betrayed his cousin, Aromar Chekavar. For this master, Chandu is an example of the type of kalari master who possesses a tamasa constitution. The ideal kalarippayattu teacher 'has a satvika constitution. If the master has a truthful constitution, it will be a blessing for the student. But, this master asked me rhetorically as he spoke from bitter personal experience, 'if some masters *do* possess a dark constitution, what will not happen? There will be a split (*sthanabramsam*) between student and master. Everything will become confused (*alangolappeduka*)!'

These examples illustrate two apparently contradictory assumptions: practice is one means of fundamentally altering one's basic, inherent nature or gunam and behaviour; however, one's fundamental nature and behaviour is understood to be given by one's gunam. Among many Hindus, all life is ranked unequally according to the relative proportion of the three gunam and the corresponding 'behavioural code (*dharma*) held appropriate to the disposition of those *gun*[am]' (Davis 1976: 6).[139] Gunam has been defined as 'property' or 'quality' (Gundert 1982: 332); 'radical material substances' (Davis 1976: 6); or 'subtle qualities, attributes, or strands' (Marriott 1980: 1). The three gunam include goodness or truth (satva), passion (rajasa), and darkness (tamasa). As Marvin Davis has observed, they are the

> 'stuff' of which the universe is made. Together they are the constituent elements of all matter; not the attributes of matter, but the three modes in which matter itself is constituted.
>
> Physical nature and behavioural codes are not (. . .) distinct and separate features . . . Hindus regard the natural and the cultural as cognitively

non-dualistic features. Each is immanent in the other; each is inseparable from the other; each is a reflection of and realization of the other (1976: 6–8).

It is still often assumed that all persons belong to specific jati defined by the inhering qualities of one's substance and accompanying behavioural code. As one older master told me, 'The three gunam are according to sastra. Brahmans are satva; ksatriyas are rajasa; and Nayars as sudras are usually associated with tamasa.' Although fundamentally tamasa by birth, as we have seen, Nayars and other practitioners of kalarippayattu must possess the rajasa element as a manifestation of the energetic, active quality necessary to develop a strong will characteristic of a vira bhava, and likewise the satva characteristic of mental calm—both are needed to remain determined, yet calm, in the face of combat. Moore notes that

> the *rajasik* quality of Nayars is seen in the idea of their fitness for war, the suitability of their natures for substances like liquor and meat, and their constant propensity to outbursts of anger . . . ' and that 'a move in the direction of *satva* is always possible (1983: 438).

One's fundamental gunam is determined at birth according to the substances mixed by the couple, the specific time of birth, and the influence of the stars and the gods (Marriott 1980: 5).[140] As Gurukkal Govindankutty Nayar said, 'in every person the combination of the three gunam varies'—among those of the satva type, there will be those with a predominance of each, i.e. of goodness, energetic or dark substance:

> Arjuna as the Son of Indra is predominantly rajasa, but with all his meditational practices he tended to gain satva. Bhima as the son of Vayu has strength and power. His power is more from his strength than skill. Therefore he is more tamasa than Arjuna, and there is also an element of the demon in his skill.

Although the fundamental combination of gunam is thought to be determined at birth, it is still possible to alter one's gunam. Govindankutty Nayar explained:

> It is possible to alter the three gunam. But, if a person has a predominance of one of the gunam he will do all things with that personality.

> You can alter the three gunam through one's karma, or through the nature of one's actions. Kalarippayattu is one way of altering the gunam but it

depends on the involvement of the person practising. If you watch three different students in the kalari you can see change in some but in others there will be no change.

He illustrated his point with the following story:

> One man who was hideous was always hurting others while practising kalarippayattu. He was a tamasa type. Others will be gentle and quiet, and some may even be too satva to practise the martial art. Only after a very very long practice the gunam may begin to change. There are two reasons for the change: when one gets more self-confidence, he becomes softer and is less prone to anger (associated with tamasa)—the mind becomes much calmer. One becomes calmer because of practice, especially through breath control. And when one's behaviour changes, his gunam changes. Just as vratam (simple forms of meditation/concentration) brings more of the satva aspect, so in my experience does kalarippayattu practice.

Since 'a person's gunam attains its mature and relatively permanent state between the ages of three and twelve' (Daniel 1984a: 141), students who begin their training at the traditional age of seven are considered more likely to manifest a change toward satva in their basic gunam complex, i.e. training will more likely affect the type of person they become. Since more students today begin their training at an older age, their gunam complex is more solidified and their behaviour less open to change. Some teachers watch for signs of a tamasa type of student.

> In my experience I can usually see a tamasa because he has no patience. Immediately he goes outside (the kalari) and tries everything (contrary to instructions). He's overpolite the first day, trying to please and offer the guru everything. If I find a student who has these (tamasa) qualities, I will send him away. It won't go right and won't be right for the art as well.

A tamasa student may misuse his knowledge and fly in the face of the code of ethics and behaviour traditionally circumscribing use of kalarippayattu.

> A tamasa person will lose his temper and be out of control. He will experience failure because he will have no control over his emotions. The master must be more discriminating. In the process of selecting (students to progress in training), there must be an evolution of character going on. To make someone a master in full, it would be difficult for someone who is tamasa. For such a person, the second time anything goes wrong in class, he'll just walk away, cursing his students!

The ideal student of kalarippayattu gains control of his emotions, and through increasing development of mental calm and courage becomes 'concentrated with a strong will'. The student should develop the intuitive ability to follow the common code of conduct traditionally assumed by the kalarippayattu practitioner—today, to only use these potentially deadly techniques when life is in danger, and never to become an unprovoked aggressor. Although from a Tamil, ati murai text, the following illustrates the explicit nature of commonplace instructions about when and how to act in the event of an unprovoked attack:

> If somebody comes to attack you, salute him with humility and evade his attack. God will save you from the first blow, and you should forgive him for this first attack. If the enemy attacks you a second time, evade the attack with techniques and take your master in your mind. Even then, if the enemy tries to hit you a third time, watch his movements carefully and, that insistent fool will come and fall into your lap.[141]

Some masters downplay the reading of kalarippayattu as involved with the goddess' heated 'fury' discussed above. One master explained that 'the basic aspect (bhava) of the kalari is as an educational institution, so the goddess here is not so hot, cruel or frenzied'. This particular interpretation and the description of practitioners as having a calm, satvika mental state is a brahmanically influenced idealized discourse of the self and person constituted by practice. This is a further example of the domestication and homogenization of traditional martial practice where the 'furious' aspect of the goddess is converted into uniform mode of satvika devotionism.

As an idealized discourse, there are numerous historical and contemporary examples of practitioners who transgress or fail to actualize this experiential and behavioural ideal, as the examples of Chandu and Tacholi Otenan make clear. As discussed in Chapter 2, Tacholi Otenan is perhaps the best historical example of the potentially erratic, rajasic personality whose use of the martial practitioner's powers is as capricious as the nature of that constellation of powers itself. Other highly volatile personalities practise kalarippayattu today.

At one kalari I visited regularly in 1983, one Tiyya practitioner in his mid-twenties from a relatively poor family was perceived by his main (Nayar) teacher as a 'trouble-maker' who broke the rules and discipline required of students. Students were traditionally instructed not to practise outside the kalari or to ever show/teach the techniques to others. When the teacher found out that the student was practising *and* teaching some local boys outside his kalari, and the student resisted the master's attempts to discipline him, they fell out. The student left the kalari, sought out a new teacher of his own caste who revealed many secrets to him, and began teaching at his home. A brash, energetic and self-confident young man, he began to invent his own techniques of practice which emphasized kalarippayattu as a practical self-defence system, and took in students whom he trained next to his house. He began to compete with his old teacher for students, and both of them would field teams at local Onam celebrations. The 'upstart's' students performed impressive displays of self-defence techniques which excited public attention. Like Otenan, he used his personal dynamism and charismatic energy (rajasic quality) as a means of personal and social empowerment. Unlike Ekalavya, this student refused to capitulate to the power and authority of his master.

A clear ideology is at work in the interpretation of gunam which emphasizes control as the ideal behavioural model. Masters taught and served at the behest of local rulers. From the master's position within society and the kalari, he is given the power to read a particular student's behaviour as tamasa, and thereby to determine whether the student gains access to the potentially lethal techniques and 'secrets' of practice by means of which one gains access to potentially deadly powers of practice. What Tacholi and his numerous contemporary counterparts illustrate is how any set of martial techniques and the powers to which pratice leads are circumscribed, shaped and actualized by the idiosyncratic temperament of the individual.

KALARIPPAYATTU AS A 'TRADITIONAL ART' AND ARTISTIC DISCIPLINE

In Chapter 2 I discussed kalarippayattu as an encapsulation of Kerala's mytho-historical heritage and the role it played in the formation of a distinctly Malayali identity. I also discussed how kalarippayattu is often figured as a 'traditional art' and carrier of the Kerala heritage which must be practised according to its 'traditional ways'. For practitioners who want to maintain the 'traditions' discussed above, kalarippayattu training is still a difficult and long-term process, and students are not introduced to 'practical' techniques until late in their training. This does not lend itself to easy marketing today, especially with young people. Chandran Gurukkal commented how

> Youngsters are very enthusiastic about studying self-defence, but kalarippayattu is not so easily learned. For this at least twelve years are

required. Do young people have the time? Are they even willing? Everyone wants to catch a fish without wetting his hands. Today, someone who goes to a kalari for one year tries to become a guru! (Ajay 1993: 1).

In this view the beauty of kalarippayattu forms, the positive, health-giving experience of its practice, and its potential as a source for use in other arts are often emphasized. This paradigm has been especially important at several successful kalari that give numerous stage demonstrations, and have attracted a number of non-Malayali actors and dancers who attend short and longer-term courses of training in order to use kalarippayattu as a basic psycho-physiological discipline for artistic practice. As part of the 'theatre of roots' movement during the 1970s, noted Kerala theatre director Kavalam Narayana Panikkar began using kalarippayattu along with other traditional Kerala dance and theatre forms to train members of his modern theatre company, 'Sopanam', so that they could create a uniquely Indian-based performance style and aesthetic. Numerous other Indian and non-Indian dance and theatre practitioners, myself included, have used kalarippayattu as a basic training regime (Zarrilli 1993, 1995; Manavendranath 1995; Krishnadas 1995), and/or as a base technique for new Indian dance. The latter has been especially important in the work of two noted contemporary choreographers, Madras-based Chandralekha (Bharucha 1995), and more recently Daksha Seth whose entire company trains in kalarippayattu in the C.V.N. Kalari, Thiruvananthapuram, on a daily basis. In this paradigm kalarippayattu is understood to provide a set of pre-expressive psycho-physiological techniques to develop full-body awareness to then be used in dance or theatre performance. The emphasis on long-term training in the preliminary body-exercises to produce body-awareness is understood as the *raison d' être* of kalarippayattu, and therefore those who share this perspective are not troubled by the years it can take to be introduced to practical self-defence techniques.

Although the most visible public interpretration of kalarippayattu today, this reading has not gone uncontested, nor is it universally accepted by all practitioners. Within Kerala a handful of kalarippayattu practitioners are aware of the larger international world of Asian martial arts and the calibre of world-class practice of other martial arts. A few among them, such as C. Mohammed Sherif, are attempting to maintain the traditional progression of practice and all its techniques, including self-defence forms, but ensure that when kalarippayattu is demonstrated in an international martial arts venue, its practical fighting efficacy and the power of its techniques are emphasized. For these practitioners many of the assumptions discussed here are not only important, but applied to daily practice and demonstrations.

While serving as a vehicle for establishing the Kerala heritage as an heroic Malayali identity, the narrative of kalarippayattu as encapsulating the Kerala heritage has also served as an ironic, anachronistic presence. When juxtaposed with the dynamic, action-packed power of live or cinema versions of karate emphasizing the apparent usefulness of the latter as a practical self-defence art, the demonstration-oriented version of body control exercises and manipulation of 'outdated' weapons, appears anachronistic to many young Malayali males. If over the past thirty to forty years many Malayalis have read kalarippayattu and its traditions as the epitome of Malayali manhood and/or of its heritage, many youth are eschewing that version of manhood today. They opt instead to practise those East Asian martial arts, especially karate, which in their 'street wise' versions better fit a transnational cosmopolitan image to which they aspire. When I asked one fourteen-year-old Malayali boy why he had started studying karate and not kalarippayattu, he simply shrugged his shoulders with disbelief that I was even asking.

I think that these discourses of kalarippayattu as producing a 'healthy body', a calm satvika disposition, and being a 'traditional' art are drawn as much from class considerations as from a brahmanical ideal. 'Fitness' is increasingly a concern of India and Kerala's growing middle classes, and modern theatre and dance are both products of this middle class. And kalarippayattu as a representation of Kerala history attracts those middle class parents seeking an identity for their children, especially among Nayars. Bryan S. Turner notes that

> . . . according to Bourdieu, while the middle class prefers fitness, the working class develops bodies which exhibit male strength. We can thus see that the body is brought into fashion and consumer culture as a mark of distinction, as a symbolic representation of class differences, as a field for gender differentiation, and as a potentiality which must be managed in the process of ageing in order for the individual to remain part of the scene (1992: 47).

To conclude this chapter, I present examples of how two Malayali practitioners, one in Thiruvananthapuram and one in Malaysia, have creatively negotiated 'traditional' and 'practical' discourses and paradigms of practice, and how the 'tradition' is incorporating harder self-defence techniques into its repertory.

KALARIPPAYATTU FOR THE PAN-ASIAN 'JET-SET' GENERATION: THE SELF-DEFENCE PARADIGM

Like a number of masters interested in kalarippayattu as a practical martial art, Ustaz Haji Hamzah Haji Abu's International Kalri-Payat Dynamic Self-Defence Institute in Kuala Lumpur, Malaysia, has repositioned the body of the kalarippayattu practitioner to fit a street-wise self-defence paradigm. Born into a family tradition of practising kalarippayattu, Ustaz Hamzah followed both his father and grandfather, and, in 1948 at the age of six, took his first lesson in kalarippayattu on the same day he began class in a traditional Muslim school. In a special training space at his family home in Malappuram district in central Kerala, his first teacher (Master Kunnachan Veetil Bavo from Andathode, Malappuram district), father, grandfather, and all the other adult males of the family gathered to bless both him and his father's sister's son, who began training together. His training began by applying oil to his body, putting on the kacca wrapped to support his navel region, receiving a light massage to the whole body, and then performing a few preliminary exercises. To mark this largely ceremonial occasion there were readings from the Koran and a goat was slaughtered for a family feast. Thereafter, in the mornings he received his religious education, and in the evenings his martial training.

Between the ages of six and fifteen, Hamzah trained under eleven different teachers including Muslims, Christians and Hindus. He describes himself as 'crazy for kalarippayattu', paying masters to come to his house to teach him techniques. Just before leaving for Malaysia at the age of sixteen in 1958, he learned a few of the most secretive kalarippayattu techniques—location, attack and defence of some of the vital spots.

Hamzah describes how at first he was 'spellbound by the number of martial arts practised' in Kuala Lumpur—the Malaysian art of silat, Chinese kungfu, Japanese judo, Korean taekwan-do, and various forms of karate. Hamzah saw these arts at demonstrations, in their training halls, as well as in their representations in popular magazines and films. After two years of this exposure to other martial arts, Hamzah concluded that 'kalarippayattu was far superior to' them all.

The landscape of Hamzah's imagination, like millions of others caught up in migration prompted by an increasingly global economy, was altered by his move to Kuala Lumpur. Anthropologist Arjun Appadurai uses the term *ethnoscape* to describe 'the changing social, territorial, and cultural reproduction of group identity' characteristic of Hamzah's new location, and of the way in which his relocation was crucial in his re-imagination of kalarippayattu (1991: 191):

> The landscapes of group identity—the ethnoscapes–around the world are no longer familiar anthropological objects, insofar as groups are no longer tightly territorialized, spatially bounded, historically unselfconscious, or culturally homogeneous.
>
> By *ethnoscape*, I mean the lanscape of persons who make up the shifting world in which we live: tourists, immigrants, refugees, exiles, guest-workers, and other moving groups and persons . . . (ibid.: 191–2)

Amidst this shifting, intercultural experience, the martial art of Hamzah's youth was juxtaposed with a global concatenation of images, discourses and paradigms of martial practice available in Kuala Lumpur—an experience through which he began to revision kalarippayattu. From the many images, discourses, and paradigms available from both Kerala and Kuala Lumpur, the principal one that crystallized this revisioning may be characterized as a practical, street-wise, self-defence paradigm of the cosmopolitan 'man-of-action', represented graphically in the ubiquitous figure of the martial arts practitioner displaying his strength, expertise, power and agency as he executes an extended high kick or fights off multiple attackers. Hamzah became convinced that if kalarippayattu was reinvented to fit this self-defence paradigm, it could compete for attention and students in the cosmopolitan Kuala Lumpur martial arts market-place.

From Revisioning to Practice: 'Re-elaborating' Kalarippayattu for a New Public

In 1960 Hamzah began a long process of 're-elaborating' kalarippayattu for a new Kuala Lumpur public that led to the 1974 opening of the first kalarippayattu training centre outside of Kerala, India. I borrow semiotician Patrice Pavis' term 're-elaboration' to describe the process of transformation which takes place when a tradition or practice is altered for a new context (1989: 38).[142] In this instance, Hamzah gradually re-elaborated all aspects of kalarippayattu for a more global, cosmopolitan public including its organization, pedagogical structure, techniques, accoutrements of practice and the narrative and images used to present and represent the art. This process of re-elaboration and transformation repositioned not only the practitioner's body, but also the notions of agency and power implicit in that body's practice. By the time of my visit in 1984, both Hamzah's style and his narrative history about its development had become crystallized as a practice and as a history. It is the story of the invention of this new style that I now relate.

In 1960 when Hamzah decided to bring kalarippayattu to this new public, he returned to Kerala for eleven months of training under three different teachers and became 'enlightened in (the practical aspects of) kalarippayattu'. During this trip and when he returned again in 1965 and 1967, Hamzah learned over one hundred locks, releases and counters to weapons attacks, how to fight off two, three or four opponents at a time, as well as numerous disarming tactics. Focusing exclusively on practical applications for fighting—especially locks and escapes—he took no interest in the preliminary exercises, advanced weapons training or esoteric ritual or meditational dimensions of practice.

In 1974, Hamzah reorganized kalarippayattu to make it 'international' by purging it of what he perceived to be its local, outmoded aspects—the preliminary exercises, massage and breathing techniques associated with the royal sage. He foregrounded the practical self-defence techniques which would appeal to his cosmopolitan public—techniques associated with the raw strength and power of a Bhima. Hamzah is clear about his reasons for these changes:

> If a diamond is kept in the ground, people will ignore it. They will only be interested in a polished and cut stone. Kalarippayattu is like that. There would have been no interest in the old style of this martial art. Today people will not be interested in the (body control) exercises. People want to learn things very fast. If I followed the Kerala style (of teaching), people would leave after two weeks. I don't think this would work (in Kuala Lumpur).
>
> In Kerala, the teachers are very protective. Some are angry with me for bringing (all these practical techniques) out into the open and making them available to all. The thinking in Kerala is very short-sighted. People in Kerala only know their own world and not the world outside. I felt it was my duty to teach what I know and help people believe in kalarippayattu's greatness.

Hamzah's vision of kalarippayattu shaped the raw strength and power of a Bhima into an urban, cosmpolitan, street-wise art in which precision, speed of execution and learning, and practical application in a street encounter are most important. He separated poses and steps from longer body-exercise sequences which in the traditional context are understood to lead to healthful congruence of the humours, and recombined them for purely offensive or defensive purposes. He joined basic stances and steps with more advanced kalarippayattu bare hand techniques including locks, throws, releases and tricks, i.e. techniques which, 'if you're really in a fight', allow you to 'counter or cheat an opponent'.

Hamzah also added approximately a hundred throws learned from studying Indian wrestling during one of his return trips to Kerala—a tradition associated in particular with Bhima and Hanuman (Alter 1992: passim). He organized combinations and sequences of moves specifically for self-defence, counter-attack, or disarming an opponent in five major categories: locks, blows, throws, steps and 'general dynamic techniques' or combinations (Figure 8.1).

Hamzah crafted a narrative to describe his reconstituted kalarippayattu, proclaiming that all its techniques are

> based on actual attack and counter-attacks from the very beginning with no imaginary movements or punches in the air. Kalari-Payat is a direct method of combat. Each one of the thousands of Kalari-Payat techniques is a complete finishing tactic, which enables the person to get into the enemy and put him under control . . . Kalari-Payat is a training to fight with the arts of chops, blows, kicks, punches, squeezes, locks, throws, sweeps breaking technique, fallen-down (sic) techniques and steps, movings and pressure-point tactics, also vital-point attacks, all methods of sticks, all ranges of weapons, swords, shields, axe, daggers, ropes, etc. and all releasing techniques.
>
> Kalari-Payat . . . is taught strictly for self-defence . . . (and is) aimed to equip its practitioner with devastating combat tactics that can apply in real defence (Hamzah n.d.: 1)

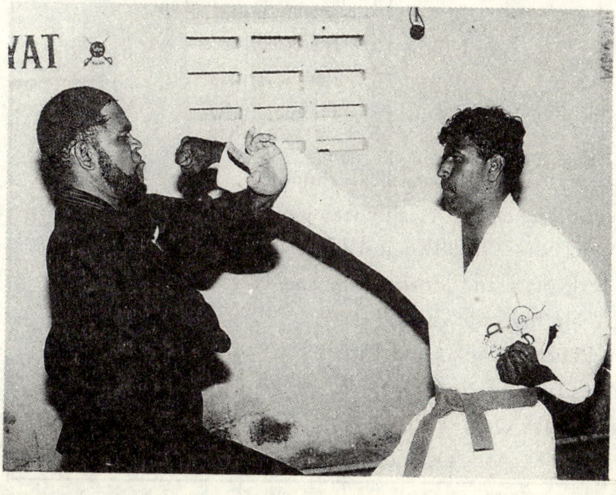

Figure 8.1: Ustaz Hamzah (left) demonstrates a left-hand block of a punch delivered by one of his black belt students in Kuala Lumpur, Malaysia.

For Hamzah self-defence, traditionally deferred until the end of training, is systematically taught from the first day. This reorganization of training around a self-defence paradigm separated the long-term psycho-physiological effects of practice from fighting applications—a repositioning of the body which emphasizes not the long-term health benefits of practice, but the short-term usefulness of its techniques to street fighting.

Fig. 8.2: Ustaz Hamzah's 'yellow belt' syllabus.

International Kalari-Payat
Dynamic Self-Defence Institute
World Headquarters, Malaysia
Yellow Best Syllabus

a. *Locks*

1) Wrist Belt
2) Hand Lock–One
3) Wrist Twist–One
4) Hair Lock–One
5) Elbow Ring–One
6) Eagle Lock–One
7) Leg Scissor
8) Hair Strangle
9) Ankle Break–One
10) Elbow Twin–One
11) Rear Wrist
12) Strangle Close
13) Body Lock–One
14) Helpless–One
15) Elbow Break–One

b. *Blows*

1) Palm Heel–One
2) Neck Chop–One
3) Proper Nose–One
4) Knuckle Chin
5) Side Heel
6) Hammer Blow
7) Light Finger
8) Middle Jab
9) Strangle Chop
10) Front Kick M–One
11) Front Kick M–Two
12) Instep Temple–One
13) Instep Temple–Two
14) Instep Arm
15) Helmet Blow

c. General Dynamic Techniques

1) Physical Mental and Health Training
2) Counter Set—One, Two and Three
3) All Style Steps and Moving One and Two
4) Eagle Fly and Triple Kicks
5) Step Punches Chokes and Kicks
6) Chumadadi One
7) Tiger Attack One
8) Multiple Weapons Defences

Hamzah also organized his techniques into a hierarchically ordered and visually marked set of ranks based on the *dan* grade model used in many modern Japanese and Korean martial disciplines (Draeger 1974) (Figure 8.2: 'Yellow Belt Syllabus'). Students wear white karate-style uniform embroidered with the most visible symbol associated with kalarippayattu in Kerala—the sword and shield.

Hamzah's marking and ordering of training may be contrasted with dress in traditional kalari where, as we have seen, students wear either the long hand-wide red cloth (*kacca*) or the white lengoti. Both provide an important degree of support in the lower abdomen while leaving the practitioner's body completely exposed so that oil can be liberally applied to promote health-giving stimulation of the body of humours and saps during exercise. The virtually unclothed body can move fluidly, unencumbered by potentially restrictive clothing. These traditional kalarippayattu wrapped cloths are unmarked and give no sign of relative rank.

The karate-style belted uniform covers the entire body, precludes application of traditional oils and makes performing the body control exercises difficult since to some degree it inhibits kalarippayattu's free-flowing movements. In self-defence forms where the karate-style uniform is used, many throws are based on grasping the opponent by the upper jacket. Unlike the unmarked kalarippayattu cloths, the karate belt marks the rank which a practitioner holds. Perhaps most important, for many young men the karate uniform is associated with a cinema image of the martial arts expert—a man of action like Bruce Lee with a taut, tough tight body who controls the world around him.

Just as the clothing of the traditional kalarippayattu student is unmarked, so is his progress through training visibly unmarked. We have seen that advancement is a gradual process which depends on a master's intuitive reading not only of a student's progress in physical execution of techniques, but also in spiritual and behavioural terms. A master is said to 'know (each student's) mind from the countenance of his face'. Consequently, advancement is not literally marked by external signs, but demonstrated by the techniques a student practises.

Hamzah's students advance through the graded ranks, hierarchically ordered by belt colour [white (beginner), yellow, green, red, brown and black (first through eight dan)], when he passes a formal examination covering a printed syllabus. Passing an examination permits the student to wear the next higher grade belt, and to move on to the more advanced set of techniques he must master to obtain the next belt.

To pass a belt examination a student must perform required locks, blows, multiple defences, throws or steps. The Green Belt examination consists of sixteen locks scored at five points each, and five multiple defences scored at four points each for a total of hundred points. Two judges (holders of a Black Belt) score each technique awarding one to five points. A student scoring between 95–100 receives a special A level grade, from 90–95 A level, 80–90 B level, 70–80 C level. The minimum passing grade is C. If any student receives three Cs in moving up the ranks, he will 'never be permitted to become an instructor'. If a student fails an examination, he is permitted to retake the examination after one month.[143] To obtain a black belt the student must also submit an essay explaining his understanding of the art. These essays include a discussion of the behavioural, moral, health and/or spiritual aspects of practice.

Malaysian students, like many of their Kerala counterparts, pay a monthly fee [$30 (in 1983) for regular classes held three days a week, and $50 for special classes in which they receive more individual attention]. But unlike Kerala, in Malaysia students are also charged an examination fee for each rank test (yellow, $20; green, $30; red, $40; brown, $50; 1st dan black, $120; 2nd dan black, $200; 3rd dan black, $300; above, 4th–8th $400–$800). It takes approximately four to six months for the typical student to progress sufficiently to pass a rank test. In Hamzah's system it is possible for some students to receive a 1st dan black belt in as little as eighteen months. When one passes one becomes a sub-instructor. Only those with advanced dan black belts are permitted to teach independently, and the title 'Mahaguru' is given on passing the 8th dan black belt examination.

Although Hamzah also learned some special breath-control/meditational techniques[144] and some treatment and revival techniques which were traditionally considered an essential part of a master's repertoire of skills, he no longer practises them. If injuries occur, instead of administering treatment himself with kalarippayattu's traditional hands-on medical treatment, he 'prefers to go to the hospital because it is faster and more effective than the traditional therapy. Ayurvedic treatment takes too long. It was fine for that age, but it is too slow for today's world.'

While Hamzah's version of kalarippayattu is the first I know to have fully conformed to a transnational self-defence paradigm, it is by no means the only one. A number of other practitioner/teachers in Kerala and throughout India have either transformed kalarippayattu itself into a form of self-defence similar to Hamzah's or borrowed parts of it to create hybrids.[145]

Over the years Hamzah's system has slowly gained public attention and a healthy number of students in Malaysia. In 1985 he reported having three hundred students in his six Kalari Payat centres in west Malaysia, some of them located in the tea estates with large populations of south Indians. Students range in age from ten to forty and are primarily long-term south Indian immigrants to Malaysia. Public recognition has come from the Malaysian government which has included demonstrations at national cultural days, and Film Nagara made a short film on Kalari Payat. An invitation was issued to Hamzah to co-represent Malaysia at the International Martial Arts Demonstration organized by the Singapore Martial Arts Instructors Association in 1986.

Hamzah's reorganization of kalarippayattu into a graded, ranked system which can be taught quickly and with practical results, as well as his representations of kalarippayattu, make two interrelated appeals: (1) the first is to a youthful, modern, fast-paced, cosmopolitan sensibility, i.e. the art is effective and can be learned and used quickly; and (2) the training is 'scientific', i.e. it is systematically organized so that the student will not waste time. Such a scientific system is represented as 'international'. By being 'international' Hamzah's kalarippayattu can cross cultural and national boundaries—it is a paradigm of practice which is intended to be geographically interchangeable. By de-emphasizing local, territorially specific, indigenous aspects of practice, martial practice transcends 'specific territorial boundaries and identities' (Appadurai 1991: 192). The transnational territory which Hamzah's kalarippayattu inhabits is itself a newly created and imagined territory—a theatricalized cosmopolitan space inhabited by a character common to martial arts action films, the man-of-action.

Images of the Kalarippayattu 'Man-in-Action: Clean Bowling Over the Jet Set Generation'

In 1974 Hamzah put his first students through an intensive three-month course at the conclusion of which he staged a two-hour public demonstration to attract public attention. At the same time he mounted 'a massive publicity campaign' for the first stage demonstration. Since then he has regularly produced his own brochures and advertisements.

Hamzah places advertisements in a variety of publications including the English-language *Movieland*, a popular film magazine. Typical of other issues, the April 1981 edition features numerous photographs and articles on American television reruns ('Ex-brunette Loni hits'; 'WKRP's other woman Jan Smithers fought to keep playing shy Bailey'; 'Nancy Allen the

Actress with the very sensually shaped figure'), Tamil and Hindi films with shorts on various stars, and semi-sensational colour photo cover stories such as Padmini Kolhapure as 'the girl who stunned India with a kiss'.[146] In this issue Hamzah's advertisement for his Self-Defence Institute appears below a photograph of an embrace between Tamil actors Rajnikanth and Madhavi in their new film, *Thillu Mullu*, and next to an advertisement for the health medicine, 'Rejuvenal'. Hamzah's advertisements always feature an action-filled photograph of a bare hand or weapons technique (Figure 8.3), usually of one combatant fighting off multiple attackers and with one of them caught in a mid-air leap, kick, attack or defence. Advertisement copy includes a variety of come-ons aimed at specific groups of potential students or employers. Most important is the appeal to the young man-about-town enamoured of the James Bond or Bruce Lee type figure for whom the advertisement asserts: 'Defend yourself in times of danger and surprise attacks.' For the image-conscious young man, the advertisement promises that you can 'Build a strong healthy body'. Appealing to a modern, fast-paced life-style, one can enroll in "Crash Training" Available for People on the Move'. Hamzah also provides 'Special Rates for Ladies and Children', and invites the 'Attention (of) All Movie Producers and Directors: Stunt Services and Dynamic Fighting Techniques Can Be Provided'.

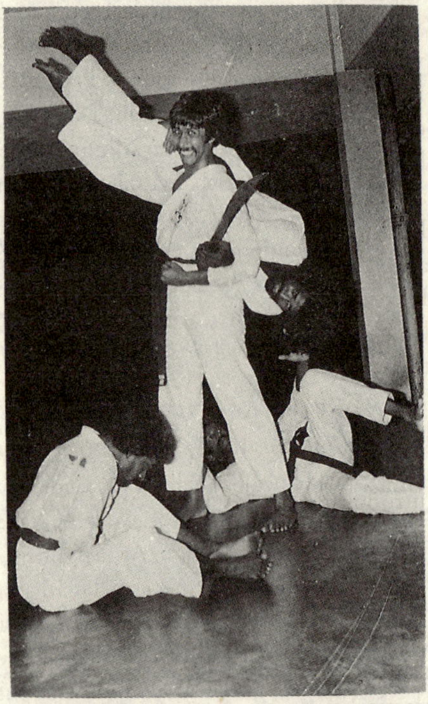

The adjacent advertisement for 'Rejuvenal', a 'preparation (which) contains some vitamins and herbs . . . manufactured in West Germany', appeals to the same energetic, active life-on-the-go audience. In terms that might just as easily have been written about his kalarippayattu classes, Rejuvenal claims to 'Help you in Health and Vitality . . . to lead a healthy, vigorous and active

Figure 8.3 : An action-packed photograph typical of those used to advertise kalarippayattu *as an effective street-wise self-defence martial art.*

life . . . restores robustness and maintains vitality . . . relieves irritability, lack of concentration, unrest and general debility'.

Hamzah recycles his version of the origins and practice of kalarippayattu through all available media. *The Malay Mail* of 31 August 1985 featured a two-page colour photo spread in the Saturday 'Lifestyle' section sandwiched between the day's television schedule/highlights and reviews of two fantasy/adventure films, 'Mad Max Beyond Thunderdome' and 'Buckeraoo Banzai'. In addition to history, this article included student testimonials about the benefits of practice. Ten-year-old David Amirthajar Samuel tells how 'this training is good for me as I feel healthier now and it has also built up my stamina', while Raja Mohammed 'has become a bolder person since taking up lessons'. The Mahaguru himself is featured in a colour photo/text insert spanning the two-page spread which presents a capsule biography of his training, and the story of how he introduced the art to Malaysia.

An important journalistic leitmotif is establishing kalarippayattu's superiority to karate. This strategy is illustrated in articles covering the 1986 visit of twenty-four-year-old Malayali black belt karate teacher, K.T. Hakeem, who came to take a crash course with Hamzah. Hakeem's story was featured in the 30 April 1986 issue of *Malaysia Post* and the 15–21 June 1986 issue of *Weekend Review* published by the *Hindustan Times*, New Delhi. Both have action photographs of the young mustachioed Malayali male executing a high kick while fighting off attackers. The *Malaysian Post* headlines tout Kalari Payat as putting 'Karate in the shade', while the *Weekend Review* article sells Hakeem as a 'New Star on Kalari Horizon'. They tell how Hakeem decided to '"give something extra" to those who got trained (in karate) under him', i.e. 'he thought a dash of kalari training would enable them to face any challenging situation with true grit and sure-fire success'. The newspaper accounts emphasize how extraordinary it is that Hakeem left his native Kerala, home of kalarippayattu, to study the art with Hamzah in Malaysia, 'the Mahaguru who had modernized (kalarippayattu) and introduced a few innovations which included a grading system and a uniform. The jet-set generations were clean-bowled over by all these.'

As seen in the *New Thrill* photo spread covering my visit, my presence in Kuala Lumpur proved an equal catalyst for publicity. At a special belt-grading function to which a number of reporters and photographers had been invited, I performed a few basic kalarippayattu exercises, and one practical application of a basic technique in which I threw one of Hamzah's advanced black-belt students. My performance of this escape was well documented by the photographer and became the subject of several feature stories.

Both Hakeem and I were multivalent symbols for Hamzah. As a Malayali holding a black-belt in karate, Hakeem's decision to submit himself to kalarippayattu training under Hamzah could be read as the wayward native Malayali who went outside his own culture to study karate returning 'home' to a better art of self-defence. As a karate master Hakeem already could be read as a 'man of action' who controls his world. By studying kalarippayattu he would be better able to exert such control. As an American from the home of the entertainment industry, I could also be read as a cosmopolitan 'man of the world'. Popular action film characters James Bond, Bruce Lee, Chuck Norris or their popular Asian cinema counterparts are all dynamic male figures who vanquish their opponents with techniques choreographed from an eclectic variety of Asian and/or Western fighting techniques.

As a scholar, my presence implicitly legitimized the importance and study of self-defence, and Hamzah's kalarippayattu specifically. As a practitioner trained in Kerala I could also be read as embodying the tradition of which they were a part. Although our styles were different, we could be read as practising the 'same art'. My presence was understood as simultaneously pointing backward to the place of kalarippayattu's origins in Kerala, as well as forward to the cosmopolitan present. Hamzah's intuitive insistence that I show 'at least one practical tactic' provided the essential link between the traditional exercises I knew and Hamzah's practically oriented modern self-defence form. My demonstration was a sign of 'authentic' practice (self-defence) which valorized his own. Besides, it was good theatre, and made for good publicity.

Reading the Presentations and Representations: Issues of Power, Control, Sex, Violence and Virility

The *New Thrill* tabloid picture spread in which I appeared, with its hyped title, 'Deadly Art of Locks and Throws', is one obvious print medium example of what Richard Schechner has called the theatricalization of news—a phenomenon on the increase 'because the public and those who exploit the public want increased theatricalization, which means simplification, quick arousal, and satisfactory resolution of the excitement' (1985: 318). Titillating headlines and photographs arouse the (male) reader's curiosity and draw him into the world of the tabloid where short 'news' stories simplify complex issues. A series of short, simplified sets of visual and print images are juxtaposed one against another. Much like the 1984 issue in which I appeared, the 21 June 1980 issue of *New Thrill* featured stories on a 'Strip Tease Queen', criminal violence, a ghost story and kalarippayattu.

As the eye travels from one image or brief narrative to the next, the sets of images/texts demand to be read intertextually for the possible meanings created by their juxtaposition. The tabloid, like its mass media counterparts, quickly juxtaposes and thereby links virility, sex and violence. In the Malaysian example, 'the unknown' is an important fourth text and set of images serially joined to the other three self-consciously joined under the tabloid's banner of exploring the 'unknown, mysterious, and exciting'. In these brief, spectacularized narratives what all four realms share is a test of a man's personal and interpersonal boundaries and behaviours. Virility, sex, violence and the supernatural are all concerned with power—with who controls what and/or whom. All three invite the male reader to vicariously enter the fantasy (if not the actuality) of arousal (sexual, physical or spiritual) associated with each dangerous encounter with an other. Each arousal provides its own brand of 'excitement', and the excitement is present in the encounter with what remains other, and is therefore unknown and mysterious. The image of the male projected here, and supported in many of the popular action-packed martial arts movies, is a highly gendered fantasy in which the 'virile' man controls his environment and all those around him either by the force of attraction, or literally by exercising force. These representations of sex, violence and the supernatural take the male reader outside his normative social and interpersonal boundaries and appear to be as potentially exciting as they are dangerous.

The image of the male which emerges from these pages is that of a controlling figure—the virile, self-confident, man-in-control. He is usually pictured with a taut, attractive and powerful physique in action and described as energetic, dynamic and therefore 'healthy'. If he can control his body and confront physical danger, he should be able to control everything in his world. To envision oneself as a Bruce Lee or Hakim, executing a dynamic high kick, is to enter the fantasy, if not the actuality, of having power and control over one's environment. This man-of-action is what Appadurai calls a 'mediascape', i.e. an 'image-centred, narrative-based account of strips of reality . . .' offering 'a series of elements (such as characters, plots and textual forms) out of which scripts can be formed of imagined lives' (1990: 9).

The re-packaging, mediation and transnationalization of kalarippayattu to fit the cosmopolitan self-defence paradigm has transformed it from a complex, embedded, local (martial, therapeutic and fighting) art where its powers are ritually, ethically, spiritually and socially circumscribed into a spectacular and melodramatic one where its powers are either decontextualized or recontextualized.[147] In these short mediated image/texts, each arena within which power is asserted is divorced from its complex local context. Indigenous arts like kalarippayattu, or a spiritual art like Master Tan's control of spirits residing in banana trees, were traditionally grounded in their local context. One experienced such arts and their practitioners, not through a mediated representation of them, but either immediately within the local context where the master demonstrated his powers in practice, or through performative means of celebrating the warrior's heroic demeanour like ballad, drama or dance. A particular master's power and control was experienced and understood within a hierarchy of interactive spheres of power operative in the local setting.

Although this melodramatic subtext does not have the same fully schematized narrative found in most modern martial arts action films, the same basic elements are present: danger, attack, defence, control and power. This schematic subtextual melodrama lies behind the resonance and articulation of the representations of kalarippayattu exemplified by Hamzah's commodified self-defence version of the art pitched to the modern martial arts market-place and is present in virtually every popular martial arts magazine such as the American monthlies, *Black Belt* and *Inside Kung-Fu*. The circles of signification embed and interpenetrate all the 'traditional' versions of the Asian martial arts in their contemporary self-defence guises where distinctions between arts, cultures, histories, etc. are erased. This tendency is often found in kalarippayattu demonstrations which feature such theatrical 'feats' such as a leaping right side-kick performed over three classmates to break three clay tiles (Figure 8.4).

The result is that the practice of kalarippayattu, as a discipline for bodymind development and to raise the subtle 'powers' necessary to enter combat is erased. The bodymind and the results of long-term practice toward a particular type of accomplishment and cultivation of internal powers are repositioned. The transnational melodramatic subtext replicated in films, and action photographs and narratives locate the very real issues of power, fear, control and attack in the individual male's fantasy world, and within quite different social and ethical contexts.

The traditional boundaries intended to contain the exercise of power/control in the local Malayali context are, in modern media, shifted as they juxtapose new images.[148] The suggestive titles and photographic images of masters of self-defence dynamically fighting off three opponents are divorced from a contextualizing narrative which might situate the potential exercise of violence within a particular context and thereby circumscribe the violence depicted. Titles like 'Deadly Art of Locks and Throws', foreground and theatricalize violence rather than explore the elements of self and/or social

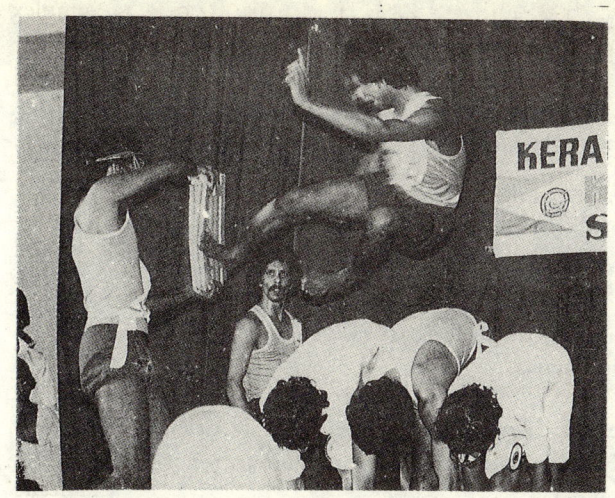

Figure 8.4 : The increasing theatricalization of kalarippayattu *is evident at demonstrations such as this one in 1983 at Palakkad where one student performed this leaping right side-kick over three class-mates to break three clay tiles.*

control which ideally circumscribed the use of methods of committing violent acts. As Joshua Meyrowitz asserts in *No Sense of Place*, the blurring by modern media of 'distinctions between here and there, live and mediated, and personal and public' is contributing to an increasing sense of placelessness, i.e. the divorce of mediated meanings from the particularity of their present, lived context (1985: 308). This decontextualization of images of the exercise of power/control does not address issues of responsibility for the exercise of power.

Ideals, Images and Intent

As Foucault points out, central to any technology of the self or power are 'modes of training and modification of individuals, not only in the obvious sense of acquiring certain skills but also in the sense of acquiring certain attitudes' (1988: 198). While exploiting every media possibility for presenting his form of self-defence through images which contribute to the representation of the practitioner as a physically fit, confident, dynamic, man-on-the-go, able to control his environment and do so violently, Hamzah simultaneously asserts the fundamental ethical principle which governs the more traditional paradigms of practice he was taught in his own training as a young boy, and which is intended to constrain the potential for violence of the self-defence practitioner. He insists that all of his students observe 'the oath that had to be taken privately with one's master and one's own god: I promise I will not misuse this and will only use it for self-defence. If I misuse it I will face the displeasure of my master and will be dismissed from further training.'

When each student fills out an application form for admission to training, the student and his/her two sponsors agree to

> abide by the rules and regulations and conditions stipulated by the International Kalari-Payat self-defence.
>
> I also understand that this art is to be used for the sole purpose of self-defence and not for any purpose of evil design. And if any evil deed motivated by evil design is done by me then the entire responsibility is with me and I shall solely bear the consequence thereof.
>
> Persons who have any criminal record or with misconduct are not allowed to continue the training.

Each student ideally achieves not only the ability to defend himself with potentially deadly force, but also the moral authority not to misuse the power he has acquired.

Hamzah's students speak and write with great conviction about how their practice of the art has helped them. In his required three hundred word essay for the first dan Black Belt examination of 1981, one student reflected on the multiple benefits of his three years of experience in training:

> I have found (the training) to be an excellent form of physical fitness and self-defence. In the beginners class, I had minor problems like body aching and over-tiredness, but eventually with continued practise (sic) I began to feel better, strong, and more eager to keep on practising. I passed my different belt gradings in stages from white to yellow, green, red, and then to brown belt. By now my legs and hands ha[d] become stronger and powerful and they have turned into a lethal weapon. I have never had the opportunity to test my self-defence skill since I have never indulged myself in any form of violence and since I would walk away or talk myself out of any fight even if the odds were to my credit. By the practise of Kalari, I have learned to control myself, my movements and to respect others. Kalari Payat teaches you to be prepared to defence (sic) yourself from sudden attacks, it gives you patience, the ability to be punctual, to have confidence in what you do and discipline. It also frees us from chronic illness.

The 1977 testimony of another student also belies the image he and other black-belts create in their action photographs featured in newspaper stories and in advertisements for the school. He tells how

> before I started practising I was hot tempered, aggressive, bulky and hunchy in shape. But now I have found that patience and calmness are two

beautiful aspects of life. Moreover my body is well formed and I am always looking forward enthusiastically to life. I can firmly say that this art builds one up not only in physique but also in character.

In 1979 another black-belt candidate wrote,

> After a few years a Kalari-Payat exponent changes for the better in both physique and character. He becomes humble and is able to think more clearly. He is confident of himself and gentle in the treatment of others around him.

These testimonies self-consciously speak of pacification of violent temperaments, of calm and self-control. Read against the assertive, aggressive, violent images of the cosmopolitan man-of-action, they clearly reflect the ambiguity implicit in practising a bodily discipline like the martial arts which can serve equally as a pathway to self-realization and/or to domination. It is a slippery path that is constantly being negotiated by each teacher and student in every arena of training and practice.

THE INDIAN SCHOOL OF MARTIAL ARTS: NEGOTIATING THE PAST IN THE PRESENT

I conclude with a final case-study of one kalarippayattu practitioner, Balachandran Master, whose life has been a creative negotiation of the relationship between the self-defence paradigm of martial practice, 'traditional' kalarippayattu, and the important discursive formations of kingship, sacrifice, and heroic honour implicit in Kerala history and its 'heritage'. As early as 1983, many incredulous youth uninterested in 'traditional' kalarippayattu flocked to teachers like Balachandran Master. Retired from the Indian navy, and making good use of the hard style self-defence training received there, he opened his 'Indian School of Martial Arts' (ISMA). Although trained in some kalarippayattu as a youth and from a Nayar family which traditionally practised kalarippayattu in the service of the Maharaja of Travancore, he had never undergone a traditional long-term apprenticeship. Similar to Hamzah, he developed his own composite style of 'hard' martial arts practice, and created maroon karate-style uniforms. Classes were run on military lines, and Balachandran often took on the persona of a drill seargent as he put students through their paces.

Balachandran initially gained legitimization 'with his fists'—a symbol (clenched fists over crossed swords and shields) that he chose as his school logo. His willingness to fight, to literally test the efficacy and usefulness of his techniques 'on the streets', as well as the military toughness of his training, attracted a devoted group of male and female students from a variety of socio-economic groups, religions and castes.

At the same time that Balachandran was teaching his hard, composite style of martial arts, he began to visit traditional masters in the area to see what techniques he might pick up from them and add to his new composite style of 'Indian Martial Arts'. He gradually became more and more interested in the value of traditional south Indian martial techniques, learned techniques from a number of varma ati masters in particular, and invited them to come and teach his students their techniques. As a Nayar by birth and from a family that historically was in service to the Travancore Raja, he also became more and more interested in the traditions of kalarippayattu practice, in reconstructing the 'lost' southern Kerala Nayar traditions, and in the more internal, subtle, meditational aspects of the system. Drawing on the antique tradition of gaining authority through meditation and/or moral perfection derived from the Buddhist, Jain and yoga traditions of personal perfection through renunciation and action, Balachandran gradually redefined himself personally as a warrior/sage/teacher. He has increasingly withdrawn from the public to focus on mentoring his students, foremost among whom is his son, and meditation.

Gradually, Balachandran began to develop a unique vision for bringing under one roof both his very practical, hard, eclectic, self-defence oriented martial art with a more traditional version of kalarippayattu. He drew up plans for creating a new martial arts centre on his own property whose design would be based on traditional Kerala and kalarippayattu architectural principles and house on three levels a traditional pit-style kalari, a concrete-floored 'gym' for his composite hard style, and a third floor meditation hall overlooking the Sage Agastya Muni's mountain.

While in Thiruvananthapuram in 1993, I attended the inauguration of this new kalari. The ritual inauguration of the kalari was in all respects a traditional Hindu temple festival which by its ritual action established this new kalari as part of Kerala and kalarippayattu's glorious traditional heritage. It included those symbols and rites pointing to continuities with the past including a caparisoned elephant, temple percussion orchestra, young girls holding lamps and rice stalks symbolizing prosperity and students of the kalari parading along the decorated alley which gives entry, holding swords and shields. Gone were the maroon karate-style uniforms with which Balachandran had begun training at ISMA, replaced now with traditional Malayali dress.

At the centre of the ceremonies was the active role played by the current Maharaja of Travancore. Greeted by the traditional orchestra, lamps and other symbols of well-being and prosperity, at the entrance to the closed doors of the kalari, Balachandran bathed the Maharaja's feet before he opened the doors and stepped in, thereby officially inaugurating the new building. Most important was the Maharaja's presentation of a sword from the royal household arsenal (Figure 8.6) to Balachandran in the kalari—a (recuperative) enactment of the traditional royal investiture of Nayar knighthood discussed in Chapter 2.

This commemorative performance of royal knighthood was a symbolic, and very public, legitimization of Balachandran's incorporation of the street with both the palace and the kalari of his Nayar origins—a recuperation of the Nayar heritage of kalarippayattu practice in old Travancore. As a rite which explicitly referred to 'prototypical persons and events' having historical, mythological, as well as contemporary existence (Connerton 1989: 61), this 'commemorative ceremony' linked kingship, history and the heroic in a present martial practice that points both backward to the heroic past, as well as forward to the cosmopolitan, street-wise present. This dialogic engagement of the past in the present is how meanings as well as practices are (re)constituted between practice *per se*, and the discursive formations which inform and shape a practice in any given present. Like other reformers such as C.V. Narayanan Nayar before him, Balachandran is both recuperating a 'lost' past—in this case the southern Kerala Nayar tradition of practice—and creating a new style of practice from the amalgam of ati tada techniques learned from Nadar and Sambavar asans in old Travancore, 'northern' kalari techniques, his own hard-style combat training, and his gleanings from a variety of traditional texts he has gathered which may have vestiges of the old styles of Nayar kalarippayattu training. Balachandran recently invited Sadasivan Asan (whose father was a Nayar) to teach his son, Girish, two forms of kalarippayattu training which may be indigenous to the south and are close to the ati tada techniques described earlier—'Hanuman fight' (*Hanuman ankam*) and 'Bali's way of fighting' (*Balivali ankam*). This new composite style is being created on Girish's young body for future generations of practitioners at ISMA.

Practice itself and the subjectivity it helps create are not static, but rather open to manipulation and interpretation in the interplay between the constantly altering horizons of individual subjectivities; the interplay between the metaphors, images, and representations of the body culturally available; the interpretation of the body, experience and practice articulated by individual masters; and the socio-political and economic environments.

No matter how 'esoteric' the techniques, no matter how 'subtle' the powers, no matter how apparently controlled the bodymind, all such martial and meditational powers are actualized by persons who are more or less responsible for the use or abuse of those powers in particular socio-political circumstances. This is nowhere more evident than in the unfortunate fact that a few masters and some students from both the Hindu and Muslim communities in Kerala began as early as 1983 to use kalarippayattu to train students for communal violence against the other community. To reiterate a point that Kondo makes, kalarippayattu becomes one means of 'crafting' a particular self and therefore is a 'culturally, historically specific pathway . . . to self-realization . . . (and/or) domination' (Kondo 1990: 305). The kalarippayattu student training toward self-control, restraint and actualization of the internal energy in a kalari where Muslims, Christians and Hindus are all welcome to train together today will be a very different experience from the kalarippayattu student secretively trained in an exclusively Muslim or Hindu fundamentalist environment where hatred may be bred even though the same techniques may be taught. Sometimes the 'self' crafted and the use to which that self puts its putative martial powers and practice are for a larger good.

Appendix I

Texts in the Kalarippayattu Tradition

Although kalarippayattu is an embodied form of practice learned through hands-on manipulation and oral correction, 'texts' play a central role in that process both literally and symbolically. The symbolic importance of texts is marked each year in kalari celebrating Navaratri Mahotsavam (Chapter 3) which inaugurates a yearly cycle of training. A typical set of texts worshipped by one master on Navaratri includes:

kalari vidya ('kalari art')—a manual of exercises and techniques in the *dronambillil sampradayam*;

marmmabhyasam ('techniques of the vital spots')—a manual which records techniques for attacking and defending the body's vital spots;

marmmaprayogam ('application to the vital spots')—a manual of locks and methods of application to the body's vital spots;

marmmacikitsa ('treatment for the vital spots')—a manual of emergency counterapplications and treatment for injuries to the body's vital spots;

vadakkam pattukal ('northern ballads')—a contemporary printed collection of the traditional oral ballads of northern Kerala about the exploits of local heroes.

Several are original palm-leaf manuscripts passed on within a family, several are handwritten notebooks copied from originals not in this master's possession, and the *vadakkam pattukal* is a printed book purchased from a local bookstore. The information within the texts is of four types: (1) records of specific martial techniques or related information on practice; (2) information on such things as construction of a kalari, deities or ritual practice; (3) records of martial mythology or legends; and (4) methods of treatment and recipes for medicinal preparations.

MANUALS OF PRACTICE

This master's *kalari vidya* text is typical of those recording verbal commands (*vayttari*). They may be titled or untitled. The oldest manuals are palm-leaf *grandam* written in archaic Malayalam; however, most masters today possess handwritten notebooks. Several traditional manuscripts are in library collections (*Mallayuddhakrama*, *Verumkaipidutham*, and *Ayudhabhyasam* are in the Madras University library manuscript collection). A few have appeared in print, such as *Rangabhyasam* (published by the Madras Government Oriental Manuscript Series). These titles are similar to those in the possession of practising masters.

During the 1970s cheap popular paperback editions of these manuals began to appear in print (Velayudhan n.d.). Sreedharan Nayar's Malayalam book on kalarippayattu (1963) also includes a complete set of verbal commands for techniques taught in his own kalari. Similarly, Balakrishnan's publications (Malayalam, 1994; English, 1995) include a complete set of verbal commands for techniques taught at the C.V.N. Kalari, Thiruvananthapuram.

A particular text may be a loose collection of sections of technical information on a variety of subjects, or confine itself to one specific type of techniques, such as empty-hand attacks and defences (*verumkaipiduttam*) or a manual of mantras.

Technical manuals record details for specific techniques. They list, word-by-word, the vayttari for each set of techniques. They are usually organized from simplest to most complex. The texts serve as a permanent reference manual, or as one master explained, for consultation 'to clarify doubts I have'. This is especially the case with advanced techniques taught to a few students. Verbal commands for weapons techniques only record the student's side of execution and were traditionally kept secret.

Techniques are authoritatively written in the embodied practice of the gurukkal. But since each lineage of practice or teacher has his own interpretation and style of 'correct' practice for every verbal command, the master is the most appropriate 'reader' of his own texts. The 'authoritative text' in the living tradition is not the grandam *per se* which is placed before Sarasvati on Navaratri, but the master's embodied practice.

TEXTS ON THE VITAL SPOTS

Although numerous palm-leaf and hand copied manuscripts dealing with the vital spots have been collected in government manuscript libraries and some have even been published (see Nadar 1968; Nadar n.d.; Selvaraj 1984; Nair 1957), given the variability of interpretation here again individual masters differ in their interpretations. As Ananda Wood asserts,

> the direct instruction of an experienced teacher is necessary to interpret such theoretical texts practically. A theoretical text is fairly meaningless without such a teacher who knows the practical skills and techniques himself. For example, a vital spot may be described in a text as located two named measures below the nipple, but the lack of a standard measure corresponding to the name in the text would mean that an experienced practitioner would be required to interpret the text and point out the spot (1985: 115).

There are an increasing number of reference texts about the vital spots available to Ayurvedic medical practitioners and/or kalarippayattu practitioners.

Appendix II

Interviews, Personal Correspondence—Kalarippayattu and Varma Ati Masters

The list is arranged geographically from north to south by district with the year[s] of interview[s] in (19xx). (*) indicates a master of varma ati. During interviews, some masters occasionally read or allowed me to copy sections of their texts with me. These texts are discussed in Appendix I, and are listed at the end of the Bibliography and References Cited. Interviews were also held with approximately seventy-five students at selected kalari listed below.

KANNUR DISTRICT

P.P. Narayanan Gurukkal (1983)
C.S. Kalari Sangham, Thayinery
P.O. Payannur, PIN-670307

K. Achuthan Gurukkal (1983)
P.O. Eruvatty
Kozhur via Kadirur

C. Mohammed Sherif (1983, 1985, 1989, 1993, 1995)
Kerala Kalarippayattu Academy
Pillyar Kovil Road, PIN-670001

Abdul Kadar Asan (1985)
c/o C. Mohammed Sherif (no address available)
K.K. Chandrashekharan Gurukkal (1985)
Elimata

Kalathil Krishnan Vaidyar (1989)
P.O. Alavil

K. Kunhikannan Gurukkal (1989)
Poyyayil House
Palathai, near Panoor

I.P. Assainar Gurukkal (1983)
(no address available)

Sreejayan v. Gurukkal (1989)
Kerala Kalari Sangham
Shantinilayam
P.O. Champad, Tellicherry

K. Chandran Gurukkal (1989)
Azhicode Street
P.O. Azhicode, PIN-670009

Sreebharath Kalari (1983)
(founded by T. Sreedharan Nayar)
Baliapatam
P.O. Chirakkal, PIN-670011

N.V. Narayanan Nayar (1983)
C.V.N. Kalari, Post Vadakkumpad
Madathumbhagam, Tellicherry

Kallada Balakrishnan (1983)
Bright Screen Painters
Puttiyakaramba, P.O. Alavil

KOZHIKODE DISTRICT

Gurukkal C.M.M. Vaidyar (1983, 1989)
Shafi Dawa Khana
Ayurveda Nursing Home
Choorakkodi Kalari Abhighata Chikilsalayam
P.O. Chelavoor

M.K. Bhaskaran Gurukkal (1983)
Udaya Kalari Sangham
Chombala, PIN-673308

K.K. Krishnan (1983)
Iykia Kerala Kalari Sangham
P.O. Vengalam via Elathur

K.T. Achuthan Gurukkal (1983)
Hindustan Kalari Sangam
Jail Road, PIN-673004

E.P. Kunnu (1983)
Nasrattul Islam Kalari Sangham
Kulannara Padam
P.O. Phoruk College, PIN-673632

P. Dasan Gurukkal (1983)
C.V.N. Kalari, Putiyangadi Branch
Putiyangadi P.O. via West Hill, PIN-673021

Karunan Gurukkal (1983)
Kadathanadu Chekor Kalari Sangham
Puthuppanam, Badagara, PIN-673105

K.V. Choyikutty (1983)
Durga Kalari Sangham
Kottooli, PIN-673016

K.V. Chandu, Secretary (1983)
Kadathanad Udaya Kalari Sangam
Naripatta P.O.

T.K. Madhavan Gurukkal (1983)
P.O. Vengalam, via Elathur

WYNAD DISTRICT

Thomas Muttam (1983)
Muttathu Kalarisangham
Fathima Mansil
Kaniyampatta P.O., via Kalpatta

MALLAPPURAM DISTRICT

V.K. Madhava Panikkar (deceased) (1983)
V.K.M. Kalari, Changaramkulam
P.O. Nannamukku, PIN-679575

K.M. Hamzah Gurukkal (1983)
Post Moorkinada, via Kollathur

PALAKKAD DISTRICT

S. Jayakumar (1983)
House 15/390, Kunnthurmadu
Palakkad 13

C.C. Velayadan Asan (deceased) (1983)

P.M. Neelakandhan Namboodiripad (1983)
Poomuli Mana, Peringode P.O.
PIN-679535

B. Kunhi Moideen Gurukkal (1983)
18/198 Hidayathil Islam
Kalari Sangam, Poolakkad
Puduppali St., Palakkad

K. Narayanan Nayar Gurukkal (1983, 1989)
C.V.N. Kalari, Kunnathur Medu
Palakkad 13

Haji N.M. Kutty (1983)
Kerala Samstana Kayikabhyasa Kalari Sangam
Vysia Street, Palakkad 1

TRISSUR DISTRICT

C. Sankaranarayanan Menon Gurukkal (1983)
Sree Narayanan Guru Smaraka Vallabhatta Kalari Sangham
Koottungal, Chavakkad, PIN-680506

P.K. Balan Gurukkal (1983)
P.K.B. Kalaris
Thozhiyoor via Kootapadi
PIN-680505

Sakhav P.V. Mohamedunni Gurukkal (1983)
Navajeevan Kalari Sangham
P.O. Punnayurkulam, PIN-679561

C.T. Balamenon Gurukkal (1983)
V.K.M. Kalari, Kizhoor North
Kozhoor P.O. via Kunnamkulam,
PIN-680523

P.S. Higgins Master (1983)
P.K. Kalari Sangham
Pracheena Bharath
Dhanavyavasaya Buildings
P.O. Road, PIN-680001

K.O. Varghese Gurukkal (1983)
V.K.M. Kalari, Kizhoor South
Kunnamkulam

KOTTAYAM AND QUILON

E.P. Vasu Gurukkal (1985, 1989)
C.V.N. Kalari
Kaduthuruthy, Kottayam 686604

A.K. Prakasan Gurukkal (1993)
K.P. Nivas, Kalumtadum P.O.
Quilon 4

THIRUVANANTHAPURAM DISTRICT

Gurukkal Govindankutty Nayar
(1976–7, 1980, 1983, 1985, 1988–9, 1993, 1995)
C.V.N. Kalari, East Fort
Thiruvananthapuram 695023

*D. Chellayyan Asan (1989)
Marmachikilsalayam, Kallara P.O.

*Sadasivan Asan (1989)
(no address available)

*Moolachal Narayanan Asan (1989)
Mekkamandapam P.O.
Kanyakumari District 629166

*Raju Asan (1989)
Vizhinjam

*S. Krishnankutty Nayar (1985)
S.K.N. Kalari Sangham
Chempoor, Mudakal P.O. Attingal

*S. Alisan Kunju (1983)
Amir Ali Kalari Sangam
Chayam, Vithura P.O.
Culvert Jun ction via Nedumangad

*A. Kumaran (1983)
Attathara Veedu, Changaramkulam
Post Nannamukku, PIN-679575

*Masters David and Richard Strathern (1989)
M.R.K. Kalarisangam
C.P. 9/490 Darsannagar, Perurkada P.O.

*Kottakkal Kunnasan (1983)
K.K. Kalari Sangham,
Idakadathi P.O., via Mukkuolthuthara

N. Musthafa Asan (1983)
Islamic Centre
Manacaud Mosque, Kovalam Rd.

*Kunnan Asan K. (1983)
K.K.N. Kalari, Kakkamula,
Kalliyoor, P.O. Neman

*K.K. Muthu Asan (1983)
K.K.M. Kalari Sangham
Attukal, Chullimanoor P.O.
Nedumangad

*Swamiappan Nayar (1983)
(no address available)

Balachandran Master (1983, 1989, 1993)
Indian School of Martial Arts
Cotton Hill

MALAYSIA

Ustaz Haji Hamzah Haji Abu (1983)
428, Kg. Champoran, Ampang
Selangor, Kuala Lumpur

ADDITIONAL INTERVIEWS AND PERSONAL CORRESPONDENCE

Renshi K. Mohanan (1983)
Kaju-Kado Karate
Latha Nivas, Kunnumpuram, M.G. Rd.
Thiruvananthapuram 695 001

S. Srinivasan (1983)
Director and Chief Instructor
Okinawa School of Karate
YMCA Tourist Hostel
Jai Singh Rd., New Delhi-110001

Venganoor Viswadev (1983)
11, Kerala Hindu Mission Buildings
Statue, Thiruvananthapuram 695 001

Murkot Kunhappa (1983)
Associate Editor
Malayala Manorama
Kozhikode

Dr. Gnanadhas (1989)
Kattaukadai, Palapallam P.O.
Kanyakumari 629159

Desmond Netto (1989)
Thiruvananthapuram

C. Moses Thilak (1983, 1989)
Madras

K.K. Gopalakrishnan (1989)
Kannur

R. Perumal Raju (1993)
Salem, Tamil Nadu

Endnotes

PREFACE

1. Chakravarty (1972) and Majumdar (1960) focus on battle strategies. Pant (1978) is the only historical study to focus on martial techniques.

2. Manuals of practice include Nayar (1963) and Balakrishnan (1994, 1995).

3. The earliest and most detailed colonial account is that of the Portuguese explorer, Duarte Barbosa (c. 1518). Fawcett (1901) and Thurston (1909, Vol. V) include some information on kalarippayattu in their accounts of the Nayars. Raghavan (1929, 1932, 1947) provides information about the social and historical context of martial practice. C.V. Narayanan Nair's brief 1933 essay provides an overview of some of the techniques. Sreedharan Nayar (1957, 1963, 1983, Malayalam) provides the most detailed information on traditional techniques.

CHAPTER 1

4. In 1983 Hamzah was the only individual who had established a viable permanent centre for kalarippayattu training outside India. Hamzah initiated our correspondence in 1980 when he responded to an article in *The Drama Review* (Zarrilli 1979).

5. The pen name Mai-Pen-Rai is an atypical Malay one not likely known to the Malay reader except those who frequent Thailand. For those who do cross the border, anthropologist Mary Grow informs me that *mai pen rai* ('never mind; it doesn't matter') is a typical Thai expression of an ideal state of 'cool heartedness'. At least among those who have visited Hatyai, the irony of using 'never mind' as a pen name for a story on prostitution is obvious.

6. I use 'mode of cultural praxis' rather than 'genre of cultural performance'. When Milton Singer first used 'cultural performance', he applied it to discrete items of performance which encapsulate and exhibit 'elementary constituents of the culture' (1972: 7). The postmodern turn in anthropology has problematized the modernist notion of culture as a relatively stable category, as well as of cultural performances as 'encapsulating' 'elementary constituents.'

It implies a fixed essence rather than the fluid process of creating meaning characteristic of any act of performance, or of cultural praxis. As a 'performance' ethnography I assume with Fabian that '"Performance" seem[s] to be a more adequate description both of the ways people realize their culture and of the method by which an ethnographer produces knowledge about that culture' (1990: 18). For Fabian performance is an appropriate metaphor for an epistemology of ethnography where 'ethnography is essentially, not incidentally, communicative or dialogical; conversational, not observation' (ibid.: 4). This move is intended to shift from simply 'collecting data and information about another culture' where the ethnographer is 'the emissary of the dominant power (unwittingly or not)', to becoming a performative ethnographer where 'the ethnographer does not call the tune but plays along' (ibid.: 18–9).

7. Although Eugenio Barba's theatre anthropology is problematic in some ways, his distinction between 'extra-daily' and daily activities/practices is useful since it calls attention to the similarities and differences between the habitualized modes of daily practice and virtuosic modes of embodied practice which are the focus of this ethnography (1991).

8. Mauss pointed out that 'body techniques' such as handshakes, winks, salutes, attention, walking, etc. not only require an organic foundation, but are also socially learned and variable across societies (1973).

9. Lakoff and Johnson assert the importance of bodily experience in shaping cultural metaphors (1980: passim).

10. On performance as practice see Foster (1996), Ness (1992), and Novack (1990). On martial arts see Dann (1978) on Japanese kendo, Alter (1992) on Indian wrestling, and Lewis on capoeira (1992).

11. Kondo problematizes our Western notion of self as 'unitary substance and consciousness', and in its singular place situates the self as plurally located according to context (1990: 304). On self and person, see Shweder and LeVine (1984), Kirkpatrick and White (1985), Mauss (1973), Carrithers *et al.* (1985).

12. Feminist theorist Judith Butler asserts that the body is 'a variable boundary, a surface whose permeability is politically regulated' (1993: 139).

13. This sense of the 'individual body-self' is distinguished from 'the social concept of the individual as 'person', a construct of 'jural rights and moral accountability' which is a 'uniquely Western notion of the individual as a quasi-sacred, legal, moral, and psychological entity whose rights are limited only by the rights of other equally autonomous individuals' (ibid.). The importance of taking into account self-consciousness as well as culture-specific understanding of 'individuality' has recently been persuasively argued by Cohen (1994), and by Mines (1994) in the context of South Asian studies.

14. Richard Jenkins discusses how Bourdieu fails to adequately account for change, innovation, and the role of subjectivity as constitutive of practice *as a process* (1992: 96–7). Margaret Drewal has clearly articulated this more processual,

performative approach which assumes that both 'society and human beings are performative, always already processually under construction' (1991: 4).

15. By paradigm I mean the model, pattern, schema, or assumptions implicit in any bodily practice. I assume with Lakoff and Johnson (1980) that structures, conceptual schema or paradigms are implicit both in how we think about what we do and in our everyday practices. Mark Johnson defines an image schema as a 'recurring, dynamic pattern of our perceptual interactions and motor programs that gives coherence and structure to our experience' (1987: xiv).

16. Hastrup argues for an understanding of the 'body-in-life' as not only a limit or 'site of resistance', but also as a 'site of transcendence' and/or 'potentiality which is elaborated and developed in social relations' (1995: 5). The assertion of practice as a potential site for transcendence/transformation or a positive sense of 'cultivation' (Yuasa 1987: passim), as well as for the more habitualized, conforming mode of disciplining the body discussed by Foucault (1977: passim), is an important corrective to an overly deterministic view that disciplining the body necessarily creates 'docile bodies'. This monograph illustrates how the same techniques have been and are being used to negotiate a variety of positions of social and/or political location.

17. This strategy is also informed by Keesing's assertion that 'cultures as texts . . . are differently read, differently construed, by men and women, young and old, experts and nonexperts . . . cultures do not simply constitute webs of significance, systems of meaning that orient humans to one another and their world. They constitute ideologies, disguising human, political, and economic realities as cosmically ordained . . . Cultures are webs of mystification as well as signification' (1987: 161). Inden (1986) provides an historical account of orientalist constructions of an essentialized India.

18. I follow Shaner's (1985) use of the compound bodymind to refer to the simultaneous presence of both body-aspect and mind-aspect in all experience.

19. Although certainly characteristic of American male sports, this aggressive approach to one's body-in-training is not restricted to Americans. Many Malayalis suffer the same problems recounted here with the same results—unnecessary tension.

20. It is difficult to describe my experience in languages that neither objectify nor, as in the above paragraphs, to some degree romantically subjectify my own experience with that thin gloss of self-congratulation that is so problematic. In performance rather than in narratives, I can demonstrate this bodymind 'connection' and then demystify it by commenting on it.

21. Between 1976 and 1995, I lived in Kerala for a total of approximately six years and visited thirty-eight kalaris (Appendix I). Of these twenty-nine were run by Hindu masters, six by Muslims and three by Christians.

22. See Manavendranath (1995) and Krishnandas (1995). As I complete final revisions to this manuscript in Thiruvananthapuram, two acting students from the Delhi National School of Drama are in residence at the C.V.N. Kalari undergoing an intensive two-month course of study.

CHAPTER 2

23. Although M.D. Raghavan (1947) suggested that kalari was derived from the Sanskrit *khalurika*, Burrow concludes that khalurika ('parade ground, arena') and its Sanskrit root, khala- ('threshing floor') are Dravidian loan words (1947; see also 1946). According to the St Petersburg Lexicon, the first occurence of khalurika is in Hemacandra's *Abhidanacintamani*, dated about the twelfth century. A cognate is the Tulu *garadi* which refers to small shrines where worship of local heroes is held today. On garadi see Babu and Kotian (1990).

24. The *vadakkan pattukal* are the orally transmitted folk ballads singing the deeds of local heroes of the north Malabar region of Kerala which date from approximately the fourteenth century.

25. On the basis of subcultural variation, A.K.B. Pillai argues persuasively for dividing Kerala into three regions, i.e. northern Kerala (north of the Korapuzha river), central Kerala (extending from the Korapuzha to the Kallada river), and southern Kerala (from the Kallada to south of Suchindram Temple). The degree of brahman hegemony varied by region, but was most evident in central and northern Kerala, and much less in the south (1987: 19).

26. Lakshmi Bayi's list of arts patronized by the Travancore royal court at annual temple festivals never mentions kalarippayattu, but rather lists a wide variety of skills practised by Nayars and developed in their kalari including *kanakkambu aivu* (the art of throwing special sticks at the body's vital spots), *karanccattam* (somersaults), *kuntam payattu* (spear fight), *nokku vidya* (the art of looking, perhaps at the body's vital spots), *vattatil cattam* (acrobatic feats), *valerum kalavidya* (the art of throwing a sword to cut a banana log), *valum paricayum dandippu* (combat with sword and shield) (1995: 261–6).

27. As Nagam Aiya records in the *Travancore State Manual*, Kuruppu was a title which denotes an ancient section of Nayars charged with specific functions including 'instructors in arms to the Royal family of Travancore . . .' (1906: II, 368–9).

28. Nagam Aiya notes that the word Nadar was used as a title granted to some families of Shanars by the ancient Travancore kings (1906: 393). The Shanars were traditionally Hindus living in Tinnevelly and the southern taluks of Travancore of Dravidian origin and speakers of Tamil who may at one time have been rulers. During the last few centuries, a number of Nadars in the southern taluks of Travancore up to Thiruvananthapuram converted to Christianity, and, given their historical practice of fighting arts, some have claimed to be ksatriyas (ibid.: 398; see also Templeman 1996).

29. An anologous example of linguistic and genre blurring would be to ignore historical, regional, and technical differences and lump Kerala's Mohiniattam and Tamil Nadu's bharatanatyam with a common title.

30. K.K.N. Kurup (1977) establishes the continuity of this ancient Sangam practice with the deification of local medieval Kerala heroes still worshipped in teyyam in north Malabar.

31. Chakravarty points out that 'the popular notion that the military profession was the exclusive monopoly of the ksatriya caste is wholly without foundation' (1972: 78–9).

32. A.K.B. Pillai attributes the transformation from patrilineal to matrilineal descent and the development of significant differences in marriage relationships among Nayars and royal lineages to the period of the hundred-year war (1987: 15). The matrilineal system first appeared 'in Northern Kerala and the upper part of Central Kerala, where the Namputiri Brahmins were most powerful, and among caste groups from which the Namputiris took wives' (1987: 80–1; Pillai 1970: 309–10).

33. Yatra brahmans traditionally performed yatrakali—an entertainment which included the demonstration of martial skills. Yatrakali texts record verbal commands (vayttari) identical to those used in kalarippayattu practice.

34. Chakravarty concludes that Dhanur Vedic literature existed before the epics 'reached their present form' (1972: x).

35. Translations of *Agni Purana* include those by M.N. Dutt Shastri (1967) and Gangadharan (1985). Selected portions of the Dhanur Veda chapters and the *Bhrat Sarngadhara Paddhati* have been translated for me by Gautam Dasgupta (1986), whose assistance is gratefully acknowledged.

36. Other passages in *Agni Purana* include information on rituals performed by brahman priests to protect and/or cause success in battle (M.N. Dutt Shastri 1967: 840, 539); construction of forts (Gangadharan 1985: 576–8); instructions for military expeditions (Gangadharan 1985: 594); and battle Formations and troop deployments (Gangadharan 1985: 612–15; 629–35). See also Chakravarti.

37. On the Nayars see Gough (1952, 1961), Mencher (1962), Fuller (1976), Jeffrey (1976), Moore (1983) and A.K.B. Pillai (1987).

38. 'Nayar' is derived from the Sanskrit 'Nayaka', 'leader'. M.G.S. Narayanan notes that similar titles were developed from 'Nayaka' in Maharashtra, Andhra, Tuluva as well as Kerala. 'The warrior classes in these regions are known as *Nayak, Nayadu, Nayga,* and *Nayar* respectively' (1972: 463–4). Early scholars mistakenly asserted that the Nayars were 'immigrants, who were amongst the first invaders of Malabar' (Thurston 1975: V, 284).

39. Jacobus Canter Visscher, Chaplain at Cochin between 1717 and 1723 provides a description of Nayar occupations: 'some of them are lords of their own

territories, possessing royal power, but most of them merely hold their estates in fief from their prince, whom they are bound to serve in war, and to protect his dominions, for which service they receive no pay, but are maintained when employed out of the country. They generally own Pulleahs, whom they have inherited with their property, and who cultivate the soil. There are also several Nairs who are employed in constant attendance upon their Rajahs, whose retinue they form' (K.P.P. Menon 1986: III, 2).

40. Kerala is infamous for being among the most rigidly stratified and hierarchically ordered societies in South Asia. Whether a *particular* practitioner gained access to particular techniques and therefore to particular powers depended on one's location within the social hierarchy and kalari. The *Mahabharata* story of the low caste Ekalavya who was unable to study the martial arts because of his low birth, but who secretly learned by observing Drona teaching the princely Arjuna, illustrates this fact. When Drona discovered Ekalavya, he requested he give his right thumb as his 'gift' to his teacher.

41. Dating between the fifteenth and eighteenth centuries, the ballads focus on families which lived in the great Kadathanatu area of north Malabar. Traditionally sung by agricultural labourers while planting paddy, authorship is anonymous and the language of the ballads is simple (Devi 1975: iii; also Menon 1957 and Raghavan 1932).

42. The story of Unniarcha tells how she was so well trained in kalarippayattu that it was she rather than her husband who fought off a group of thugs who confronted them as they travelled to a temple festival.

43. Fuller traces how sovereignty is actualized at the 'local level' where 'the Indian village is "a reduced version" of the kingdom' and 'there is a homology between the function of dominance at village level and the royal function at the level of a larger territory . . .' 'The king's counterpart in the village is the headman' (1992: 139). In the larger households, the eldest male or *karanavan*, in essence serves as 'lord' of the extended family.

44. In areas where both Christians and Nayars practised, Gouvea records the fact that they often trained together under whoever the local master (Panikkar) happened to be (Zacharia 1994: 54).

45. K.V. Krishna Ayyar notes that the children of the Zamorin of Kozhikode received instruction in kalarippayattu from the specially appointed Tamme Panikkar (1938: 7). As the spiritual authority presiding over the royal kalari, the Tamme Panikkar also served important ritual functions relating to the transfer of power among the royal family. When first taking office a Zamorin had to perform the rituals of sharpening and receiving the sword as a symbol of his secular power. During a period of fourteen-day pollution, the Zamorin was unable to touch the sword and shield. When the period of pollution ended 'after worshipping the precious heirloom the Zamorin goes to his *kalari* . . . Under the guidance of the Tamme Panikkar . . . he bows before each of the twenty-seven deities presiding over the *kalari*, after which he receives his sword from the Panikkar' (ibid.: 22).

46. Among matrilineal Nayars children would remain in their mother's household and therefore followed the occupational tradition of their uncles. In families with a tradition of teaching kalarippayattu, nephews would train with their uncles. As the nuclear family emerged in the early twentieth century, it has become common for traditions like kalarippayattu to be passed down primarily from father to son rather than uncle to nephew.

47. Specific ranks, family names, native places and diocese of Christian practitioners are known.

48. Narayanan asserts that these units follow the tradition of the royal bodyguards prescribed in the *Arthasastra* and appointed 'from the families of hereditary servants with high connections, good education, firm loyalty, and long service' (1977: 99).

49. Gouvea confirms the same tradition among Christians (Anthony 1981: 117).

50. Barbosa records a slightly different form of the ritual induction in Kozhikode where the oath and arming take place in the kalari (1921: II, 47).

51. A. Sreedharan Menon (1967: 96) notes that 'an important and underlying cause of the struggle between [Kozhikode and Kochi] was the difference in caste between the Zamorin who was a Nayar, and the ksatriya ruler of Kochi who possessed a higher ritual and social status.

52. The Ilavas may have migrated to Kerala from Sri Lanka—a tradition supported by the northern ballads (Menon, C.A. 1935: 430). Raghavan has established the historical link between Kerala and Ceylon during the Cera period (1964: 133–9). Based on the Devi Ankam cloths which depict duels similar to those of Kerala, there is evidence for a highly evolved system of martial training which included jumping and acrobatics, wrestling and boxing, single stick, club fighting, sword-and-shield combat, fencing, fighting on horse, managing an elephant and archery [Deraniyagala (1937, 1942, 1944–6, 1951), Davy (1821), de Silva (1971), Hart (1975)]. There must have been some traffic in martial techniques between the Cera empire and the island nation leading to the immigration of *chekors* and their martial techniques which eventually became part of kalarippayattu.

53. All quotations are from van Buitenen (1973: 296–303).

54. There is an obvious Sanskritic bias in this hierarchical ordering of martial techniques—a ranking which reflects the transmission of pollution associated with touching and distance. Since one can kill an enemy from the greatest distance with the bow and arrow, one can kill without becoming polluted. The Tamil emphasis upon power being transmitted through sacred swords is reflected in kalarippayattu's emphasis upon sword and shield as their premier weapons.

55. Mahabali is the celebrated emperor of the Asuras, son of Virocana and grandson of Prahlada. According to the *puranas* Mahabali was expelled from his throne by Vamana, the dwarf incarnation of Visnu.

56. The fourth decree of the Synod of Diamper prohibited Christians from sharing in displays of arms associated at Onam (Zacharia 1981: 85).

57. Elias discusses the Olympic game-contests 'as an exercise for war and war as an exercise for these contests' (1972: 100). The line between combat and exercise was similarly blurred in Kerala.

58. On kalarippayattu and cultural performances see Zarrilli (1986).

59. See Fuller (1976), Jeffrey (1976, 1993) and Gough (1952).

60. Ati tata and its related system of medicine (Chapter 6) continued to be practised by many traditional Nadar families.

61. Murkot Kunhappa recalls that during his youth between 1900 and 1920 there were as many as seventy-five kalari operating in and about the town of Tellicherry in north Malabar alone (Kunhappa 1984: 31).

62. Poet Vallathol spearheaded the Kerala revival when he founded the Kerala Kalamandalam in 1930—the first public institution for teaching traditional arts. He first championed Kathakali dance-drama, languishing from the loss of patronage (Zarrilli 1984b).

63. C.V. Narayanan Nayar's father was Chittarathu Othayothu Kunjunni Nambiar, magistrate of Puthooramsam. Recognizing the son's abilities in sports, and prompted in part by a birth defect, the father brought Karnaran Gurukkal to live on their family property near which a kalari was constructed, and provided patronage for his son's lessons in kalarippayattu. Karnaran Gurukkal was from a traditional Chekavar family of Mukkali.

Another important figure during this period was Narayanan Nayar's main rival for public attention, Chirakkal T. Sreedharan Nayar, a member of the Chirakkal royal family. Sreedharan Nayar was also a serious student of kalarippayattu and its history, and he has published three important books in Malayalam documenting kalarippayattu techniques (1957, 1963, 1983).

64. C.V. Narayanan Nayar's 1933 account of the training illustrates how codified this style had become. His training in European fencing probably influenced some of the techniques, especially dagger.

65. Sridharan Champad provides a fanciful description of one of the first performances at Payyoli:

Narayanan Nayar came to the stage alone. Everyone was watching him. Narayanan Nayar jumped upwards like a bird flying. There was a mango tree branch about eleven feet above and slanting toward the stage. Raising himself up, Narayanan Nayar gave a jumping kick to the mango tree branch with his right foot. Leaves rained down continuously as the spectators cheered. Happiness and wonder filled the audience (1984: 54).

66. Transcribed from the film at the South Asian Area Center, University of Chicago.

67. A variety of popular entertainment genres have made the northern ballads commonplace in Kerala including cheap paperbacks, comic books, as well as theatre and film adaptations. In 1964 Kadathanat Raju of Badagara wrote *Aromar Chekavar*. It was produced by Raju Theatres and staged by three leading masters of the Badagara area: Bhaskaran Gurukkal, Karunan Gurukkal and Raghavan Gurukkal. Such dramas remained popular through the 1970s, but since then interest in such dramas has declined considerably with the introduction of television in 1983.

68. Kaviraj argues that the question of whether nation or region is prior is a false one since 'the region, though culturally more homogeneous, is as much an historical construction as the nation is. More startlingly, in some cases, the formation of a linguistic region is not of much greater antiquity than the coming of an anti-colonial consciousness, for the rise of a distinct regional language was related to some developments linked to colonialism' (1993: 23).

69. In 1988 the seventeen officially sanctioned associations receiving support from the Kerala Sports Council were: aquatics, ball badminton, amateur boxing, billiards, bridge, cycling, football, kabaddi, kalarippayattu, kho-kho, mountaineering, rifle, volleyball, weight lifting, women's cricket, wrestling, women's football.

70. Governance was based on a constitution accepted by the Sports Council in which there was a General Body consisting of one representative from each district association of kalari and the office bearers, while the day-to-day administration was to be carried on by the Executive Committee ('Constitution of the Kerala Kalarippayat Association', 1958). The Executive Committee consists of the seven office-bearers and three representatives from three district associations. Kalari wishing to affiliate in 1958 paid an annual fee of Rs 10. By any standards, the funds available for dispersal have always been meagre.

71. Since 1958 a total of 121 kalari have been registered as members of the Association, but in 1985 only 100 of the 121 were still officially affiliated. Of the 121, 85 were 'northern' and 36 'southern'. Of the 85 northern, 68 were still active and affiliated. Of the 36 southern, 32 were still active.

72. There was one attempt to re-establish the Tamil art of varma ati under one of its original names as a completely separate Adi Tata Association.

73. The varma ati requirements are even more stringent, stating that 'only the person who has undergone a minimum of eight years training including the treatment methods can be the master. He must have a minimum age of 25 years.'

74. An English version of the book was published in 1995 with the title, *Kalarippayattu: The Ancient Martial Art of Kerala*.

75. In 1980 kalarippayattu (along with Manipuri thang ta) travelled abroad for the first time since 1937, under the auspices of the Indian Council for Cultural Relations as part of its 'Martial Dances of India' programme for the 5th Asian

Arts Festival in Hong Kong, thus gaining for kalarippayattu a secure place in the national government's catalogue of cultural performances encapsulating India's antique heritage and suitable for export abroad. Kalarippayattu has subsequently been included as a regular item in India's national 'cultural diplomacy' strategy which has taken the form of a series of international Festivals of India. Since 1982, when the policy was first forged and a Festival of India was held in England, Festivals have also been held in France, the United States, Sweden ('India Manifestation'), concluding with the massive 1988 Festival of India in the USSR. Approximately Rs 22.68 crore were spent on the five festivals. Kalarippayattu was included as part of the official programmes at three of the festivals (England, France and the USSR). Competition to participate in tours has further politicized masters into factions and interest groups.

CHAPTER 3

76. Traditionally there were two kinds of kalari—payattu kalari for training and treatment, and *anka* kalari for duels. Only payattu kalari exists. The ankakalari was either a platform constructed especially for a duel, or may have been an enclosed larger version of a training kalari. Kalari is a term also used for training in a variety of traditional arts (Zarrilli 1986–7; Freeman 1991: 386–7).

77. For variations see C.T.S. Nayar 1963: 4.

78. Since land reform, the obligation of caring for permanent kalari deities has made some property less desirable to purchase. One teacher explained: 'There was a kalari where no training went on any longer, but where the lamps still had to be lit daily. Nobody dares buy this land where permanent kalari have existed because of the obligation to the deities of the kalari.' This obligation is not simply ritual or legal, but substantive. As Moore said regarding houses, '(. . .) the nature of past inhabitants becomes so indelibly combined with the house that such a nature remains even if the inhabitants should leave' (1983: 470).

This importance is witnessed in the transcript of a legal dispute over division of property on which a kalari was located. It was decided: 'Where under a family compact, property belonging to a Taravad is dedicated to the *kalari* or household deity, the property thenceforth ceases to be property of the Tarawad except, or otherwise than, as representing the *kalari* or household deity, and can be encumbered, if at all, only for purposes essential to the *kalari* (. . .) that is, for the proper expenses of keeping up the worship of the family (or kalari) deity'. (Linda Moore, personal communication, 'Nachi Kurumpa vs. Mathevan Kannan', *Travancore Law Reports:* Keralaodayam Press, 1896: 72–3).

Permanent deities *are* occasionally removed through a special ritual process of removal.

79. In her form as Bhadrakali, the 'fierce virgin' is the heroine of mudiyettu, one of a series of ritual arts and possession performances based on the legend of 'the killing of Darika' performed in Bhagavati temples during annual temple festivals (see Caldwell 1995).

80. In rituals such as mudiyettu, teyyam, and Ayappan tiyatta, the deity's sword is the literal vehicle through which the power of the deity passes directly into the oracular vehicle whose state of possession, dance, etc., is a manifestation of the visitation of the god.

81. For a discussion of popular notions of sakti in Chirakkal, northern Kerala, see Ayrookuzhiel's sociological study (1983: 21–42).

82. Regarding Bhairava, Virabhadra and other single goddesses, see Fuller (1993: 225ff.).

83. Danielou explains how 'the regent of the southwestern direction is Misery (Nirrta) ... and also the lord-of-the-directions (Dikpala)' worshipped 'to gain victory over their enemies (*Bhagavata Purana* 2.3.9) (...)' (1964: 137–8).

Caldwell provides another interpretation of the significance southwest/northeast associated with the goddess in Kerala: 'The NE ... represents the peak of the hot, dry season ... the SW ... corner, epitomizes the cool, dry, fertile energies of life. The SE and NW quarters ... (corresponding) to the solstices, represent the liminal, transitional periods' (1995: 330) ... 'The earth goddess in the season of Meenam is a virgin—infertile, menstrual, hot, desirous, and angry ...; in Kanni, she is an erotic wife, wet, cool, and fertile, impregnated by continual infusions of semen ... These two seasonal poles of the year ... reflect the continuous cycle of life and death in the landscape of the goddess. In the Dravidian worldview, neither pole can exist without the other (ibid.: 363).

84. See Caldwell's discussion of the relationship between Bhagavati and serpents (1995: 358–62), and also Neff.

85. Those who practise ati murai usually call their masters by the singular, asan. Muslims often go by asan though a few have the title gurukkal.

86. A sixth offering, *nivedyam*, can be the use of gestures (mudra), usually a cow's udder, given for Amritam.

87. The central role of Saraswati in Navaratri celebrations is especially evident in Thiruvananthapuram where the Maharaja of Travancore traditionally participated in celebrations honouring Saraswati.

88. Fuller notes that ayudha puja is conducted in many parts of India on the ninth day of the festival, and then is often repeated on the tenth day (1992: 120).

89. The area in front of Ganapadi is purified with water. A floor drawing (kalam) is created, inside which is the firepit. The offerings include ingredients which

delight Ganapadi. After the homam the pujari conducts brief puja for Sarasvati, Durga, and Mahalakshmi, and each of the kalari deities.

90. Given the sanskritization of puja, this flower offering is probably a recent substitution for blood sacrifices.

91. Certainly the goddess in her fierce form as Durga or Bhagavati, played an even more important role in kalarippayattu Navaratri celebrations in the past. Navaratri as an articulation of divine and kingly power is implicit in these celebrations, but may have been explicit in Kerala courts of the past. For a description of the elaborate celebrations at the Mysore court, see Fuller (1992: 114–17).

CHAPTER 4

92. The body is also the primary vehicle of the Tamil Siddha tradition where 'the human body is conceived as the boat to cross the ocean of life' (Ganapathy 1993: 63).

93. My citation of particular texts makes no claim that these particular texts were necessarily sources from which martial practitioners derived their assumptions about the body and/or power.

94. The body is understood to be composed of five elements or substances (the *panchabhutas*): *prithvi, ap, tejas,* vayu, and *akasha* which through proportionate condensation meet the various 'needs and requirements of different structures and functions of the body' (Kurup and Raghunathan 1974: 68). The three basic humours are known as *dhatu* 'since they sustain and support the body, when within proper measure and when in a state of equilibrium . . . But when they are in imbalance and cause disease they are also known as *dhosas*' (ibid.).

95. Under appropriate conditions sweating (svedana) preserves health, and may also be a treatment for disease. Sweating treatments are discussed at length in the classic text of Ayurveda, the *Caraka Samhita* (*Sutrasthana*, XIV). In contemporary Ayurvedic practice, of the eight *niragnisvedana* treatments which achieve sweat or heating without application of heat *per se,* three are forms of exercise: physical activities (like kalarippayattu), yoga and physiotherapies including massage.

96. Kutty is the past tense of *kuttuka*, 'to pierce or stab' (Gundert 1982: 262).

97. The best known martial example of blind trust and devotion for one's master is the story of Ekalavya from the *Mahabharata*. Ekalavya, the son of Kiranyadhanus, king of Nisadas (the lowest of the 'mixed castes'), became Drona's secret pupil when Drona refused to teach him because of his low birth. When Arjuna saw Ekalavya practising in the woods and recognized that Ekalavya's skills were superior to his own, he complained to Drona. When Drona asked for his fees, Ekalavya was overjoyed, and said, 'What shall I give

you? Command me; for there is nothing . . . that I will not give my teacher.' Drona replied, ' . . . I would like to have the thumb of your right hand.' The devoted Ekalavya cut off his thumb and gave it to Drona. Although usually read from the point of view of the teacher, it can be read from Ekalavya's point of view as an example of the injustice implicit in their relationship.

98. Bow and arrow were part of kalarippayattu but died out long ago.

CHAPTER 5

99. Two other terms for channels appeared in the Vedas, *dhamani* and *hira* (later *sira*). Classical Ayurveda's understanding of the body's channels is primarily as dhamani and sira; however, as early as 'the epoch of the *Atharvaveda*, the mystical speculations on the similarity of the *nadi* of the human body with the cosmic regions had already commenced. But in this respect Ayurvedic medicine has not preserved the heritage, which has been passed on, in its entirety, first to the later Vedic texts and then to the texts of Yoga and Tantra (Filliozat 1964: 159).

100. On the microcosmic level the spinal column corresponds to Siva's embodiment of the central axis of the cosmos (see Kramrisch 1981: 439–40).

101. Gupta et al. define mudra as 'specific positions of the body made by using the hands, fingers, toes, heels, and even the tongue to close several or all inlets and cavities of one's body (. . . as an important aid) for successfully regulating the vital breath (*pranayama*)' (1979: 166).

102. The English, 'scientific', is used to describe the result of 'correct' performance.

103. Balam means overt physical strength. Wherever there is sakti there is strength (balam); however, it is not always the case that where there is balam, there is power or sakti.

104. Varenne makes a similar distinction: 'Yoga, like all Hinduism's traditional disciplines, is a continuous progress (. . . therefore) we can be sure that *dharana* is in some sense 'higher' (that is more intense, more efficacious) than *ekagrata*. Where the latter was merely the fixing of mental activity on to a single point, *dharana* must appear as a motionless meditation, a silent collecting together of the mind's powers' (1976: 120).

105. Gupta et al. note that pranava or 'aum' repetition is often considered the 'greatest of all seed-mantras' (1979: 180).

106. '. . . "the breaths are counted; every breath that goes out without remembering him is dead, but every breath that goes out in recollecting the Lord is alive and is connected with Him"' (Schimmel 1975: 173).

CHAPTER 6

107. Chattambi Swamigal is said to have attained mastery in 'all the sastras in Tamil', and to have learned both yoga sastra and the vital spots from a siddha in Maruthwamala on his way back to Travancore from Kalladakurichi in Tamil Nadu.

108. *Varma Oti Murivu Cara Cuttiram* tells a teacher not to teach this 'to anyone who is short tempered or cruel, but at the same time, I tell you, teach this to one who is pious and has patience' (19.4, trans. James Deva Kamala Arumal Raj with the author's assistance).

109. According to Hindu belief, from the beginning of Brahma's creation to the destruction of all the worlds is only one of Brahma's days—a Kalpa. Encompassed by a Kalpa are the cycles through which the world passes— great Yugas or ages, each lasting twelve thousand years of the gods or 4,320,000 human years. According to Hopkins, the final Kali Yuga lasts 'only 1,800 years of the gods. During this period *dharma* steadily declines from its natural perfection in the *Krita Yuga*. In the *Kali Yuga* unrighteousness is rampant, men are weak and unable to follow their proper duties, rulers plunder their subjects, students disobey their parents and teachers . . .' (1971: 101)

110. The *Dhanur Veda* chapters of the *Agni Purana* contain no specific information on the vital spots; however, we can assume that the weapons techniques described there were used to attack these deadly spots.

111. See Ros (1995) for a discussion of the possible relationship between the vital spots and an Ayurvedic form of acupuncture.

112. Although this conception of the humoral body is used for combat injuries and/or other traumas that require surgical intervention, a fundamentally different concept of healing is used as well. Zimmermann notes that the surgical understanding of the body in the classical texts lies outside the usual twofold scheme of medical therapy by purifying (*sodhana*), and by quieting (*samana*) (1980: 103). One is 'an *operative* art, which includes the rational observation of anatomical facts and the fulfilment of practical tasks' and the other is '*expectant* medicine' based on the concept of humours and saps (Zimmermann 1978a: 100). Both concepts operate complementarily within the martial master's repertory.

113. Similarly the 'wrestlers' of north India traditionally practised bonesetting and massage for 'bruises, swelling, joint pain, fractures and other forms of injury . . . associated with fighting' (Lambert 1991 personal correspondence; Alter 1992: passim).

114. See Appendix I.

115. Within the Tamil Siddha yoga tradition, 'the only way to make the soul immortal is to make the body immortal also, and this is what the Siddha yogis aimed to do' (Trawick 1983: 938). This practice toward immortality is

reflected in some texts like *Varma Oti Murivu Cara Cuttiram*. The nature of the breath (prana) is to 'gradually lose four lives' with each cycle. From this defect, death arises. James Devi Raj explained that a normal cycle includes an inhalation and exhalation. Air is inspired from the area eight *viral* (the width of the fingers) from the nose, while during normal expiration the air goes to an area twelve finger widths from the nose. Consequently, with each breath we are understood to 'lose' four finger widths of breath. This is the meaning of 'losing four lives' with each cycle of breath. The text also records how 'this defect is corrected (in the yogi) and his vital points will not be affected'—by becoming accomplished in pranayama, the Siddha yogi's breath is evened out, becoming twelve-by-twelve finger widths (*viral*) so that with each breath he does not lose 'four lives'.

116. Classification is given as either a flesh, bone, tendon, vein, artery or joint vital spot.

117. Translated by C. Mohammed Sherif with the author's assistance. *Marmmrahasyangal* records *talahrttu* as 'at the centre of the sole (of the foot or palm).'

118. One *can* is equal to eight *angulam*—the length of the top of the thumb from its tip to the knuckle.

119. C. Mohammed Sherif has credibly hypothesized that the Susruta-based texts/techniques are derived from the practice of weapons-bearing soldiers and physicians who served as part of an army in service to a ruler, while the *abhyasa marmmam* techniques might be attributed to early Buddhists. The Buddhists developed empty-hand techniques to defend themselves, and immediate counter-applications to revive their attackers, thereby protecting themselves while fulfilling their religious vow not to kill. When Buddhism was suppressed this system of practice was absorbed into the kalarippayattu tradition as a complement to the weapons system of the traditional warrior.

120. Sometimes the number is 116. Moolachal Asan includes a 109th spot 'located inside which you cannot touch', and a 110th in the eyes.

121. Since 6 of the 12 are double, the number is 18.

122. Some practitioners also identify kochu or ullu varmam, i.e. unnamed 'catch' spots located in the muscles. If penetrated or hit they produce a painful contraction.

123. Kalam means 'time', but refers to those spots whose symptoms recur after initial revival and treatment have been administered.

124. Translated by Usha and Moses Thilak with the author's assistance.

125. Chandran Gurukkal explained that 'Dhyanamurti is a form of Kali in her peaceful guise. There is a particular verse (*sloka*) which is recited which describes her in this form. When chanted, the picture comes into your mind.'

126. In 1993 his library included Cirakkal T. Sreedharanan Nayar's *Marmmadarppanam, Better Judo, Amazing Secrets of Psychic Healing, Speaking of Acupuncture, Why Be Afraid* and *Health and Healing in Yoga*.

127. Salim either neglected to mention or did not observe what I noticed. The first of the five of Prakasan's students to sink senseless to the floor during the thirty-five minute demonstration kept opening his eyes to see what was happening.

CHAPTER 7

128. *Caritam* may be translated as behaviour, good conduct, action, law, or rule. The title may be translated as 'Rugmaamgada's Rule' or 'Rugmaamgada's Law', implying the king's steadfast/good conduct. The play is based on Chapter 21 of the *Padma Purana*.

129. The *Natyasastra* originally identified eight basic states of being: the erotic, love or pleasure; the comic, mirthful or derision; pathos or sadness; the furious, anger or wrath; the heroic or vigorous; fearful or terrible; repulsive or disgust; and the wondrous or marvellous. The twelfth-century commentator, Abhinavagupta, added a ninth—at-onement or serenity—accepted in the Kathakali tradition. *Bhava* is the state of being/doing of the character or actor; *rasa* is the audience's experience of the character's state or condition.

130. The use of *vadham*, literally, 'killing', is significant since it reflects the performative act of killing.

131. *Dharmamgada* literally means 'the mace (gada) of the law or duty (dharma).'

132. All quotations are from the translation by V.R. Prabodhachandran Nayar, M.P. Sankaran Namboodiri and Phillip B. Zarrilli.

133. This form of Visnu is especially sacred to Malayalis who worship Padmanabha at Sri Padmanabhaswamy Temple at Thiruvananthapuram.

134. When a Kathakali drama is performed, the performance is not limited to the literary text as originally authored (Zarrilli 1984, Chapter 6). The literary text is only the beginning place in the history of a performance text which expands through the addition of performative interpolations (*ilakiyattam*) based on the source text, or contracts through editing—each of which reveals the particular historical 'anxieties and concerns' of Kathakali's patron-connoisseurs.

Interpolations in the literary text provide opportunities for the most heralded senior Kathakali actor-dancers to display aspects of their virtuosic performative abilities–such as Arjuna's choreographic *tour de force* describing Devaloka in *Kalakeyavadham*, or the mimetic dynamism of Bhima in *Kalyanasaugandhikam* enacting the fight between an elephant, python, and lion. Rugmamgada's *attam* is similar to the histrionic demands of the role of Nala in *Nala Caritam*, *both* of which focus on the inner state of the character.

135. Other readings of the drama are also possible. The play could be read as enacting the conflict between eighteenth-century Vaisnavite devotionalism and the violent/dangerous powers of Dravidian tantric Saktism. As in Mantavappali Ittiraricca Menon's Santanagopalam, devotion to Visnu prevails (see Zarrilli 1994b: passim). This contrast is clearly marked in the differences between mudiyettu which enacts the goddess' violent fury and Krisnattam where Vaisnavite erotic lyricism predominates (Caldwell 1995: 327).

136. Hart (1975, 1979), Hiltebeitel (1988, 1991) and Caldwell (1995) discuss the antique association of hair with 'power' in Dravidian culture. 'This inheritance is still seen in the loosening of women's hair during state of spirit possession, as well as in the *veliccappatu's* (oracle) running of the fingers of his left hand through his long, loosened hair while in trance at Bhagavati temples. The running of the fingers through the hair, especially female hair, infuses the body with wild, natural sacred power' (Caldwell 1995: 184–5).

137. This state is clearly marked in *yakshagana tenkutittu* and, as David Gitomer records, in *The Catastrophe of the Braid* where Bhima is associated with ogres and demons: 'Bhima's interactions with the race of cannibalistic ogres in the epic lie behind his adharmic violence and voraciousness' (1998: 287–8). In *The Catastrophe* as well as in the *yakshagana tenkutittu* version of the killing of Dushasana, an ogre must possess Bhima in order for him to drink blood:

> Bloodfield says, 'My master wolfbelly has vowed to drink the blood of Dushasana. But I, the appointed ogre, must enter the body and do the drinking for him' (ibid.: 94).

> In both *yakshagana tenkutittu* and *The Catastrophe,* 'the depiction of *bibhatsa rasa*, the disgusting, often becomes comic, and emerges as a species of *hasya rasa:* the raksasas of the *Venisamhara* function as vidushakas (buffoons) in a play where there is no vidusaka' (ibid.: 286).

138. This reading of the dynamics of 'raudra' as a state of heightened acuity from which dire consequences result is ubiquitous in Kerala, and has symbolic importance in the world the communists have created to enhance consciousness about radical social change. In Bhaasi's *Memories in Hiding* the main character, Ceennan, during the Suranand Revolution in Kerala where many peasants and party workers died at the hands of the police, undergoes a transformation from lifelong acceptance of his social position in service to his landlord/oppressor, to a state where his fury 'explodes': 'Tamburaan! (*He stares at the landlord and stands up straight. The landlord is puzzled by the expression on his face. Nannu Naayar (the landlord's bodyguard) becomes afraid. Ceennan stares at him for a moment. In a firm declaration*) I no longer have a Tamuraan! I am no longer a slave!' (Act 4, Scene 1, 1995: 55). In the Kerala People's Art Club production, Ceenan is bathed in red light during this scene. A number of articulations exist between the goddess/terror/fury and the radical/ revolutionary leftist movement in Kerala—the association of red with the 'heated' nature of the goddess, her fury and necessary bloodletting; the 'terror'

society witnesses when the 'people' rise up in righteous/divine 'fury'; and the 'blood' it is necessary to shed to assuage this fury.

This reading is supported by the fact that just before this scene of revolt, in Act 3, Scene 4 during the chaotic melée in which the police are attacking the agricultural labourers and their families, Bhaasi has 'kathakali drumming from the nearby (Bhagavati) temple' during a performance of *The Killing of Duryodhana* playing in the background. With Dussassana and Duryodhana both having been killed, the drumming from the performance comes to an end just as the fighting 'decreases and ends'.

CHAPTER 8

139. See Carter (1982), E.V. Daniel (1983, 1984), Davis (1976), Mahadevan (1967) and Nikhilananda (1967).

140. *Gunam* type determined at birth is still considered important by most Malayalis today, especially when considering a suitable marriage partner.

141. Regarding those who have used kalarippayattu to train Hindus or Muslims for potential communal violence, once master said, 'Those who use kalarippayattu techniques for communal purposes are not teaching kalarippayattu! They are only teaching its techniques. You can call this kalarippayattu only when the practice follows these traditional rules and rituals. When taken out of the traditional context (the use of the techniques for dharmic purposes), and without the spiritual side of practice, it cannot be called kalarippayattu. It should only be described as learning fighting techniques!'

142. Hamzah inhabits an intercultural ethnoscape where there is no target 'culture', although there definitely is a target public.

143. The Kerala Kalarippayat Association has instituted annual competitions. Students compete for awards in the preliminary exercises and weapons practice. Weapons are wielded only with students from the same school. There is no free-style competition. Senior masters serve as judges who make awards based on style and form. Although student participants train hard for the annual competition, the awards *per se* are not linked to advancement within a particular kalari.

144. Hamzah learned special breath control/meditation techniques for two months. He was required to be celibate, fast and completely separate himself from the material world. In the first stage of meditation he was required to sit still, focusing his eyes straight ahead, and his mind on god. From this simple sitting exercise he progressed to more complex forms.

145. Two of these innovators, Renshi K. Mohanan and Balachandran Master, are located in Thiruvananthapuram. Each has fashioned his own composite self-defence styles. Mohanan is founder of Kaju-Kado Karate, a combination of

karate (ka-), judo (-ju-), kalari (-ka-), and aikido (-do). Trained as a youth in kalarippayattu in college he took up the 'rough, very practical, full contact' Japanese karate. He devised a composite style which he feels is effective for street fighting. Balachandran Master is discussed below.

146. The cover story title refers to how Padmini 'Sweet 16 and never been kissed . . . decided that Prince Charles was just too, too desirable to be allowed to pass by without a pair of cherry-red lips being pressed against his cheek. So the star of India's film industry — "Kiss Oomph" to her fans—stepped forward in the Bombay Studios and kissed her hero . . .' The story comes complete with a colour photograph of Padmini and Prince Charles.

147. Other contemporary contexts such as the demonstration stage are also transforming kalarippayattu in radical, though different ways. The emphasis on training students exclusively for stage demonstrations makes kalarippayattu into a beautiful, fluid, dance-like art; however, for those most interested in the art as a martial art, this style has lost its *raison d' être*.

148. Spectacle and melodrama were an important part of the subtext of many traditional performative representations of the 'heroic' warrior. They were embedded within a socio-cultural fabric that ideally restrained and constrained the powers of the practitioner. This ideal, its melodramatic spectacularization, and its 'failure' are all seen in the case of Tacholi Otenan who, as noted earlier, subdued the recalcitrant Kunki by attacking her vital spots and then raped her.

Bibliography

Achutanandan, K.V.
    1973. *24 Vadakkan Pattukal* (Malayalam). Kunnamkulam: A&C Stores.
Aiya, Nagam
    1906. *Travancore State Manual.* Trivandrum: Government Press.
Ajay
    1993. 'Where is the time when Unniarcha's Urumi will shine?', *Malayala Manorama*, 15 August, pp. 1, 3, 'Sunday Supplement' (Malayalam).
Alper, Harvey P., (ed.)
    1989. *Mantra.* Albany: State University of New York Press.
Alter, Joseph S.
    1992. *The Wrestler's Body: Identity and Ideology in North India.* Berkeley: University of California Press.
Anderson, Benedict
    1983. *Imagined Communities.* London: Verso.
Appadurai, Arjun
    1990. 'Disjuncture and Difference in the Global Cultural Economy', *Public Culture*, 2, 2: 1–24.
    1991. 'Global Ethnoscapes: Notes and Queries for a Transnational Anthropology', *Recapturing Anthropology*, Richard G. Fox (ed.). Santa Fe: School of American Research Press, 191–210.
Appadurai, Arjun and Breckenridge, Carol A.
    1988. 'Why Public Culture?', *Public Culture*, 1, 1: 5–9.
Arunachalam, Thiru M.
    1977. 'The Siddha Cult in Tamilnad', *Bulletin of the Institute of Traditional Cultures,* Madras, 85–117.
Arvind, V.
    1983. 'Master of the Games', *The Sun*: 6, 45: 16–17.
Awasthi, Suresh
    1982–3. 'Kerala's Martial Art, Kalarippayattu', *Namaskaar*, 12–18.

Ayrookuzhiel, A.M. Abraham
- 1983. *The Sacred in Popular Hinduism.* Madras: Christian Literature Society.

Ayyar, K.V. Krishna
- 1928–32. 'The Kerala Mamakam', *Kerala Society Papers*, 2, Series 6: 324–30.
- 1938. *The Zamorins of Calicut.* Calicut: Norman Printing.
- 1966. *A Short History of Kerala.* Ernakulam: Pai & Co.

Ayyar, Rah Bahadur L.K. Anantakrishna
- 1926. *The Anthropology of the Syrian Christians.* Ernakulam: Cochin Government Press.

Babb, Lawrence A.
- 1975. *The Divine Hierarchy: Popular Hinduism in Central India.* New York: Columbia University Press.

Babu, Bananje, and Mohan Kotian
- 1990. *Tulunada Garodigala Samskritika Adyayana.* Udipi: Sree Brahma Baidarkala Samakritika Adyayaya Pratisthana.

Balakrishnan, P.
- 1994. *Kalarippayattu: Keralattile Prachina Ayodaya Mura.* Bangalore: S.N. Process.
- 1995. *Kalarippayattu: The Ancient Martial Art of Kerala.* Trivandrum: C.V.N. Kalari.

Balaratnam, L.K.
- 1942. 'Games and Pastimes of Kerala', *Modern Review: A Monthly Review & Miscellany*, 72, 3: 265–8.

Barba, Eugenio and Nicola Savarese
- 1991. *A Dictionary of Theatre Anthropology: The Secret Art of the Performer.* London: Routledge, 1991.

Barbosa, Duarte
- 1989. (1921) *The Book of Duarte Barbosa*, Vol. II. Trans. Mansel Longworth Dames. New Delhi: Asian Educational Services.

Bauman, Richard
- 1977. *Verbal Art as Performance.* Prospect Heights, IL.

Bayi, Gouri Lakshmi
- 1995. *Sree Padmanabha Swamy Temple.* Bombay: Bharatiya Vidya Bhavan.

Beck, Brenda
- 1976. 'The symbolic merger of body, space and cosmos in Hindu Tamil Nadu', *Contributions to Indian Sociology*, 10, 2: 213–43.

Bhaasi, Tooppil
- 1995. *Memories in Hiding.* Calcutta: Seagull Press.

Bhabha, Homi K. (ed.)
    1990. *National and Narration*. London: Routledge Press.

Bharata
    1956. *Natyasastra* Vol. I, ed. and trans. M. Ghosh. Calcutta: Manisha Granthalaya.
    1961. *Natyasastra* Vol. II, ed. and trans. M. Ghosh. Calcutta: Asiatic Society.

Bharucha, Rustom
    1995. *Chandralekha: Woman Dance Resistance*. New Delhi: Indus.

Bhishagratna, K.K. (ed. and trans.)
    1963. *The Susruta Samhita, Vol. II*. Varanasi: Chowkhamba Sanskrit Series.

Blacking, John (ed.)
    1977. *The Anthropology of the Body*. London: Academic Press.
    1985. 'Movement, dance, music and the Venda girls' initiation cycle', in P. Spencer (ed.), *Society and the Dance*, Cambridge: Cambridge University Press.

Blundell, Valda, John Shepherd and Ian Taylor. (eds.)
    1993. *Relocating Cultural Studies*. London: Routledge Press.

Bourdieu, Pierre
    1977. *Outline of a Theory of Practice*. Cambridge: Cambridge University Press.
    1990a. *The Logic of Practice*. Cambridge: Polity.
    1990b. *In Other Words: Essays Towards a Reflexive Sociology*. Cambridge: Polity.
    1993. *The Field of Cultural Production*. New York: Columbia University Press.

Breckenridge, Carol A. (ed.)
    1995. *Consuming Modernity: Public Culture in a South Asian World*. Minneapolis: University of Minnesota Press.

Briggs, G.W.
    1973. *Goraknath and the Kanphata Yogis*. Delhi: Motilal Banarsidass.

Bruckner, Heidrun, Lothar Lutze and Aditya Malik (eds.)
    1993. *Flags of Fame: Studies in South Asian Folk Culture*. New Delhi: Manohar.

Bruner, Edward M.
    1986. 'Ethnography as Narrative', in *Victor W. Turner and Edward M. Bruner* (eds.) *The Anthropology of Experience*, Urbana: University of Illinois Press, 139–55.

Burrow, T.
    1946. 'Loanwords in Sanskrit', *Transactions of the Philological Society* 1–30.

1947. 'Dravidian Studies VII: Further Dravidian Words in Sanskrit', *Bulletin of the School of Oriental and African Studies* (London University), 12, Part 1, 365–96.

Burrow, T. and M.B. Emeneau

1943–6. 'Dravidian Studies III: Two Developments of Initial k-in Drivian', *Bulletin of the School of Oriental and African Studies* (London University), 9, 122–39.

1961. *A Dravidian Etymological Dictionary.* Oxford: Clarendon Press.

Butler, Judith

1989. *Gender Trouble.* London: Routledge Press.

1993. *Bodies that Matter.* London: Routlege Press.

Caldwell, Sarah Lee

1995. 'Oh Terrifying Mother: The Mudiyettu Ritual Drama of Kerala, South India', unpublished Ph.D. dissertation, Berkeley: Department of Anthropology, University of California.

Carrithers, M., S. Collins and S. Lukes

1985. *The Category of the Person.* Cambridge: Cambridge University Press.

Carter, Anthony T.

1982. 'Hierarchy and the Concept of the Person in Western India', in Akos Ostor, Lina Fruzzetti, and Steven Barnett (eds.), *Concepts of Person: Kinship, Caste, and Marriage in India.* Cambridge: Harvard University Press, 118–42.

Chakravarty, P.C.

1972 (1941). *The Art of Warfare in Ancient India.* Delhi. (Dacca: University of Dacca, Bulletin # 21).

Champad, Sridharan

1984. *Mahacharithamala: C.V. Narayanan Nayar.* Kottayam: Kairali Children's Book Trust.

Charaka

1949. *Charaka Samhita* (Vols I–VI), Shree Gulab Kunverba Ayurvedic Society (ed.), Jamnagar.

Clifford, James (ed.)

1986. *Writing Culture.* Berkeley: University of California Press.

Cohen, Anthony P.

1994. *Self Consciousness: An Alternative Anthropology of Identity.* London: Routledge Press.

Comaroff, John and Jean

1992. *Ethnography and the Historical Imagination.* Boulder: Westview Press.

Connerton, Paul

1989. *How Societies Remember.* Cambridge: Cambridge University Press.

Cromwell, L.G.
    1981. 'The Root of Power', *Social Analysis*, 7: 50–71.
Daniel, E.V.
    1984a. *Fluid Signs: Being a Person the Tamil Way.* Berkeley: University of California Press.
    1984b. 'The Pulse as an Icon in Siddha Medicine', *Contributions to Asian Studies*, 18: 115–26.
Danielou, Alain
    1964. *Hindu Polytheism.* New York: Bollingen Foundation.
Dann, Jeffrey Lewis
    1978. '*Kendo* in Japanese Martial Culture: Swordsmanship as Self-Cultivation', unpublished Ph.D. dissertation, University of Washington, Department of Anthropology.
Dasgupta, Gautam (trans.)
    1993a. 'Dhanur Veda' (Chapters 249–52) in *Agni Purana*, unpulished translation (*Agnipurana of Maharsi Vedavyasa*. Varanasi: Chowkhambra Sanskrit Series, 1966).
    1993b. Bhasa's *Karnabharan*, unpublished translation of lines 102–15 (*Karnabharan* by Bhasa. Mysore: Samskrita Sahitya Sadana, 1961).
Dash, Vidya Bhagwan.
    1992. *Massage Therapy in Ayurveda.* New Delhi: Concept.
David, Kenneth (ed.)
    1977. *The New Wind: Changing Identities in South Asia.* The Hague: Mouton.
Davis, M.
    1976. 'A Philosophy of Hindu Rank from Rural West Bengal', *Journal of Asian Studies*, 36, 1: 5–24.
de Certeau, Michel
    1984. *The Practice of Everyday Life.* Berkeley: University of California Press.
Deraniyagala, P.E.P.
    1937. 'The Two Deva Angam Cloths of Hanguranketa Maha Devale', *Journal of the Royal Anthropological Society* (Ceylon Branch), 34, 90: 88–102.
    1941. 'Some Medieval Representations of Sinhala Wrestlers and Gladiators', *Journal of the Royal Anthropological Society* (Ceylon Branch), 35, 94: 85–90.
    1942 'Sinhala Weapons and Armour', *Journal of the Royal Anthropological Society* (Ceylon Branch), 35, 97: 97–142.
    1944–6. 'Medieval Sinhala Wrestling', *Spolia Zeylanica*, 14: 155–6.
    1951. 'Some Sinhala Combative, Field and Aquatic Sports and Games', *Spolia Zeylanica*, 26: 179–215.

DeSilva, M.S.C.
- 1971. 'The Sinhala Army During the Portuguese, Dutch and British Periods—1505 to 1815', *Spoliz Zeylanica*, 32, 1: 79–87.

Devi, E.H.
- 1975. 'Medieval Society as Reflected in the Ballads of North Malabar', M.A. thesis, University of Calicut.
- 1976. 'The Military System of Malabar', *Journal of Kerala Studies*, 3–4: 413–20.

Draeger, Donn
- 1973a. *Classical Bujutsu*. New York: Weatherhill.
- 1973b. *Classical Budo*. New York: Weatherhill.
- 1974. *Modern Bujutsu and Budo*. New York: Weatherhill.

Draeger, Donn F. and Robert W. Smith
- 1969. *Asian Fighting Arts*. Tokyo: Kodansha.
- 1980. *Comprehensive Asian Fighting Arts*.

Drewal, Margaret
- 1991. 'The State of Research on Performance in Africa', *African Studies Review*, 34, 3: 1–64.

Dutt Shastri, M.N. (trans.)
- 1967. *Agni Puranam*. Varanasi: Chowkhamba Sanskrit Series.

Eck, Diana L.
- 1981. *Darsan: Seeing the Divine Image in India*. Chambersburg: Anima.

Eliade, Mircea
- 1958. *Yoga, Immortality, and Freedom*. Princeton: Princeton University Press.
- 1975. *Patanjali and Yoga*. New York: Schocken Books.

Elias, Norbert
- 1972. 'The Genesis of Sport as a Sociological Problem', in Eric Dunming (ed.), *Sport: Readings from a Sociological Perspective*, Toronto: University of Toronto Press.

Emeneau, Murray B.
- 1954. 'Linguistic Prehistory of India', *American Philosophical Society, Proceedings*, 98: 282–92.

Fabian, Johannes
- 1990. *Performance and Power: Ethnographic Explorations through Proverbial Wisdom and Theater in Shaba, Zaire*. Madison: University of Wisconsin Press.

Fairs and Festivals of Kerala, Part VIIB (I). *Census of India* 1966 (1961, VII, *Kerala*).

Fawcett, E.
- 1901. *Nayars of Malabar*. (Madras) *Government Museum Bulletin*, 3, 3.

Fedorova, Mariana.
> 1989. 'The Theory of Marmans–A Reconstruction According to Classic Texts', unpublished paper delivered at the 1989 IASTAM Conference, Bombay.

Feher, Michel (ed.)
> 1989. *Zone: Fragments for a History of the Human Body, Parts I, II, III.* New York: Urzone.

Ferguson, Donald (ed.)
> 1908. 'The History of Ceylon, from the Earliest Times to 1600 A.D., as related by Joan de Barros and Diogo do Couto', *Journal of the Royal Anthropological Society* (Ceylon Branch), 20, 60.

Fernandes, Eddie
> 1982 'The Bruce Lees of India', *Indian Express*, 21 March.

Filliozat, J.
> 1964. *The Classical Doctrine of Indian Medicine: Its Origins and its Greek Parallels.* Delhi: Munshiram Manoharlal.

Fiske, John
> 1989. *Understanding Popular Culture.* Boston: Unwin Hyman.
> 1993. *Power Plays Power Works.* London: Verso.

Foster, Susan Leigh (ed.)
> 1996. *Corporealities: Dancing Knowledge, Culture and Power.* London: Routledge Press.

Foster, William (ed.)
> 1968 *Early Travels in India 1583–1619.* Bombay: S. Chand.

Fox, Richard G. (ed.)
> 1991. *Recapturing Anthropology.* Sante Fe: School of American Research Press.

Foucault, Michel
> 1977. *Discipline and Punish.* London: Allen Lane.
> 1988. 'Technologies of the Self', in Luther H. Martin (ed.), *Technologies of the Self: A Seminar with Michel Foucault.* Amherst: University of Massachusetts Press.

Freeman, J. Richardson
> 1991. 'Purity and Violence: Sacred Power in the Teyyam Worship of Malabar', unpublished Ph.D. dissertation, University of Pennsylvania.
> 1993. 'Performing Possession: Ritual and Consciousness in the Teyyam Complex of Northern Kerala', in Heidrun Bruckner, Lothar Lutze and Aditya Malik (eds.), *Flags of Fame: Studies in South Asian Folk Culture* New Delhi: Manohar, 109–38.

Fuller, C.J.
> 1976. *The Nayars Today.* Cambridge: Cambridge University Press.

1992. *The Camphor Flame: Popular Hinduism and Society in India.* Princeton: Princeton University Press.

Ganapathy, T.N.
    1993. *The Philosophy of the Tamil Siddhas.* New Delhi: Indian Council of Philosophical Research.

Gangadharan, N. (trans.)
    1985. *Agni Purana*, Part II, Chapters 101–251; Part III, Chapters 252–311. *Ancient Indian Tradition and Mythology,* J.L. Shastri (ed.), 28. Delhi: Motilal Banarsidass.

Gellner, Ernest
    1983. *Nations and Nationalism.* Ithaca: Cornell University Press.

Gitomer, David
    1998. *The Catastrophe of the Braid: The Mahabharata in Classical Drama.* New York: Oxford University Press.

Giyani, S.D.
    1964. *Agni-Purana, A Study.* Varanasi: Chowkhamba Sanskrit Series.

Gladstone, J.W.
    1985. 'Caste, Religion and People's Movements in Kerala with particular reference to South Kerala', *Religion and Society*, 32, 1: 24–35.

Gode, P.K.
    1955. 'History of the Practice of Massage in Ancient and Medieval India', *Annals of the Bhandarkar Oriental Research Institute*, 36: 85–113.

Gough, Kathleen
    1952. 'Changing Kinship Usages in the Setting of Political and Economic Change among the Nayars of Malabar', *Journal of the Royal Anthropological Institute*, 82: 71–88.
    1959a. 'Cults of the Dead among the Nayars', in Milton Singer (ed.), *Traditional India: Structure and Change*, Philadelphia: American Folklore Society, 446–78.
    1959b. 'The Nayars and the Definition of Marriage', *Journal of the Royal Anthropological Institute*, 89: 23–34.

Gough, Kathleen and D.M. Schneider (eds.)
    1961. *Matrilineal Kinship.* Berkeley: University of California Press.

Grey, Edward (ed.)
    1956. *The Travels of Pietro Della Valle in India.* New York: Burt Franklin.

Gundert, Rev. H.
    1982. (1872). *A Malayalam and English Dictionary.* New Delhi: Asian Educational Services.

Gupta S., D.J. Hoens and T. Goudriaan
    1979. *Hindu Tantrism.* Leiden: E.J. Brill.

Hardy, F.
- 1983. *Viraha-bhakti: The Early History of Krsna Devotion in South India*. Oxford: Oxford University Press.

Hart, George L.
- 1975. *The Poems of Ancient Tamil: their Milieu and their Sanskrit Counterparts*. Berkeley: University of California Press.
- 1979. *Poets of the Tamil Anthologies: Ancient Poems of Love and War*. Princeton: Princeton University Press.

Hastrup, Kirsten.
- 1995. 'Incorporated Knowledge', *Mime Journal*, 2–9.

Hiltebeitel, Alf
- 1976. *The Ritual of Battle: Krishna in the Mahabharata*. Ithaca: Cornell University Press.
- 1988. *The Cult of Draupadi, Vol. I*. Chicago: University of Chicago Press.
- 1991. *The Cult of Draupadi, Vol. II*. Chicago: University of Chicago Press.

Hobsbawm, E.J.
- 1990. *Nations and Nationalism since 1780*. Cambridge: Cambridge University Press.

Hobsbawm, Eric and Terence Ranger (eds.)
- 1983. *The Invention of Tradition*. Cambridge: Cambridge University Press.

Hopkins, Thomas J.
- 1971. *The Hindu Religious Tradition*. Encino: Dickenson.

Huang, Pierre and Ming Wong
- 1977. *Oriental Methods of Mental and Physical Fitness*. Donald N. Smith (trans.). New York: Funk and Wagnalls.

Inden, Ronald
- 1986. 'Orientalist Constructions of India', *Modern Asian Studies*, 20, 3: 401–46.

Innes, C.A.
- 1951. *Malabar*. Madras: Government Press.

Irschick, Eugene F.
- 1994. *Dialogue and History: Constructing South India, 1795–1895*. Berkeley: University of California Press.

Iyer, K. Bharata.
- 1955. *Kathakali*. London: Luzac.

Iyer, L.A. Krishna
- 1937. *The Travancore Tribes and Castes*, Vol. I. Trivandrum: Government Press.

Iyer, L.K.A. Krishna
- 1968. *Social History of Kerala*. Madras: Book Centre.

Iyer, T.G. Ramamurthi.
    1981 (1933). *The Handbook of Indian Medicine: The Gems of the Siddha System*. Delhi: Sri Satguru.

Jackson, Gary Brian
    1975. 'Kendo: On a Japanese Psychology of Life', unpublished Ph.D. dissertation, Department of Anthropology, University of California-Irvine.

Jackson, Michael
    1989. *Paths Toward a Clearing: Radical Empiricism and Ethnographic Inquiry*. Bloomington: Indiana University Press.

Jaggi, O.P.
    1973a. *History of Science and Technology in India, Vol. 4, Indian System of Medicine*. Delhi: Atma Ram & Sons.
    1973b. *History of Science and Technology in India, Vol. 3, Folk Medicine*. Delhi: Atma Ram & Sons.

Jeffrey, R.
    1976. *The Decline of Nayar Dominance*. Sussex: Sussex University Press.
    1993. *Politics, Women and Well-being: How Kerala Became 'a Model'*. Oxford: Oxford University Press.

Jenks, Chris (ed.)
    1993. *Cultural Reproduction*. London: Routledge Press.

Jenkins, Richard
    1992. *Pierre Bourdieu*. London: Routledge Press.

Johnson, Don Hanlon
    1992. (1983) *Body: Recovering our Sensual Wisdom*. Berkeley: North Atlantic Books.
    1994. *Body, Spirit and Democracy*. Berkeley: North Atlantic Books.

Johnson, Mark
    1987. *The Body in the Mind: The Bodily Basis of Meaning, Imagination, and Reason*. Chicago: University of Chicago Press.

Johnson, Richard
    1986. 'What is Cultural Studies Anyway?', *Social Text*, 16: 38–80.

Jones, Betty True
    1983. 'Kathakali Dance-Drama: An Historical Perspective', Bonnie C. Wade (ed.), *Performing Arts in India*. Berkeley: Center for South and Southeast Asia Studies, University of California, 14–44.

Jones, Betty True and Clifford R.
    1970. *Kathakali*. New York: Theatre Arts Books.

Jones, Clifford R.
- 1981. 'Dhulicitra: Historical Perspectives on Art and Ritual', in Joanne G. Williams (ed.), *Kaladarsana: American Studies in the Art of India*, Leiden: E.J. Brill, 69–75.

Kailasapathy, K.
- 1968. *Tamil Heroic Poetry*. Oxford: Clarendon Press.

Kakar, S.
- 1982. *Shamans, Mystics, and Doctors*. Chicago: University of Chicago Press.

Kapferer, Bruce
- 1986. 'Performance and the Structuring of Meaning and Experience', in Victor W. Turner and Edward M. Bruner (eds.), *The Anthropology of Experience*, Urbana: University of Illinois Press, 188–206.

Kareem, C.K.
- 1973. *Kerala under Haidar Ali and Tippu Sultan*. Cochin: Paico.

Kasulis, Thomas P. (ed.), with Roger T. Ames and Wimal Dissanayake
- 1993. *Self as Body in Asian Theory and Practice*. Albany: State University of New York Press.

Katiyar, Arun
- 1983. 'Enter the Super Corps!', *Bombay*: 4, 21 (June–July), 40–3.

Kaviraj, Sudipta
- 1993. 'The Imaginary Institution of India', in Partha Chatterjee and Gyanendra Pandey (eds.), *Subaltem Studies* VII, Delhi: Oxford University Press, 1–39.

Keat, Russell
- 1986. 'The Human Body in Social Theory: Reich, Foucault, and the Repressive Hypothesis', *Radical Philosophy*, 42, 24–32.

Kersenboom, Saskia C.
- 1990. 'Devadasi Murai', *Sangeet Natak*, 96: 44–54.

Kersenboom-Story, S.C.
- 1987. *Nityasumangali*. Delhi: Motilal Banarsidass.

Kesaven, Veluthat
- 1976. 'Aryan Brahman Settlements of Ancient Kerala', 27th Indian History Congress, University of Calicut, 24–7.

Keshwani, N.H. (ed.)
- 1974. *The Science of Medicine and Physiological Concepts in Ancient and Medieval India*. New Delhi: National Book Trust.

Kiyota, Minoru
- 1989. *Kendo: Its History, Philosophy and Means to Personal Growth*. Madison: Center for South Asian Studies, University of Wisconsin-Madison.

Kiyota, M. and H. Kinoshita
　1990. *Japanese Martial Arts and American Sports*. Tokyo: Nihon University.

Kleinman, Arthur
　1980. *Patients and Healers in the Context of Culture*. Berkeley: University of California Press.

Kondo, Dorrine K.
　1990. *Crafting Selves*. Chicago: University of Chicago Press.

Kramrisch, S.
　1981. *The Presence of Siva*. Princeton: Princeton University Press.

Krishnadas, K.P.
　1995. 'Kalaripayyat', in 'Crossovers: Explorations across Disciplines, Martial Arts', *Seagull Theatre Quarterly*, 8: 17–18.

Kunhappa, Murkot.
　1984. 'The Significance of Kalari Payattu: An Insider's Point of View' (manuscript).

Kunju, A.P. Ibrahim
　1975. *Studies in Medieval Kerala History*. Trivandrum: Kerala Historical Society.

Kuppuswamy, B.
　1993. *Source Book of Ancient Indian Psychology*. Delhi: Konark.

Kurup, K.K.N.
　1973. *The Cult of Teyyam and Hero Worship in Kerala*. Indian Folklore Series, No. 21. Calcutta: Indian Publications.
　1975. *Ali Rajas of Cannannore*. Trivandrum: College Book House.
　1977. *Aryan and Dravidian Elements in Malabar Folklore*. Trivandrum: Kerala Historical Society.

Kurup, P.N.V. and K. Raghunathan
　1974. 'Human Physiology in Ayurveda', in N.H. Keswani (ed.): *The Science of Medicine and Physiological Concepts in Ancient and Medieval India*. New Delhi: All India Institute of Medical Sciences.

Kutumbiah, P.
　1962. *Ancient Indian Medicine*. Bombay: Orient Longman.

Lach, Donald F.
　1965. *Asia in the Making of Europe, Vol. I*. Chicago: University of Chicago Press.

Laderman, Carol
　1991. *Taming the Wind of Desire: Psychology, Medicine, and Aesthetics in Malay Shamanistic Performance*. Berkeley: University of California Press.

Lakoff, George
　1987. *Women, Fire, and Dangerous Things*. Chicago: University of Chicago Press.

Lakoff, George and Mark Johnson
- 1980. *Metaphors We Live by*. Chicago: University of Chicago Press.

Lambert, Helen
- 1991. Personal Correspondence, August 1.
- 1992. 'The Cultural Logic of Indian Medicine: Prognosis and Etiology in Rajasthani Popular Therapeutics', *Social Science and Medicine*, 34, 10: 1069–76.

Leder, Drew
- 1990. *The Absent Body*. Chicago: University of Chicago Press.

Leslie, Charles (ed.)
- 1976. *Asian Medical Systems*. Berkeley: University of California Press.

Lewis, J. Lowell
- 1992. *Ring of Liberation: Deceptive Discourse in Brazilian Capoeira*. Chicago: University of Chicago Press.

Lindenbaum, Shirley and Margaret Lock (eds.)
- 1993. *Knowledge, Power, and Practice: The Anthropology of Medicine and Everyday Life*. Berkeley: University of California Press.

Lock, M. and N. Scheper-Hughes
- 1990. 'A Critical-Interpretive Approach in Medical Anthropology: Rituals and Routines of Discipline and Dissent', in T.M. Johnson and C.F. Sargent (eds.), *Medical Anthropology: Contemporary Theory and Method*. New York: Praeger, 47–72.

Logan, William
- 1951. (1887) *Malabar*. Madras: Government Press (reprint).

Lorenzen, D.
- 1978. 'Warrior Ascetics in Indian History', *Journal of the American Oriental Society*, 98: 61–75.

Majumdar, Bimal Kanti
- 1960. *The Military System in Ancient India*. Calcutta: Firma K.K. Mukhopadhyay.

Majumdar, R.C.
- 1950. *Encyclopaedia of Indian Physical Culture*. Baroda: Good Companions.

Maliszewski, Michael
- 1987. 'Martial Arts: An Overview', in Mircea Eliade (ed.), *The Encyclopedia of Religion*, Vol. 9. New York: Macmillan, 224–8.
- 1992. 'Meditative-Religious Traditions of Fighting Arts and Martial Ways', *Journal of Asian Martial Arts*, 1, 3: 1–104.

Mammen, M.P.
- 1975. 'Traditional Kerala Society', *Journal of Kerala Studies*, 11, 3: 269–92.

Manavendranath, K.C.
    1995   'Blueprint for an Actor', *Seagull Theatre Quarterly*, 8: 4–12.

Marglin, Frederique A.
    1985. *Wives of the God-King: The Rituals of the Devadasis of Puri*. Delhi: Oxford University Press.

Marriott, McKim
    1976. 'Hindu Transactions; Diversity without Dualism', in Bruce Kapferer (ed.), *Transaction and Meaning: Directions in the Anthropology of Exchange and Symbolic Behavior*. Philadelphia: Institute for the Study of Human Issues, 109–42.
    1977. (Remarks in) 'Symposium: Changing Identities in South Asia', in Kenneth A. David (ed.), *The New Wind: Changing Identities in South Asia*. Chicago: Aldine, 227–38.
    1980. 'The Open Hindu Person and Interpersonal Fluidity', manuscript read at Session 19, 'The Indian Self', 21 March, Association for Asian Studies.
    1990. (ed.), *India through Hindu Categories*. New Delhi: Sage.

Mathew, K.S.
    1979. *Society in Medieval Malabar*. Kottayam: Jaffe Books.

Mauss, M.
    1973. 'Techniques of the Body', *Economy and Society*, 2, 1: 70–88.

Mayer, Adrian C.
    1952. *Land and Society in Malabar*. Oxford: Oxford University Press.

Mencher, Joan P.
    1962. 'Changing Familial Roles among South Malabar Nayars', *Southwestern Journal of Anthropology*, 18: 230–45.
    1963. 'Growing up in South Malabar', *Human Organization*, 22: 54–65.
    1964. 'Possession, Dance, and Religion in North Malabar, Kerala, India', *International Congress of Anthropological and Ethnological Sciences*, 9: 340–5.
    1965a. 'The Nayars of South Malabar', in M.F. Nimkoff (ed.), *Comparative Family Systems*. Boston: Houghton Mifflin, 163–91.
    1965b. 'Social and Economic Change in India: The Namboodiri Brahmins', in *American Philosophical Society Yearbook 1964*, Philadelphia, 398–402.
    1966a. 'Kerala and Madras: A Comparative Study of Ecology and Social Structure', *Ethnology*, 5, 2: 135–71.
    1966b. 'Namboodiri Brahmins: An Analysis of a Traditional Elite in Kerala', *Journal of Asian and African Studies*, 1, 3: 183–96.
    1974. 'The Caste System Upside-down, or the Not-so-mysterious East', *Current Anthropology*, 15, 4: 469–78.

1975. 'Viewing Hierarchy from the Bottom up', in A. Beteille and T.N. Madan (eds.), *Encounter and Experience: Personal Accounts of Fieldwork*, Delhi: Vikas, 114–130.

Mencher, Joan P. and H. Goldberg

1967. 'Kinship and Marriage Regulations among the Namboodiri Brahmans of Kerala', *Man*, 2, 1: 87–106.

Mencher, Joan P. and K. Raman Unni

1975. 'Anthropological and Sociological Research in Kerala: Past, Present, and Future Directions', in Burton Stein (ed.), *Essays on South India*. Honolulu: University of Hawaii Press.

Menon, A. Sreedhara

1967. *A Survey of Kerala History*. Kottayam: Sahitya Pravarthaka Cooperative Society.

1979. *Social and Cultural History of Kerala*. New Delhi: Sterling.

Menon, C.A.

1911. *Cochin State Manual*. Ernakulan: Cochin Government Press.

1935. *Ballads of North Malabar*. Madras: University of Madras.

Menon, K.P.K.

1967. *Chattambi Swamigal. The Great Scholar-Saint of Kerala, 1853–1924*. Reproduced in Ananda E. Wood, *Knowledge before Printing and after*. Delhi: Oxford University Press, 1985: 134–72.

Menon, K.P.P.

1986. *History of Kerala*, ed. T.K.K. Menon. New Delhi: Asian Educational Services.

Menon, Mantavapalli Ittirariccha

2000. *Rugmamgada Caritam (King Rugmamgada's Law)*, trans. V.R. Prabodhachandran Nair, M.P. Sankaran Namboodiri and Phillip B. Zarrilli, *When Gods and Demons Come to Play: Kathakali Dance-Drama in Performance and Context*. London: Routledge.

Meyrowitz, Joshua

1985. *No Sense of Place*. New York: Oxford University Press.

Miller, Eric J.

1954. 'Caste and Territory in Malabar', *American Anthropologist*, 410–20.

1955. 'Village Structure in North Kerala', in M.N. Srinivas (ed.), *India's Villages*, New York Asia.

Mines, Mattison

1994. *Public Faces, Private Voices: Community and Individuality in South India*. Berkeley: University of California Press.

Monier-Williams, M.

1899. *A Sanskrit English Dictionary*. Oxford: The Clarendon Press.

Moore, Melinda A.

    1982. 'Nalukettu: The House as Microcosm', unpublished paper presented at the 11th Annual Conference on South Asia, Madison, Wisconsin.

    1983. 'Taravad: House, Land, and Relationship in a Matrilineal Hindu Society', Ph.D. dissertation, University of Chicago.

    1990. 'The Kerala House as a Hindu Cosmos', in McKim Marriott (ed.), *India Through Hindu Categories*, New Delhi: Sage, 169–202.

Mooss, Vayaskara N.S.

    1983. *Ayurvedic Treatments of Kerala*. Kottayam: Vaidyasarathy Press.

Mujumdar, D.C. (ed.)

    1950. *Encyclopaedia of Indian Physical Culture*. Baroda: Good Companion.

Mullassery, Prassannan G.

    1965 (1977). *Kalarippayattum Kayyamkaliyum* (Malayalam). Kodungallur: Devi Printing.

Mundadan, A. Mathias

    1970. *Sixteenth Century Traditions of St. Thomas Christians*. Bangalore: Dharmaram College.

Nagatomo, Shigenori

    1992a. 'An Eastern Concept of the Body: Yuasa's Body-Scheme', in Maxine Sheets-Johnstone (ed.), *Giving the Body its Due*. Albany: State University of New York Press, 48–68.

    1992b. *Attunement through the Body*. Albany: State University of New York Press.

Nair, C.V. Narayanan

    1933. 'Fencing in Ancient Kerala', *Kerala Society Papers*, 2, 11: 347–9.

Namboodiri, M.P. Sankaran

    1983. 'bhava as expressed through the presentational techniques of *Kathakali*', in Betty True Jones (ed.), *Dance as Cultural heritage*, Vol. I. CORD: *Dance Research Annual XIV*, 194–210.

Nambudiripad, K.V.

    1976. *Malayalam Lexicon*, Vol. 3. Trivandrum: Government Press.

Narayanan, M.G.S.

    1972. 'Political and Social Constitutions of Kerala Under the Kulasekhara Empire (C 800 AD to 1124 AD), unpublished Ph.D. dissertation, University of Kerala.

    1973 *Aspects of Aryanisation in Kerala*. Trivandrum: Kerala Historical Society.

    1976a. 'The Ancient and Medieval History of Kerala', *Journal of Kerala Studies*, 3, 3–4, pp. 441–6.

    1976b. 'The Ceraman Perumals of Kerala', 27th Indian History Congress, University of Calicut, 28–34.

1977. *Reinterpretations in South Indian History*. Trivandrum: College Book House, 1977.

Nayar, Cirakkal T. Sreedharan

1957. *Marmmadarppanam*. Calicut: P. K. Brothers. (Malayalam).

1963. *Kalarippayattu*. Cannannore. (Malayalam).

1983. *Massage (Uliccil): An Old Method of Treatment* (Malayalam). Calicut: Cannannore Printing Works.

Nayar, K. Narayanan

1983. Personal manuscript.

Neff, Deborah

1987. 'Aesthetics and Power in Pambin Tullal: A Possession Ritual of Rural Kerala', *Ethnology*, 26, 1: 63–71.

Ness, Sally Ann.

1992. *Body, Movement and Culture: Kinesthetic and Visual Symbolism in a Philippine Community*. Philadelphia: University of Pennsylvania Press.

Nichter, Mark

1983. 'Paying for what Ails You: Sociocultural Issues Influencing the Ways and Means of Therapy Payments in South India', *Social Science and Medicine*, 17, 14: 957–65.

Nongmaithem, Khilton

1995. 'Thang-ta', in 'Crossovers: Explorations across Disciplines: Martial Arts in Theatre', *Seagull Theatre Quarterly*, 8: 13–17.

Nossiter, T.J.

1982. *Communism in Kerala*. Delhi.

1988. *Marxist State Governments in India*. London.

Novack, Cynthia J.

1990. *Sharing the Dance: Contact Improvisation and American Culture*. Madison: University of Wisconsin Press.

Pallath, Jaya Rani

1976. 'Mamakam', unpublished M.A. thesis, University of Calicut.

Pandian, V.

1983a. 'A Force to Reckon with', *Indian Express*, 18 September.

1983b. 'Fire without, Calm within', *Indian Express*, 4 September.

Panikkar, K.M.

1918. 'Some Aspects of Nayar Life', *Journal of the Royal Anthropological Institute*, 48: 254–93.

Pant, G.N.

1978. *Indian Archery*. Delhi: Agam Kala.

Parry, Jonathan
    1989. 'The End of the Body', in Michel Feher (ed.), *Zone: Fragments for a History of the Human Body*, Part II, New York: Urzone.

Pavis, Patrice
    1989. 'Dancing with *Faust*: A Semiotician's Reflections on Barba's Mise-en-Scene', *TDR: A Journal of Performance Studies*, 33, 3: 37–57.

Pillai, A.K.B.
    1987. *The Culture of Social Stratification/Sexism: The Nayars*. Acton, Mass.: Copley.

Pillai, Elamkulam Kunjan
    1970. *Studies in Kerala History*. Kottayam: National Book Stall.

Pillai, M.E. Manickavasagom
    1970. *Culture of the Ancient Cheras*. Kovilpatti: Manjula.

Pillai, S.T.K.
    1940. *Travancore State Manual*. Government of Travancore.

Pillai, Sooranad P.N. Kunjan
    1966. 'Onam', in *Fairs and Festivals of Kerala*, Vol. VII B (i) of *Census of India 1961, Vol. VII, Kerala*. New Delhi: Manager of Publications, Government of India.

Podipara, Placid J.
    1970. *The Thomas Christians*. Bombay: St Paul Publications.

Preston, James J.
    1985. 'Creation of the Sacred Image: Apotheosis and Destruction in Hinduism', in Joanne Punzo Waghorne and Norman Cutler (eds.), *Gods of Flesh, Gods of Stone*, 9–32.

Puthenkalam, S.J.
    1977. 'Marriage and the Family in Kerala', in George Kurian (ed.), *Journal of Comparative Family Studies Monograph Cases*. Calgary: Department of Sociology. University of Calgary.

Radhakrishnan, R. and Sridharan Chempad.
    1984. *Mahacharithamala: C.V. Narayanan Nayar*. Kottayam: Kairali Chidren's Book Trust.

Raghavan, M.D.
    1929. 'The Kalari and the Angam–Institutions of Ancient Kerala', *Man in India*, 9: 134–48.
    1932. 'A Ballad of Kerala', *The Indian Antiquary*, January, 9–12; April, 72–7; June, 112–16; August, 150–4; November, 205–11.
    1947. *Folk Plays and Dances of Kerala*. Trichur: Mangalodayan Press.
    1964. *India in Ceylonese History, Society, and Culture*. New Delhi: Asia.

Raj, J. David Manuel
- 1971. *Silambam Technique and Evaluation.* Karaikudi.
- 1975. *Silambam Fencing from India.* Karaikudi.
- 1977. 'The Origin and the Historical Development of Silambam Fencing: An Ancient Self-Defense Sport of India', Ph.D. dissertation, University of Oregon.

Raja, K. Kunjunni
- 1964. 'The Sanghakkali of Kerala', *Bulletin of the Institute of Traditional Cultures,* Madras, 169–78.

Raja, P.K.S.
- 1966. *Medieval Kerala.* Calicut: Nava Kerala Cooperative Society.

Rao, P.V. Krishna
- 1941. *Comparative Study of the Marmas.* Madras.

Rao, Ramalingeswara M.C.
- 1978. *Sreemad Bhagavadgeeta,* Meerut: Anu Prakashan.

Raphy, Sabeena
- 1964. *Cavittunatakam.* Kottayam: India Press.
- 1969. 'Chavittu-Natakam Dramatic Opera of Kerala', *Sangeet Natak,* 12: 56–73.

Reid, H. and M. Croucher
- 1983. *The Fighting Arts.* N.Y.: Simon and Schuster.

Reiker, Hans.-Ulrich (ed. and trans.)
- 1971. *The Yoga of Light: Hatha Yoga Pradipika.* Los Angeles: Dawn Horse Press.

Richards, J.F. (ed.)
- 1981. *Kingship and Authority in South Asia.* Madison: University of Wisconsin South Asian Studies Center.

Ros, Frank
- 1995. *The Lost Secrets of Ayurvedic Acupuncture.* Delhi: Motilal Banarsidass.

Rosaldo, Michelle
- 1984. 'Toward an Anthropology of Self and Feeling', in Richard A. Sweder and Rober A. LeVine (eds.), *Culture Theory: Essays on Mind, Self and Emotion.* Cambridge: Cambridge University Press, 137–57.

Rosu, Arion
- 1981. 'Les *marman* et les arts martiaux indiens', *Journal asiatique,* 259, 417–51.
- 1982. 'Le renouveau de l'Ayurveda', *Wiener Zeitschrift für die Kunde Südasiens,* 26: 59–82.

Rosu, Arion and Myriam Jobard
- 1987. 'Arts de sante et technique de massage en Inde', *Annales de Kinesitherapie,* 14, 3: 87–91.

Roy, Mira
- 1967. 'Anatomy in the Vedic Literature', *Indian Journal of the History of Science*, 2, 1: 35–46.

Roy, Ramashray
- 1985. 'Region and Nation: A Heretical View', in Paul Wallace (ed.), *Region and Nation in India*. New Delhi: American Institute of Indian Studies, 269–86.

Said, Edward
- 1978. *Orientalism*. New York: Pantheon Books.

Salim, Saslin
- 1993. 'Finger Fighter Prakasan Can Knock out Opponents from a Distance of 10 Feet', *The Week*. 28 March: 20–1.

Saram, L. Karthikeya
- 1962. 'Vijayapuri—the Capital of Iksvakus or Nagarkunakonda', *Indian History Quarterly*, 38, 4: 267–82.

Sastri, K.A. Nilakanta
- 1972. *Sangam Literature: Its Cults and Cultures*. Madras: Swathi.

Scarry, Elaine
- 1985. *The Body in Pain*. Oxford: Oxford University Press.

Schechner, Richard
- 1985. *Between Theatre and Anthropology*. Philadelphia: University of Pennsylvania Press.

Schrag, Calvin O.
- 1969. *Experience and Being*. Evanston: Northwestern University Press.

Setumadavan, Arikkattu
- 1987. Letter to the Editor, *Kerala Kaumudi*, 28 March: 5.

Shah, Umakant P.
- 1968. 'Cattanam Madham–A Gleaning from the Kuvalayamala-Kaha', *Annals of Bhandarkar Oriental Research Institute, Golden Jubilee Volume* (Poona), 250–2.

Shaner, David Edward
- 1985. *The Bodymind Experience in Japanese Buddhism*. Albany: State University of New York Press.

Shastri, Manmatha Nath Dutt.
- 1967. *Agni Puranam*. Varanasi: Chowkhamba Sanskrit Series.

Sheets-Johnstone, Maxine (ed.)
- 1992. *Giving the Body its Due*. Albany: State University of New York Press.
- 1994. *The Roots of Power: Animate Form and Gendered Bodies*. Chicago: Open Court.

Shweder, Richard A. and Robert A. LeVine
- 1984. *Culture Theory: Essays on Mind, Self, and Emotion*. London: Cambridge University Press.

Siegel, Lee
- 1991. *Net of Magic: Wonders and Deceptions in India*. Chicago: University of Chicago Press.

Singer, Milton
- 1972. *When a Great Tradition Modernizes*. New York: Praeger.
- 1981. 'On the Semiotics of Indian Identity', *American Journal of Semiotics*, 1, 1–2: 85–126.

Singh, L.M., K.K. Thakral and P.J. Deshpande
- 1970. 'Susruta's Contributions to the Fundamentals of Surgery', *Indian Journal of the History of Science*, 5, 1: 36–50.

Singh, Sarva Daman
- 1965. *Ancient Indian Warfare with Special Reference to the Vedic Period*. Leiden: E.J. Brill.

Singhal, G.D. and L.V. Guru
- 1973. *Anatomical and Obstetrical Considerations in Ancient Indian Surgery Based on Sarira-Sthana of Susruta Samhita*. Varanasi: Banaras Hindu University.

Staal, Fritz
- 1983–4 'Indian Concepts of the Body', *Somatics*, Autumn-Winter, 31–41.
- 1993. 'Indian Bodies', in Thomas P. Kasulis (ed.), *Self as Body in Asian Theory and Practice*. Albany: State University of New York Press, 59–102.

Stoller, Paul
- 1989. *The Taste of Ethnographic Things: The Senses in Anthropology*. Philadelphia: University of Pennsylvania Press.

Stoller Miller, Barbara
- 1984. *Theater of Memory: The Plays of Kalidasa*. New York: Columbia University Press.

Subramanian, N.
- 1966. *Sangam Polity*. Bombay: Asian.

Susruta
- 1981. *The Susruta Samhita* (Vols I–III). Trans. and ed. by Kaviraj Kunjalal Bhishagratna. Varanasi: Chowkhamba Sanskrit Series.

Synnott, Anthony
- 1993. *The Body Social: Symbolism, Self and Society*. London: Routledge Press.

Tacholi Otenan (Malayalam)
- 1980. Bombay: India Book House Education Trust.

Templeman, Dennis
    1996. *The Northern Nadars of Tamil Nadu*. Delhi: Oxford University Press.

Thampuran, Rama Varma Appan
    1113 (Malayalam Era) *Sangakkali*. Trissur: Mangalodayam Press.

Thatte, D.G.
    1988. *Acupuncture Marma and Other Asian Therapeutic Techniques*. Varanasi: Chaukhamba Orientalia.

Thulaseedharan, K.
    1977. *Studies in Traditional Kerala Society*. Trivandrum: College Book House.

Thurston, E.T.
    1906. *Ethnographic Notes in Southern India*. Madras: Government Press.
    1975 (1909). *Castes and Tribes of Southern India, Vol. V.* Delhi: Cosmo Publications.

Tilak, Moses
    1982. *Kalaripayat and Marma Adi (Varmam)*. Madras: Neil Publication.

T.K.A.M.
    1986. 'New Star on Kalari horizon', *Weekend Review*, 15–21 June: 15.

Trawick Egnor, Margaret
    1983. 'Death and Nurturance in Indian Systems of Healing', *Social Science and Medicine*, 17, 4: 935–45.
    1987. 'The Ayurvedic Physician as Scientist', *Social Science and Medicine*, 24, 12: 1031–50.

Turner, Bryan S.
    1992. *Regulating Bodies: Essays in Medical Sociology*. London: Routledge Press.

Turner, Graeme
    1990. *British Cultural Studies*. London: Routledge.

Turner, Victor
    1969. *The Ritual Process*. Chicago: Aldine.
    1974. *Dramas, Fields, and Metaphors*. Ithaca: Cornell University Press.
    1982. *From Ritual to Theater: The Human Seriousness of Play*. New York: Performing Arts Journal Press.

Turner, Victor W. and Edward M. Bruner (eds.)
    1986. *The Anthropology of Experience*. Urbana: University of Illinois Press.

Tyler, Stephen A.
    1987. *The Unspeakable: Discourse, Dialogue, and Rhetoric in the Postmodern World*. Madison: University of Wisconsin Press.

Vagbhata
    1938. *Astanga Sangraha*. Poona: Chitrasala Press.

van Buitenen, J.A.B.
    1973. *Mahabharata*, Vol. I. Chicago: University of Chicago Press.

Varenne, Jean
    1976. *Yoga and the Hindu Tradition*. Chicago: University of Chicago Press.

Varma, L.A. Ravi
    1932. 'Castes of Malabar', *Kerala Society Papers*, 2, 9: 171–204.
    1971. 'Yatrakali and Bhadrakali-Pattu', *Bulletin of the Rama Varma Research Institute*, 9, 1.

Vasu, Rai Bahadur Srisa Chandran (ed. and trans.)
    1975. *The Siva Samhita*. New Delhi: Oriental Books Reprint Corporation.

Vasugurukkal
    1984. *Kalarippayattu* (Malayalam manuscript).

Velayudhan, C.K.
    n.d. *Kalarippayattu and Marmmacunthaniyum*. Palghat: Shanta Bookstall.

Veluthat, Kesavan
    1976. 'Aryan Brahman Settlements of Ancient Kerala', 27th Indian History Congress, University of Calicut, 24–7.
    1978. *Brahmin Settlements in Kerala: Historical Studies*. Calicut: Calicut University, Sandhya Publications.

Vijayakumaran
    1976. 'The Author and Date of *Dronampallil Vidya*', *Journal of Kerala Studies*, 3, 3–4: 407–13.

Vogel, C.
    1965. *Vagbhata's Astangahrdayasamhita*. Wiesbaden.

Wadley, Susan S.
    1975. *Shakti: Power in the Conceptual Structure of Karimpur Religion*. University of Chicago Studies in Anthropology, Series in Social, Cultural, and Linguistic Anthropology, 2. Chicago: Department of Anthropology, University of Chicago.
    1980. (ed.) *The Powers of Tamil Women*. Syracuse: Foreign and Comparative Studies/ South Asian Series, No. 6, Maxwell School of Citizenship and Public Affairs, Syracuse University.

Warrier, M.R. Balakrishna
    1955. 'Kerala and Parasurama Tradition', *Kerala Studies*, Trivandrum: University of Kerala, 14–27.

White, Geoffrey and John Kirkpatrick (eds.)
    1985. *Person, Self and Experience: Exploring Pacific Ethnopsychologies*. Berkeley: University of California Press.

Wood, Ananda
  1985. *Knowledge before Printing and after: The Indian Tradition in Changing Kerala*. Delhi: Oxford University Press.

Yuasa, Yasuo
  1987. *The Body: Toward an Eastern Mind-Body Theory*. Albany: State University of New York Press.

Zacharia, Scaria (ed.)
  1994. *The Acts and Decress of the Synod of Diamper 1599*. Edamattam, Kerala: Indian Institute of Christian Studies.

Zarrilli, Phillip B.
  1978. '*Kalarippayattu* and the Performing Artist East and West', Ph.D. dissertation, University of Minnesota.
  1979. 'Kalarippayatt, Martial Art of Kerala', *The Drama Review*, 23, 2: 113–24.
  1984a. 'Doing the Exercise: The In-body Transmission of Performance Knowledge in a Traditional Martial Art', *Asian Theatre Journal*, 1, 2: 191–206.
  1984b. *The Kathakali Complex: Actor, Performance, Structure*. New Delhi: Abhinav.
  1986. 'From Martial Art to Performance: Kalarippayattu and Performance in Kerala, Parts 1 and 2', *Sangeet Natak*, 81–2: 5–41; 83: 14–45.
  1989a 'Three Bodies of Practice in a Traditional South Indian Martial Art', *Social Science and Medicine*, 28, 12: 1289–1310.
  1989b. 'Between Text and Embodied Practice: Writing and Reading in a South Indian Martial Tradition', in A.L. Dallapiccola (ed.), *Shastric Tradition in Indian Arts*, Stuttgart: Franz Steiner Verlag, 415–24.
  1992a. 'To Heal and/or To Harm: The Vital Spots (*Marmmam/Varmam*) in Two South Indian Martial Traditions. Part I: Focus on Kerala's *Kalarippayattu*', *Journal of Asian Martial Arts*, 1, 1: 36–67.
  1992b. 'To Heal and/or To Harm: The Vital Spots (*Marmmam/Varmam*) in Two South Indian Martial Traditions. Part II: Focus on the Tamil Art, *Varma Ati*', *Journal of Asian Martial Arts*, 1, 2: 1–15.
  1993. (ed.), *Asian Martial Arts in Actor Training*. Madison: Center for South Asia, University of Wisconsin-Madison.
  1994a. 'Actualizing "Power(s)" and "Crafting a Self" in Martial Practice: *Kalarippayattu*, a South Indian Martial Art and the Yoga and Ayurvedic Paradigms', *Journal of Asian Martial Arts*, 3, 3: 10–51.
  1994b. 'An Ocean of Possibilities: From *Lokadharmi* to *Natyadharmi* in a Kathakali *Santanagopalam*', *Comparative Drama*, 28, 67–89.
  1995a. 'The Kalarippayattu Martial Master as Header: Traditional Kerala Massage Therapies', *Journal of Asian Martial Arts*, 4, 1: 67–83.

1995b. 'Repositioning the Body, Practice, Power, and Self in an Indian Martial Art, in Carol A. Breckenridge (ed.), *Consuming Modernity: Public Culture in a South Asian World*. Minneapolis, University of Minnesota Press, 183–215.

1998. 'Back Toward the Next Millennium: [Re]Considering History, Discourses/Representations, and Positionality in the Indian Arts through Kerala's *Kalarippayattu* and *Kathakali*', in Shanta Sarbjeet Singh (ed.), *Culture in the New Millennia: Classical Dance*, New Delhi: Wiley Eastern.

2000. *Kathakali Dance-Drama: Where Gods and Demons Come to Play*. London: Routledge Press.

Zaynu'd-Din, Shaykh

1941–2. *Tuhfat-al-Mijahidin*, trans. S. Muhammed Husayn Nainar. *Annals of Oriental Research* (Madras), 6, 1: 1–112.

Zimmermann, Francis

1978a. 'From Classic Texts to Learned Practice: Methodological Remarks on the Study of Indian Medicine', *Social Science and Medicine*, 12: 97–103.

1978b. 'Introducing Western Anatomy to the Practitioners of Classical Indian Medicine: An Ethno-Historical Analysis of the Treatises by P.S. Varier in the 1920s', *Colloques Internationaux Centre National de la Recherche Scientifique, No. 582: Asie du Sud, Traditions et Changements*. Paris: Editions du Centre de la Recherche Scientifique, 1–3.

1979. 'From Tradition to Profession: Intellectual and Social Impulses behind the Professionalization of Classical Medicine in India', *Journal of the Japan Society of History of Medicine*, 25, 13.

1980. '*Rtu-satmya*: the Seasonal Cycle and the Principle of Appropriateness', *Social Science and Medicine*, 14B: 99–106.

1983. 'Remarks on the Conception of the Body in Ayurvedic Medicine', in B. Pfeiderer and G.D. Sontheimer (eds.), *South Asian Digest of Regional Writing, Vol. 8 (1979): Sources of Illness and Healing in South Asian Regional Literatures*, Heidelberg, 10–26.

1986. *Susruta Samhita*, Cikitsasthana xxiv, 38–49 (unpublished translation).

1988. 'The Jungle and the Aroma of Meats: An Ecological Theme in Hindu Medicine', *Social Science and Medicine*, 27, 3: 197–215.

Zvelebil, Kamil

1973 *The Smile of Murugan: On Tamil Literautre of South India*. Leiden: E.J. Brill.

MANUSCRIPTS

(The following manuscripts consulted are in Malayalam except as noted for Tamil. Unpublished works are from private collections.)

Chandrasekharan, T. (ed.), *Rangabhyasam*. Madras: Madras Government Oriental Manuscript Series, #22, 1952.

Grandhavari. Trivandrum: Government Press, 1973.

Granthavarimarmma cikitsa

Kalari Vaidya. Trivandrum: University of Kerala Malayalam Manuscript Series, 90, 1955.

Kulamarmmangal.

Marmmani cikitsa.

Marmmanidanam.

Marmmarahasyangal.

Nadar, M. Kunnakrishnan. *Marmmasastraphithika.* Thiruvananthapuram: Upasana Books (Malayam script of Tamily texts), n.d.

Nadar, K. Koccukrishnan. *Marmmasastrasamharam.* Thiruvananthapuram: Redyar Press (Malayalam script of Tamil texts), 1968.

Marmmayogam.

Selvaraj, S. John. *Varma Cuttiram* (Tamil). Madras: International Institute of Tamil Studies, 1984.

Varma Alavu Nool Pramanam (Tamil).

Varma Cuttiram (Tamil).

Varma Oti Murivu Cara Cuttiram (Tamil).

Other Primary Documents

Privately Published Kalarippayattu Association Documents

Kerala Kalarippayat Association: Bylaws of the Association. 1958. (date of founding, English).

Kerala Kalarippayattu Association: Rules and regulations governing *kalari* specifications, duration of training, becoming a *gurukkal*, customs and traditional weapons, exercises, massage, verbal commands for exercise sequences, rules governing annual competitions, rules and regulations regarding *atitada* clubs, and state championships. 1961 (date of adoption, Malayalam).

Kerala Samsthana Kayikabhyasa Kalarisangham. Constitution and bylaws. 1982 (date of founding, Palakkad).

Glossary

All terms are Malayalam except those marked [S] (Sanskrit) or [T] (Tamil). Many of the Malayalam terms are originally Sanskrit. Except for commonplace terms, I usually make use of the Malayalam rather than Sanskrit form of the word. At the request of the publisher diacritical marks have not been included. Commonplace usage is adopted for names of familiar deities, epics, etc.

adangal: [T] Tamil term for the twelve to sixteen vital spots to which revival techniques are applied in emergency counter applications.

adavu: the basic 'forms' of martial training.

adharam: another term for the location or 'places' where the wheels or centres (*cakra*) of the subtle body are located. These are the places along which the *kundalini sakti* (serpent power) travels once it is awakened and raised, and the places or centres for meditation.

Agastya: a sage descended from Visnu who became well-versed in the Vedas, a variety of sciences, and renowned for his use of many weapons. Agasthya is believed to have achieved many of his powers through his practice of austerities. Ati murai practitioners claim their lineage of martial, medical, and meditation practice from Agasthya who is still believed to be doing penance in the Agasthya Kuta hills (Kanyakumari district, Tamil Nadu). In the *Mahabharata,* Drona cites his own teacher as Agnivesa–a disciple of Agasthya.

akampadi: a ruler's retinue, constituted by those martial practitioners who took a vow to death on behalf of the ruler.

ankam: a special form of duel legislated to solve disputes between higher ranking castes, especially Nayars. Each party to the dispute would hire a lower ranking *chekor* of the Ilava caste to fight to the death on its behalf in a duel. Whichever fighter won the duel, 'won' the case on behalf of his sponsor.

asan: teacher.

asana: [S] basic forms or postures of *hatha yoga*, similar to poses (*vativu*) in martial practice.

asari: a relatively high-ranking expert in the science of architecture traditionally consulted when building a house or *kalari*.

ati murai: [T] literally, the 'law of hitting'. Along with *varma ati*, one of several names for the style of martial practice taught in the old Travancore region of southern Kerala and adjacent Kanyakumari district of Tamil Nadu, and practised primarily by Nadars. It is also known as 'southern' kalarippayattu today.

Ayurveda: [S] South Asia's indigenous humoral system of medicine dating from antiquity. Literally, the 'science' by knowledge of which life (*ayuh*) can be prolonged. Principles of ayurveda inform the martial practitioner's understanding of his bodymind, and the hands-on therapies which are part of his medical practice.

balam: strength, valour, vigour. Usually associated with overt physical strength like Bhima.

Bhadrakali: the violent form of the goddess, especially associated with the power of destruction and therefore of war (see Bhagavati).

Bhagavati: the best known form of the goddess. As Bhagavati the goddess encompasses a number of different personalities which range from the ferocious to the benign. The goddess or some form of Siva/Sakti in combination is worshipped as the guardian deity of the kalari.

bhava: [S] state of mind, being, disposition. Most commonly used to refer to the actor's embodiment of a character's states of being/emotion in dance-drama. Used also to refer to the 'correct form' or 'inner life' of a form in martial practice such as an animal pose.

cakra: [S] the five, six, or seven internal wheels or centres of the subtle body.

can: a basic measure between the outstretched thumb and index finger.

cattar: brahman students schooled in a variety of forms of knowledge, including martial arts, at schools attached to temples, and serving as a voluntary force defending temple and school as necessary.

caver: by the twelfth century the retinue of martial practitioners in service to a ruler were known as '*caver*'—those were pledged to die in service to their master.

chekor: a unique title given to kalarippayattu practitioners among the lower-ranking Ilava caste who fought duels (*ankam*) to the death on behalf of higher-ranking sponsors.

cittar: see *siddhi*.

cottaccan: small stick, often rounded at both ends, concealed in the hand, and used to attack the body's vital spots. A second style is more like a small club.

cumattadi: self-defence sequences combining poses, steps, kicks, and hits, usually associated with 'central' style of kalarippayattu practice.

cundu-marmmam: subtle means of attacking the body's vital spots by simply 'pointing'.

curika: the traditional double-edged sword.

cuvatu: literally, 'steps', including the steps in martial practice.

cuvatumayakkal: literally, 'wiping out the steps'—the traditional ritual exit from the kalari after training is over. The master is the last to leave and 'wipes out the steps' with a weapon.

dakshina: [S] traditional 'gifts' or 'offerings' a student gives to his teacher at the beginning and end of a course of training.

Dhanur Veda: [S] literally the 'science of the bow', Dhanur Veda encompasses all fighting arts in Indian antiquity. Considered one of the traditional eighteen branches of knowledge, Dhanur Veda was the means of education in warfare for all those called upon to fight. The earliest extant Dhanur Veda texts is chapters 249–52 of the encyclopaedic *Agni Purana* dating no earlier than the eighth century. According to tradition, kalarippayattu traces its ancestry to Dhanur Veda.

dharma: [S] law, duty, the order of things as it should be, conduct, code, or customary observance.

dhyana: [S] one of a series of ever-deeper states of actualization during meditation.

dhikr: Sufi Muslim methods of remembrance or recollection of Allah performed either silently or aloud.

ekadasi: day most sacred to lord Visnu on which his devotees fast and meditate.

ekagrata: [S] single-point focus which is ideally internalized in yoga and martial arts training/practice.

gunam: one's basic, inherent nature and behaviour. There are three basic *gunam* including goodness or truth (*satva*), passion/energy (*rajasa*) and darkness/lethargy (*tamasa*).

gurukkal: the plural of 'guru', refers not only to one's teacher, but to the teacher's teachers, and therefore the whole lineage of practice represented by the teacher. An honorific term of respect most often used in kalarippayattu. A teacher assumes the title only when he has reached a sufficient age of mastery, ability, and accomplishment.

gurutvam: having complete trust in one's master.

jivan: life, individual soul, manifest in one's 'life force' (*prana vayu*).

kacca: the long cloth wrapped around the abdominal/hip area to support the 'vital energy' of the practitioner.

kalam [T]: refers to the cleared space around homes, as well as the same space used as a threshing floor. Also refers to the patterns drawn daily with white rice powder outside the entrance to houses, especially in southern Kerala, as well as to the patterns drawn on the floor of a kalari for training/footwork in central and southern styles of practice.

kalam: literally, 'time'. An especially important concept in the esoteric understanding of when to give counter-applications after the body's vital spots have been penetrated.

kalari: a technical term for the place where the traditional Kerala martial art, kalarippayattu, is practised. Ideally it is a 'pit' dug out of the ground.

kalarippayattu: literally, 'place' where 'exercises' are practised. Kerala's traditional martial/medical art dating from at least the twelfth century.

kal etupp or *kaluyarttal*: preliminary leg exercises in martial training.

kanni mula: the southwest corner of the kalari where its guardian deity is located.

Kathakali: literally, 'story-play'. A genre of dance-drama dating from the late sixteenth century which enacts stories from the *Mahabharata, Ramayana,* and *puranas*. Kathakali's physical and training techniques originate in kalarippayattu. Its aesthetic form, hand-gestures, and facial expression are derived from Kerala's genre of enacting Sanskrit dramas in temples, *kutiyattam*.

Keralopathi: the quasi-historical Kerala brahman chronicle which records the story of the foundation of Kerala, the ascendancy of brahmans, and the role the Nayars were to play as protectors of brahmans through their practice of the martial art.

ksatriya: [S] a member of the governing or ruling order—what eventually was considered the second highest ranking caste next to the brahmans.

kuli kalari: a traditional 'pit' style kalari dug out of the ground about five feet deep with a pounded earth floor and woven palm-leaf roof.

kundalini: [S] the serpent power understood to lie sleeping and dormant within the subtle body. Once awakened in the lowest wheel or centre, she is raised through each succeeding centre until she breaks through to assume her place on top of the last centre. This power is also assumed to be present, awakened, and raised through martial practice.

laksana: from medicine, the 'signs' a physician looks for when attempting a diagnosis. Commonly used by martial masters when watching a student's practice and attempting to 'diagnose' the corrections the student needs.

lengotti: a piece of white cloth wrapped and worn around the hips and thighs, and providing support like a jock strap.

Mahabali: emperor of the Asuras (demons), son of Virocana, and grandson of Prahlada, Mahabali ruled Kerala at one time. According to the *puranas*, Mahabali was expelled from his throne by Vamana, the dwarf incarnation of Visnu. His rule is viewed as a golden age of happiness, peace, and prosperity.

Mahabharata: Along with the *Ramayana*, India's great epic which serves as a source of traditional oral narratives and teaching stories. It tells the story of the enmity and conflict between two sets of princely brothers, the Kauravas and the Pandavas. In that telling it provides much information on early martial arts in India.

Malayalam/Malayali[s]: Malayalam is the language of Kerala. A Dravidian language, Malayalam developed as a specific regional language from old Tamil and Sanskrit. The people who speak Malayalam as their native tongue and live in present-day Kerala state are often called 'Malayalis.'

Mamakam: a festival held every twelve years, this 'great' festival celebrated the descent of the goddess Ganga into the Bharatappula river in Tirunavayi, north Malabar, Kerala, which made the river as holy as the sacred Ganges. In a protracted thirteenth-century conflict, the ruler of Calicut usurped the right of the traditional Valluvanadu ruling family to oversee the festival. At each subsequent festival until 1766, the martial practitioners pledged to die on behalf of the Vellatri ruling family sacrificed themselves in battle against the ruler of Calicut's superior forces.

manasakti: literally, 'mental power'. Through practice of the martial art the master ideally gains superior mental power to be used in combat and/or daily life.

manassu: mind.

manodhiryam: a state of 'mental courage' where someone is able to face 'anything'.

mantram: usually consisting of a series of sacred words and/or syllables which may or may not be 'translatable', *mantram* are 'instruments of power' (Alper 1989: 6), often designed to accomplish a particular task.

marmma cikitsa: literally 'treatment of (injuries to) the vital spots'. The traditional methods of kalarippayattu medical treatment for injuries received during training or diseases affecting the wind humour. Especially important are a variety of 'hands-on' massage therapies. A crucial part of Ayurveda in Kerala.

marmmam: (*marman*, S; *varmam*, T): the vulnerable vital junctures or spots of the body first identified by Susruta in his *Samhita*. The spots attacked, defended and used for emergency counter-applications and revival in martial practice.

marukai: literally, 'opposite hand'—refers to the administration of a strong slap with the hand to the opposite side of the body after penetration of a vital spot. One technique of emergency counter-application to injuries to the body's vital spots.

meippayattu: literally, 'body exercises'. Combinations of kicks, steps, jumps, turns linked in a variety of set forms and constituting the basic training in kalarippayattu.

meyyabhyasam: literally, 'body art'—reference to the foundation of kalarippayattu martial practice in the 'art' of using the bodymind through daily exercise.

meyyarappatavu: literally, 'body control exercises'—the basic exercises in both kalarippayattu and Kathakali dance-drama through which the bodymind is trained.

meyyu kannakuka: literally, 'the body becomes all eyes'. Malayalam folk expression which encapsulates the ideal state of accomplishment of the martial practitioner as he is able to move, like Lord Brahma 'the thousand eyed' in any direction in response to any stimulus in his environment.

mudiettu: Kerala propitiatory ritual for the goddess Kali in her destructive form performed only at a few temples in Kerala.

mudra: special hand (or full body) configurations used in practice of yoga, with repetition of *mantram*, or in dance and dance-drama performances as a language of gesture.

nabhi mula: literally, 'root of the navel'.

nadi: [S] the channels of the subtle body.

nalika: basic time unit in astrology—the period during which one star stands, equal to 24 minutes. Important in determining when to administer counter-application for revival.

Namboodiri: the brahmans of Kerala are known as Namboodiris or Namboodiripads. Patrilineal by descent, the Namboodiris developed very close relationships with either Ksatriya or Nayar ruling families. Since only the eldest son in an extended family married a Namboodiri woman, the other sons developed long-term relationship with Nayar women.

Navaratri Mahotsavam: annual pan-Indian festival of new beginnings held for nine nights in October/November. In kalari the observance includes special offerings for weapons and serves as a beginning of a new cycle of training.

Nayar: as a distinct term, 'Nayar' first appeared in the ninth century, and by the eleventh century it was commonly used to refer to a large indigenous group of non-polluting subcastes among Kerala Hindus. Although a few families became ruling lineages (such as the Zamorin of Kozhikode), the majority of Nayars were in service occupations providing military, personal, and managerial services for higher castes. Until the twentieth century, Nayars lived in extended households, followed matrilineal descent, and children were raised in their mother's household.

nokku-marmmam: subtle means of attacking the body's vital spots by simply 'looking'.

Onam: celebration each August/September commemorating the return of the mythical Mahabali to Kerala where he ruled before his expulsion.

otta: curved wooden stick shaped like one-half of a bow or an elephant's tusk and made of tamarind wood. Used to teach empty-hand combat and attack/defence of the body's vital spots.

pacca: the green 'heroic' make-up for Kathakali dance-drama heroes such as Arjuna, Bhima and Rugmamgada.

pampin tullal: serpent worship ritual traditionally held to assure prosperity of an extended family by propitiating the serpent deities living on the family property.

Parasurama: an incarnation of Mahavisnu and by birth a brahman, from an early age he was known as Rama and learned martial arts (Dhanur Veda). He went to the Himalayas to undergo austerities to Siva to attain divine powers. After defeating the demons, Siva gave him a weapon named Parasu (axe). Thereafter he was known as Parasurama. One of his most important disciples was Drona. Practitioners of kalarippayattu claim their descent directly from Parasurama at the time of Kerala's founding when the sage reclaimed the land that is Kerala from the sea by throwing his axe. At this time he is said to have established the original 108 kalari.

Pasupata: divine weapon given by Siva to Arjuna after undergoing austerities.

payattu: from the Tamil *payil*, meaning to practise, or become trained; therefore, exercise.

phalam: fruit, results, effect.

piduttam: to grip, seize, catch, or hold. Especially refers to the retention or gripping in the lower abdominal region where the long *kacca* is tied.

pitham: the seat, pedestal, tripod, or throne representing the lineage of teachers in a kalari. The seat through which power in manifest in a variety of ritual performances as well as in martial practice.

prana or *prana vayu*: the breath(s) or wind(s) understood to circulate within the body. Also refers to the 'life force' or 'breath of life'.

pranayama: special yogic breathing which includes repetition of the following fourfold pattern: inhalation (*puraka*), retention (*kumbhaka*), exhalation (*rejaka*), retention/pause.

prasad: the 'leavings' at the end of a *puja* and considered the sanctified or blessed food of the god. When offerings have been given to a deity, whatever is left over is passed out to devotees by the *pujari*.

prayogam: 'application', especially refers to the practical application of martial exercises for offence or defence.

puja: worship of Hindu deities through daily or special/seasonal offerings pleasing to the specific deity.

pujari (tantri): the priest who gives offerings (*puja*) at Hindu temples. Brahman *pujari* are considered the most 'pure'. Also known as *tantri* since their rituals include the repetition of sacred syllables (*mantra*), the drawing of ritual diagrams, etc.—all vehicles for the manifestation of a god's power(s).

puttara: the six or seven-tiered platform topped with a 'flower' or 'bud' and carved out of the clay-earth or made of stone. Located in the southwest corner of the kalari where the guardian deity (usually Bhagavati or Bhadrakali) resides.

Ramayana: Along with the *Mahabharata*, India's great epic which serves as a source of traditional oral narratives and teaching stories. It tells the story of the trials and tribulations of Prince Rama, his brother Lakshmana, and his wife Sita.

ratheeb: collective form of spiritual awakening practised by Sufi Muslims.

raudra: 'fury', usually associated with the destructive power of the goddess, and the state of mind required to kill.

sakti: [S] (*cakti* [T]) the active principle of power/energy. When deified as Sakti, the goddess, she embodies the dangerous, unstable feminine energy and is associated with the generation of a powerful, 'furious', heated condition, and therefore inspires terror.

sampradayam: tradition, traditional method, lineage of practice or style.

sastra: [S] literally, 'science'. That which is traditional.

siddhi: [S] to become accomplished in a practice, usually through repetition, or by divine gift. Can also refer to an individual who has become accomplished as in a Siddha Yoga (*cittar* [T])—one who is accomplished in yoga.

sthanam: literally, 'place'. Also refers to the specific places in martial practice where the body is 'locked'.

sthula sarira: the physical body based on humoral theory and articulated most fully in Ayurveda.

suksma sarira: the internal subtle body associated with yoga as well as kalarippayattu, and consisting of channels (*nadi*), wheels or centres (*cakra*), and the dynamic element of the vital energy or wind (*prana vayu*) and cosmic energy (*kundalini* or Sakti).

swasam: literally, 'breathing', also refers to simple kalarippayattu-style breathing where there is continuous deep inhalation and exhalation without retention or pause.

teyyam: traditional ritual performances of northern Kerala which serves as the locally most popular form of Hinduism through which hundreds of pan-Indian and local deities are propitiated, including local heroes who trained in and fought using kalarippayattu.

uliccil: massage given with feet, hands, or bags of medicinal herbs.

urumi: five-foot long flexible sword sharpened on both sides and coiled at the waist. Used for mass combat.

vadakkan pattukal: the 'northern ballads'—traditional oral ballads recited in the fields celebrating the exploits of the kalarippayattu-trained heroes of northern Kerala.

varma ati: [T] literally, 'hitting the vital spots'. Also known as ati murai ('the law of hitting/attacking'), ati tata ('hit/defend'), the Tamil martial art closely related to kalarippayattu which is practised in the South Travancore region of Kerala and Kanyakumari district, Tamil Nadu.

vativu: the basic 'poses' in kalaripppayattu named after animals and constituting the basic building blocks of the system of training. Similar to, and perhaps in some cases based on, basic yoga postures (*asana*).

vayttari: the verbal instructions recited by the master as students perform body exercises or weapons practice.

veliccappatu: priests who serve as mediums for the goddess to speak at Bhagavati temples.

verumkai: literally, 'empty-hand' techniques of martial practice.

vira: literally, the 'heroic'.

yantra: [S] sacred diagrams understood to be one form of accessing divine power(s). In martial training these can take the form of floor patterns with esoteric, mystical significance, especially in central style practice.

yatrakali: brahman variety entertainment which included kalarippayattu demonstrations as one item in the repertory. Performed by 'degraded' Yatra brahmans who practised martial arts.

yoga: [S] from the root (*yug*) meaning 'to bind together, hold fast, or yoke'. Any ascetic, meditational, or psycho-physiological technique which achieves such a 'binding' of bodymind. A variety of yogic paths developed historically including *karma yoga* or the law of universal causality; *maya yoga* or a process of liberating oneself from cosmic illusion; *nirvana yoga* or a process of growing beyond illusion to attain at-onement with absolute reality; and *hatha yoga* or specific techniques of psycho-physiological practice.

Index

Achuttan, Gurukkal K. 118, 127–8, 134–6
Agastya 28, 184, 185, 240, 299
ankam (duel) 42–3, 299
Aromar Chekavar 42–4, 262
Arjuna 115, 127, 201, 203
astrology 168
asan (teacher) 27, 299
ati murai (varma ati) 27, 29, 58–9, 108–11, 154–8, 164–9, 184–93, 220, 262, 300
Ayurveda (see vital spots) 26–7, 84–91, 130–1, 154, 161–4, 216, 245, 265, 300
Balachandran Master 159, 187, 198–9, 239–42, 272
Barbosa, Duarte 40–1, 95–6, 144, 254
Bhadrakali 13, 69–70, 74, 264, 300
Bhagavati 13, 69, 72, 81, 146, 209, 265, 271, 300
Bhagavad Gita vii, 92, 206
Balan, Gurukkal P.K. 70–2, 74, 98, 100, 107, 133
bhava 91–3, 118, 202–3, 207–8, 220, 300
Bhima vii, 203
body/body-practices 5–9, 11, 18–19, 61, 84, 203, 209, 226–7, 256, 265, 'body as all eyes' 19, 199, 201–14, 216, 304; body of 'humours and saps' 85–91; physical body 61, 84–5, 91–4; subtle body 61, 84, 123–6, 193–7
brahmans (in Kerala) 30–2, 34
breathing/breath control 124–5, 128–39, 167–8, 266, 305
Caraka 130–1, 265
cattar (brahman students) 30–1, 300
Chandran Gurukkal 171–2, 194–7, 221–2, 268
chekor ix, 42–3, 300
Chelayan Asan 187, 189
Christian practice 37
C.V.N. Kalari (s) 22, 52–3, 64, 67–8, 73, 76, 81, 87, 95–7, 112-15, 126, 216, 222
deities (of the *kalari*) 64–76
Dhanur Veda (science of archery) 24, 33–5, 94, 209, 258, 267, 301
dharma 46, 80, 83, 301
Drona vii, 115, 127
focus *(ekagrata,* single point) 97, 126–8, 211–14, 301
gunam 209, 217–21, 271, 301

guru/gurukkal 65, 73, 76, 113–16, 301

Hamzah Haji Abu, Ustaz 1, 2, 224–39, 254, 271

Hanuman 74, 146

heroes, heroic, hero stones 29–30, 49, 73, 147–8, 201–14, 241–2, 272

humoral theory 86–91, 211, 226

Ilava (Tiyya) ix, 36, 260

kalam (floor patterns) 106–8, 148–52, 302

kalari (as place of training) 12–15, 26, 64–83, 263, 302

kalarippayattu etymology 24–6, 302; exercises/techniques 15–16, 26, 51–2, 84–7, 95–111; history 29–60; as symbol of Malayali identity 24, 54–7, 223, 239–42; organization in Kerala 57–9; poses 97–100; concept of 'correct' practice 91–4, 111–12, 116–18; texts 81–2, 164–5, 243–5; weapons 116–22

karate 4, 113, 229

Karnaran Gurukkal 95, 116

kathakali 3, 12, 49, 91, 157, 201–14, 269, 302

Kerala (State of) viii

Kerala Kalarippayattu Association 57–9, 262, 271

Keralopathi 32

kingship (in Kerala) 37–41, 56–7, 69, 80–3, 203–14, 241–2, 259

Krishnan Vaidyar, Kalathil 193–4

ksatriya 34, 36, 204–5, 218, 302

laksana (marks or sings) 64, 302

Mahabharata vii, 33, 45–6, 72, 115, 127, 203, 259, 265, 303

Mahabali 48, 260, 302

Mamakam festival 41

mantra (s) (instruments of power) 141–8, 212, 303

massage *(uliccil)* 12, 87–91, 138–9

Menon, Gurukkal Sree Narayana 39, 74

Moolachal Asan 186, 192

mudiyettu (ritual performance) 47, 70, 264

Muslim practice 36, 148–52

Nadar 27, 257

Narayanan Gurukkal, P.P. 95, 116

Navaratri Mahotsavam 79–82, 304

Nayar (caste) ix, 27, 35–9, 42–3, 50, 59, 69, 218. 257, 259, 304

Nayar, C.V. Narayanan 25, 51, 95, 116, 261

Nayar, Chirakkal T. Sreedharan 27, 29, 50, 108, 112, 159, 175, 185, 261, 269

Nayar, Gurukkal Govindankutty 14, 17–19, 20, 51–2, 57, 65–7, 70, 73, 77, 80–1, 85, 87, 89, 91–2, 94–5, 99, 102, 117, 130, 134–8, 141, 163, 182, 198, 216, 218

northern ballads *(vattakan pattukal)* 36, 42–4, 116, 257, 306

oils 88–90

Onam (harvest festival) 10, 48, 54–6, 221, 304

Panikkar, Kalarikkal Velu 66

Panikkar, Gurukkal Madhavan 176–8

Parasurama 24, 26, 72, 94, 305

Pasupata 46

performance 5, 222–3, 236–7, 254–5

pitham (tripod) 73–4, 81, 305

practice (s) 5–11, 21, 84–5ff

power 6–8, 11, 30, 44–8, 237–8; mental 201–14

Prakasan Guru, A.K. 199–200

prana vayu (energy/breath) 21, 65, 124–39

puja (worship) 13, 78–82, 265, 305

puttara 65–6, 68, 71, 78, 306

Raju Asan 110, 187–90

Raju, R. Perumal 160, 166, 197

Ramayana vii, 306

raudra ('fury') 69–71 201–14, 220, 271, 306

ritual (s) 26, 40–1, 61–83; sacrifice as ritual 203–14

sakti ('power') 65–6, 70–2, 123–53, 241–2, 306; Sakti (the goddess) 67, 70, 74–6, 139–41, 148, 212–14

Sangam age 29–30

Sherif, C. Mohammed 102, 105–6, 108, 113, 127, 150, 222, 268

Sreejayan Gurukkal 89, 98, 139, 181

Sree Narayana Guru Sangham Vallabhatta Kalari (SNGS) 22, 65, 74–6

Styles of *kalarippayattu* 26–8, 94–5; 'northern' 95–105, 168–84; 'central' 106–8, 148–50; 'southern' 108–11, 184–93

Sufi (muslim) practice 150–2

Susruta 161–3, 168–9, 171, 183–4

sword 13, 17, 26, 29, 205, 209

Tacholi Otenan 22, 43–4, 52, 54, 57, 73, 113, 220–1, 272

teyyam (ritual performance) 3, 49, 212–13, 258, 264, 306

varma ati (see *ati murai*)

Vasco da Gama 39, 50

Vasu Gurukkal 134, 146–8

Velayudan Asan, C.C. 173–4, 176

vital spots *(marmmam, Varmam)* 26, 154–200, 303

vayttari (verbal commands) 13, 20, 93, 112–13, 126, 307

yoga 34–5, 46, 85, 88, 93, 123–53, 160–1, 166, 193–7, 267, 268, 307

Zamorin of Kozhikode 37, 41